Grace Simpson

2748.♡

1045

PDR

PEOPLE'S DESK REFERENCE

for ESSENTIAL OILS

Compiled by
Essential Science Publishing

First Printing July 1999

Copyright ©1999 Essential Science Publishing

ISBN 0-943685-25-7

Printed in the United States of America 10 9 8 7 6 5 4 3 2 1

Disclaimer: The information contained in this book is for educational purposes only. It is not provided to diagnose, prescribe, or treat any condition of the body. The information in this book should not be used as a substitute for medical counseling with a healthcare professional. Neither the author nor publisher accepts responsibility for such use.

To all those who seek truth, light and wisdom.
After all, it is their hearts that turn to
the information in this book.

Table of Contents

Preface

Essential oils are the oldest and some of the most powerful therapeutic agents known to man. They have enjoyed a millennia-long history of use in healing and anointing throughout the ancient world. Oils, like frankincense, are cited repeatedly in many Judeo-Christian and Moslem religious texts and were used to cure every ailment "from gout to a broken head." Myrrh, lotus, and sandalwood oils were widely used in ancient Egyptian purification and embalming rituals. Other oils, like clove and lemon, were highly valued as antiseptics hundreds of years before the discovery of chemical germkillers.

With the advent of modern industrial biochemicals during the last two centuries, natural therapeutic agents, like essential oils, have been largely forgotten. It has been only during the last 20 years that essential oils have enjoyed a resurgence in popularity as their broad-spectrum antibacterial and therapeutic action has been rediscovered by many health-care professionals. Essential oils are some of the most concentrated natural extracts known, exerting significant antibacterial, hormonal, and psychological effects. Essential oils have the ability to penetrate cell membranes, travel throughout the blood and tissues, and enhance electrical frequencies. As we watch an essential oil work, it becomes clear that the powerful life force inherent in many essential oils gives them an unmatched ability to communicate and interact with cells in the human body.

After using them, there is no doubt that essential oils were ordained as the medicine for mankind and will be held as the medicine of our future: the missing link of modern medicine, where alopathic and holistic medicine join together for the leap into the 21st century.

Acknowledgements

We wish to acknowledge D. Gary Young, N.D., for his tremendous contribution to the rebirth of essential oils in North America. One of the pioneers in researching, cultivating, and distilling essential oils in North America, he has spent decades conducting clinical research on the ability of essential oils to combat disease and improve health. He has also developed new methods of application from which thousands of people have benefited, especially his integration of essential oils with herbal supplements and personal care products. He is certainly one of the first, if not the first, to create these types of products.

Growing up as a farmer and rancher in Idaho, Gary has a passion for the land that has driven him to become one of the leading organic growers and distillers of essential oils in North America. With over 2,000 acres of land under cultivation in North America, he has set new standards for excellence that are redefining how therapeutic-grade essential oils are produced throughout the world.

Gary's roles as a grower, distiller, researcher, and alternative care practitioner, not only give him an unsurpassed insight into essential oils but also make him an ideal spokesperson and educator on therapeutic properties of essential oils. Few people have as comprehensive a knowledge as he does. Gary regularly travels throughout the world lecturing on the powerful potential of essential oils and what it takes to produce therapeutic-grade essential oils that can consistently deliver results.

Much of the material contained in the book is derived from his research, lectures, and workshops, as well as the work of other practitioners and physicians who are at the forefront of understanding the clinical potential of essential oils to treat disease. To these researchers, the publishers are deeply indebted.

Essential Oils:
The Missing Link in Modern Medicine

Yesterday's Wisdom, Tomorrow's Destiny

Plants not only play a vital role in the ecosystem and the balance of our planet, but they also have been intimately linked to the physical, emotional, and spiritual well-being of man since the beginning of time.

The plant kingdom is still the subject of an enormous amount of research and discovery. Over 50 percent of current medicines are based on naturally-occurring compounds that are found in plants and vegetation. Each year, millions of dollars are allocated for research grants to universities searching for novel therapeutic agents that lie undiscovered in the barks, roots, and foliage of jungle canopies, river bottoms, forests, hillsides, and the vast wilderness regions throughout the world.

As the most powerful part of the plant, essential oils and plant extracts have been woven into history since time immemorial. Essential oils have been used medicinally to kill bacteria, fungi, and viruses. They have provided exquisite fragrances to balance mood, lift spirits, dispel negative emotions, and create a romantic atmosphere. They can stimulate the regeneration of tissue or stimulate nerves. They can even act to oxygenate and carry nutrients into the cells.

Today, it has become evident that we have not yet found permanent solutions for dreaded diseases, such as the Ebola virus and hantavirus, as well as new strains of tuberculosis and influenza. Essential oils may assume an increasingly important role in combating new mutations of bacteria, viruses, and fungi. More and more researchers are undertaking serious clinical studies on the use of essential oils to combat these types of diseases.

The research that Young Living Essential Oils has conducted at Weber State University as well as other documented research indicates that most viruses, fungi, or bacteria cannot live in the presence of many essential oils, especially those high in phenols, carvacrol, thymol, and terpenes. This perhaps offers a modern explanation why the Old Testament prophet Moses used aromatic substances to protect the Israelites from the ravages of the plagues that decimated the ancient Egyptians. It may also help us to understand why a notorious group of thieves who were spice traders by trade were protected from the plague as they robbed the bodies of the dead during the 14th century.

A vast body of anecdotal evidence (testimonials) suggests that those who use essential oils are less likely to contract infectious diseases. Moreover, oil users who do contract an infectious illness tend to recover faster than those using antibiotics.

Essential oils are, without question, substances that definitely deserve the respect of proper education. Users need to be fully versed in the chemistry and safety of the oils. However, this knowledge is not taught at universities in the United States. There is a disturbing lack of institutional information, knowledge, and training on essential oils, a science commonly known as aromatherapy. Only in Europe, which has a far longer history of using natural products and botanical extracts, can one obtain adequate instruction.

The European communities have a tight framework of controls and standards concerning botanical extracts and who may administer them. Only practitioners with proper training and certification can practice aromatherapy. However, in the United States, the regulatory agencies have not recognized these disciplines or mandated the type and degree of training required to distribute and apply essential oils. This means that individuals can bill themselves as "aromatherapists" after a weekend class in essential oils and apply oils to people—even though they may not have the experience or training to properly administer them. This may not only undermine and damage the credibility of the entire discipline of aromatherapy, but it can be dangerous to our society.

Essential oils are not simple substances. They are mosaics of hundreds—or even thousands—of different chemicals. The average essential oil may contain anywhere from 80 to 200 chemical constituents. An essential oil, like lavender, may contain as many as 800 different chemical constituents, many occurring in minute quantities but all contributing to the oil's therapeutic effects to some degree. To understand these constituents and their activity and function requires years of study.

Even though an essential oil may be labeled as "basil" and have the botanical name of *Ocimum basilicum*, it can have widely different therapeutic actions, depending on its chemistry. For example, basil high in linalool or fenchol is primarily used for its antiseptic properties. However, basil high in methyl chavicol is more anti-inflammatory than antiseptic. A third type, basil high in eugenol, has both anti-inflammatory and antiseptic effects.

Moreover, essential oils can be processed in different ways that may have dramatic effects on their chemistry and medicinal action. Oils that are redistilled two or three times are obviously not as potent as oils that are distilled only once. Also, oils that are subjected to high heat and pressure processing will have a distinctly simpler and inferior profile of chemical constituents, since excessive heat and temperature will fracture and break down many of the delicate aromatic compounds within the oil—some of which are responsible for its therapeutic action. Also, oils that are steam distilled are far different from those that are solvent extracted.

Of even greater concern is the risk that many oils become adulterated or "extended" by the use of synthetic chemicals. Oftentimes pure frankincense is extended by the addition of colorless, odorless solvents, such as diethylphthalate or dipropylene glycol. The only way to distinguish the authentic from the adulterated is to subject it to rigorous analytical testing using state-of-the-art gas chromatography and mass spectroscopy.

Different Schools of Application

Therapeutic treatment using essential oils follows three different models or frameworks: the French, German, and English.

The English model advocates diluting a small amount of essential oil in a vegetable oil and massaging the body for the purpose of relaxion and relieving stress.

The French prefer the ingestion (oral administration) of therapeutic-grade essential oils. A common form of internal use is to add several drops of an essential oil to a sugar cube or a piece of bread. Many French practitioners have found that taking the oils internally yields excellent benefits.

The German model recommends inhalation of the essential oil. Research has shown that the effect of fragrance and aromatic compounds on the sense of smell can exert strong effects on the brain—especially on the hypothalamus (the hormone command center of the body) and limbic system (the seat of emotions). Some essential oils high in sesquiterpenes, such as myrrh and frankincense, can dramatically increase oxygenation and activity in the brain. This may directly improve the function of many systems of the body.

Together, these models show how versatile and powerful essential oils may be. By integrating all three techniques in conjunction with Vita Flex, auricular therapy, contact therapy, spinal touch, lymphatic massage, and Raindrop Therapy, the best possible results may be obtained.

In some cases, inhalation of essential oils might be preferred over topical application if the goal was to increase growth hormone secretion, induce weight loss, or balance mood and emotions. Sandalwood, lavender, and fir oil would be outstanding used this way. In other cases, however, topical application of essential oils would produce better results, particularly in the case of spinal or muscle injuries or defects. Topically applied, rosemary is outstanding for muscles, lemongrass for ligaments, and birch for bones. For indigestion, peppermint oil taken orally may be more effective. However, this does not mean that peppermint cannot produce the same results when massaged on the stomach. In some cases, all three methods of application (topical, inhalation, and ingestion) are interchangeable and may produce the similar benefits.

The ability of essential oils to act both on the mind and body is what makes them truly unique among natural therapeutic agents. The fragrance of an essential may be very stimulating—both psychologically and physically. Similarly, the fragrance of the same essential oil may also be calming and sedating, helping to overcome anxiety or hyperactivity. On a physiological level, essential oils may stimulate immune function and regenerate damaged tissue. Essential oils may also combat infectious disease by killing viruses, bacteria, and other pathogens.

During the last 15 years, there has been extensive research and study performed worldwide at many universities to expand the knowledge of essential oils and their history.

The two most effective methods of essential oil application are cold-air diffusing and neat (undiluted) topical application. By incorporating essential oils into the disciplines of reflexology, Vita Flex, acupressure, and acupuncture, the healing response is greatly enhanced. Essential oils produce phenomenal results that, in many cases, can never be achieved by acupuncture or reflexology alone. Only one to three drops of an essential oil applied to an acupuncture meridian or Vita Flex point on the hand or foot may produce dramatic effects— sometimes within minutes.

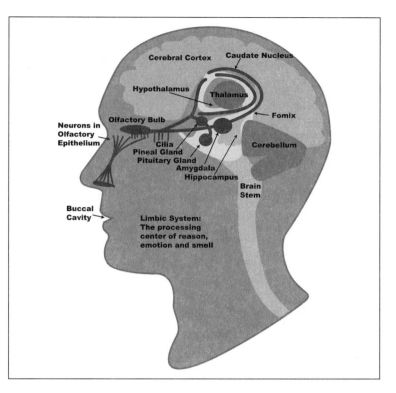

Many practitioners doubt that essential oils can produce these types of results—even though research has shown that essential oils can magnify the benefits of healing modalities, like acupuncture, by two to ten times.

Several years ago at one of the universities in Europe, a professor very well known throughout the field of aromatherapy commented that anyone who claims to cure diseases using essential oils is a quack. However, there are many people who are living proof that essential oils can be used to engineer cures and recoveries from serious illness. Essential oils have been pivotal in helping many people live pain free after many years of suffering intense pain. Many people have also witnessed firsthand how essential oils have corrected scoliosis and restored the hearing in those who are born deaf.

A lady in Palisades Park, California, developed scoliosis as a result of surviving polio as a teenager. Over 22 years ago she had fallen and dislocated her shoulder. Suffering pain and immobility, she had traveled extensively in a fruitless search to locate a practitioner who could permanently reset her shoulder. She topically applied the oils of valor, helichrysum, and birch to the shoulder. Within a short time she became pain free as the shoulder relocated. She was able to raise her arm over her head for the first time in 22 years.

When one sees such dramatic recoveries, it is difficult to discredit the value and the power of essential oils and the potential they hold.

What Is an Essential Oil?

The essential oil today is known variously as "volatile oil," "ethereal oil," "herbal oil," or perfume oil." It is occasionally referred to as an "essence" instead of an oil, a term which is better suited for describing cold-pressed oils from fruit rind, like the citrus oils.

Essential oils are chemically very complex, consisting of hundreds of different chemical compounds. Moreover, they are highly concentrated and far more potent than dried herbs. The distillation of an entire plant may produce only a single drop of essential oil.

Essential oils are also different from vegetable oils, such as corn oil, peanut oil, and olive oil. They are not greasy and do not clog the pores like vegetable oils can.

Mankind's First Medicine

For many centuries essential oils and other aromatics were used for religious rituals, the treatment of illness, and other physical and spiritual needs. Perhaps the people of ancient times had a greater understanding of essential oils than we have today.

Records dating back to 4500 B.C. describe the use of balsamic substances with aromatic properties for religious rituals and medical applications. The translation of ancient writings tell of scented barks, resins of spices, and aromatic vinegars, wines, and beers that were used in rituals, temples, astrology, embalming, and medicine. The Egyptians were masters in using essential oils and other aromatics in the embalming process. Historical records describe how one of the founders of "pharaonic" medicine was the architect Imhotep, who was the Grand Vizier of King Zeser (2780 - 2720 B.C.). Imhotep is often given credit for ushering in the use of oils, herbs, and aromatic plants for medicinal purposes. Hieroglyphics on the walls of the temples depict the blending of oils and describe hundreds of oil recipes. A sacred room in the temple of Isis on the island of Philae depicts a ritual called "Cleansing the Flesh and Blood of Evil Deities." This emotional clearing required three days of cleansing using essential oils.

Translation of ancient papyrus found in the Temple of Edfu reveal the blending of aromatic substances by the alchemist and the high priest for medicinal formulas and perfume recipes for their rituals.

The Egyptians were the first to discover the potential of fragrance. They created various aromatic blends for both personal use and for the ceremonies performed in the temples and pyramids. Many Egyptian temple carvings and reliefs describe how essential oils were used by priests and physicians in ancient ceremonies. Well before the time of Christ, the ancient Egyptians collected essential oils and placed them in alabaster vessels. These vessels were specially carved and shaped for housing scented oils. In 1922, when King Tut's tomb was opened, 350 liters of oils were discovered in alabaster jars. Plant waxes had solidified into a thickened residue around the inside of the container openings, leaving the liquefied oil in excellent condition.

In 1817, the Ebers Papyrus was discovered. It was over 870 feet long and was referred to as a medicinal scroll. Dating back to 1500 B.C., the scroll included over 800 different formulations of herbal prescriptions and remedies. Other scrolls described a high success rate in treating 81 different diseases. Many mixtures contained myrrh and honey. Myrrh is still recognized for its ability to help with infections of the skin and throat and to regenerate skin tissue. Because of its effectiveness in preventing bacterial growth, myrrh was used for embalming.

The physicians of Ionia, Attia, and Crete came to the cities of the Nile to increase their knowledge. At this time, the school of Cas was founded and was attended by Hippocrates (460 to 377 B.C.), who the Greeks, in their enthusiasm and with some exaggeration, named the "Father of Medicine."

The Romans purified their temples and political buildings by diffusing essential oils. The also used aromatics in their steam baths to both invigorate the flesh and ward off disease.

Early History of Essential Oil Extraction

Ancient cultures found that aromatic essences or oils could be extracted from the plant by a variety of methods. One of the oldest and crudest forms of extraction was known as effleurage. Raw plant material (usually stems, foliage, bark, or roots) were crushed and steeped with olive oil. In the case of cedar, the bark was stripped from the trunk and branches, ground fairly fine, soaked with olive oil, and wrapped in a wool cloth. The cloth was then burned. The heat would pull the essential oil out of the bark into the olive oil. The wool cloth was then pressed to extract the essential oil. By placing petals in goose or goat fat, the essential oil molecules would be pulled into the fat. The oil was then separated from the fat. This ancient technique was among the most primitive forms of essential oil extraction.

Other extraction techniques were also used throughout ancient cultures. Some of these included:

- Soaking plant parts in boiling water
- Pressing flower petals, roots, and leaves into fat (effleurage)

- Cold-pressing

- Soaking in alcohol

- Steam distillation by passing steam through the plant material and condensing the steam to separate the oil from the plant.

Many ancient cosmetic formulas were created from a base of goat fat. They formulated eyeliners, eyeshadows, and other cosmetics. They also stained their hair and nails with a variety of ointments and perfumes. They probably used the same aromatic oils that were used in the temples. Such temple oils were commonly poured into evaporation dishes for fragrancing the chambers associated with sacred rituals and religious rites.

The ancient Arabians were another early culture that developed and refined a process of distillation. They perfected the extraction of rose oils and rose water, which were popular in the Middle East during the Byzantine Empire (330 A.D. - 1400 A.D.).

Biblical References and Ancient References to Essential Oils

There are over 200 references to essential oils, incense, and ointments throughout the Old and New Testaments of the Bible. Aromatics, such as frankincense, myrrh, galbanum, cinnamon, cassia, rosemary, hyssop, and spikenard, were used for anointing and healing the sick. In Exodus, the Lord gave the following recipe to Moses for "a holy anointing oil":

Myrrh	"five hundred shekels" (about 1 gallon)	
Cinnamon	"two hundred and fifty shekels"	
Calamus	"two hundred and fifty shekels"	
Cassia	"five hundred shekels"	
Olive Oil	"an hin" (about 1 1/3 gallons)	

Psalms 133:2 speaks of the sweetness of brethren dwelling together in unity and says: "It is like the precious ointment upon the head, that ran down the beard, even Aaron's beard: that went down to the skirts of his garments." This is not the only reference to the anointing of Aaron as High Priest mentioning the overflowing abundance of precious oils. In Ecclesiastes 9:8 is the admonition:

"Let thy garments be always white; and let thy head lack no ointment."

The Bible lists an incident where an incense offering by Aaron stopped a plague. Numbers 16:46-50 records that Moses instructed Aaron to take a censer, add burning coals and incense, and to "go quickly into the congregation to make an atonement for them: for there is a wrath gone out from the Lord; the plague is begun." The Bible records that Aaron stood between the dead and the living and the plague was stayed. It is significant that according to the biblical and Talmudic recipes for incense, three varieties of cinnamon were included. Cinnamon is known to be highly antimicrobial, anti-infectious and antibacterial. The incense ingredient listed as "stacte" is believed to be a sweet, myrrh-related spice, which would make it anti-infectious, and antiviral as well. Whether the antibacterial nature of the incense played a part in stopping the plague or not, 14,700 Israelites died of the plague before Aaron brought forth the incense.

The wise men presented the Christ child with essential oils of frankincense and myrrh. The New Testament records the anointing of Jesus with spikenard. "And being in Bethany in the house of Simon the leper, as he sat at meat, there came a woman having an alabaster box of ointment of spikenard very precious; and she brake the box, and poured on his head" (Mark 14:3). "Then took Mary a pound of ointment of spikenard, very costly, and anointed the feet of Jesus, and wiped his feet with her hair: and the house was filled with the odour of the ointment" (John 12:3).

Other Cultures That Used Essential Oils

Throughout history, fragrant oils and spices played a prominent role in everyday life. The Qu'ran, scripture to the world's Muslims, mentions sweet-smelling sandalwood. One of the Dead Sea Scrolls on display in Israel at the Shrine of the Book Museum contains this intriguing phrase: "and he will know his children by their scent."

Napoleon is reported to have liked a cologne water made of neroli and other ingredients so much that he ordered 162 bottles of it. After conquering Jerusalem, one of the things the Crusaders brought back to Europe was attar of roses.

And the 12th century mystic, Hildegard of Bingen, used herbs and oils extensively in healing. This Benedictine nun founded her own convent and was the author of numerous works. Her book, *Physica*, has more than 200 short chapters on plants and their uses in healing.

The Rediscovery

The reintroduction of essential oils into modern medicine first became evident during the late 19th and early 20th centuries. During World War I, the use of aromatic essences in civilian and military hospitals became widespread. One physician in France, Dr. Moncière, used essential oils extensively for their antibacterial and wound-healing properties and developed several kinds of aromatic ointments.

The term "aromatherapy" was coined in 1920 by René-Maurice Gattefossé, Ph.D., a French cosmetic chemist. Widely regarded as the father of aromatherapy, Gattefossé discovered the healing powers of essential oils quite by accident. While working in his laboratory, he suffered an accident in which his hand and forearm were severely burned. To cool the wound, Dr. Gattefossé plunged his arm into a vessel that he assumed was water. The vessel actually contained pure lavender oil *(Lavendula officinalis)*. To his surprise, the pain ceased within moments. With the regular application of lavender oil, the wound healed without a scar. When he investigated the chemistry of the oil, he discovered that some chemical constituents or components had tremendous healing properties.

Dr. Gattefossé shared his studies with his colleague and friend, Jean Valnet, a medical doctor practicing in Paris. Exhausting his supply of antibiotics as a physician in Tonkin, China, during World War II, Dr. Valnet began using therapeutic-grade essential oils on patients suffering battlefield injuries. To his surprise, they exerted a powerful effect in combating and counteracting infection. He was able to save the lives of many soldiers who might otherwise have died, even with antibiotics.

Two of Dr. Valnet's students, Dr. Paul Belaiche and Dr. Jean Claude Lapraz, expanded his work. They clinically investigated the antiviral, antibacterial, antifungal, and antiseptic properties in essential oils.

How Do Essential Oils Work?

Therapeutic-Grade Essential Oils

Essential oils are the volatile liquids that are distilled from various part of plants, including seeds, bark, leaves, stems, roots, flowers, and fruit. One of the factors that determine the purity of an oil are its chemical constituents. These constituents can be affected by a vast number of variables, including: the part(s) of the plant from which the oil was produced, soil condition, fertilizer (organic or chemical), geographical region, climate, altitude, harvest season and methods, and distillation process. For example, common thyme *(Thyme vulgaris)* produces several different chemotypes (biochemically unique species), depending on the conditions of its growth, climate, and altitude. One chemotype of thyme will yield an essential oil with high levels of thymol, depending on the time of year it is distilled. The later it is distilled in the growing season (ie., midsummer or fall), the more thymol the oil will contain.

The key to producing a therapeutic-grade essential oil is to preserve as many of the delicate aromatic compounds within the essential oil as possible. Such fragile aromatic chemicals are easily destroyed by high temperature and pressure as well as contact with chemically reactive metals, such as copper or aluminum. This is why all therapeutic-grade essential oils should be distilled in stainless steel cooking chambers at low pressure and low temperature.

The plant material should also be free of pesticides, herbicides, and other agrichemicals. These can react with the essential oil during distillation to produce toxic compounds.

As we begin to understand the power of essential oils in the realm of personal, holistic healthcare, we will appreciate the necessity for obtaining the purest essential oils possible. No matter how costly pure essential oils may be, there can be no substitutes.

Although chemists have successfully recreated the main constituents and fragrances of some essential oils in the laboratory, these synthetic oils lack therapeutic benefits and may even carry risks. Why? Because essential oils contain hundreds of different chemical compounds, some of which have never been identified but which lend important therapeutic properties to the oil. Moreover, some essential oils contain molecules and isomers that are impossible to manufacture in the laboratory.

Anyone venturing into the world of aromatherapy and essential oils must use the purest quality oils available. Inferior quality or adulterated oils most likely will not produce therapeutic results and could possibly be toxic. In Europe, a set of standards has been established that outlines the chemical profile and principal constituents that a quality essential oil should have. Known as AFNOR and ISO standards, these guidelines help buyers differentiate between a therapeutic-grade essential oil and a lower grade oil with a similar chemical makeup and fragrance. All of the therapeutic effects of the essential oils in this book are based on oils that have been graded according to the AFNOR standard.

Science and Application

The essential oil of the plant and the human blood share several common properties: They fight infection, contain hormone-like compounds, and initiate regeneration. Working as the chemical defense mechanism of the plant, essential oils possess potent antibacterial, antifungal, and antiviral properties. They also ward off attacks by insects and animals. Both essential oils and human blood contain hormone-like chemicals. The ability of some essential oils to work as hormones helps them bring balance to many physiological systems of the human body. Oils like clary sage and fennel, for example, have an estrogenic action. Essential oils also play a role in initiating the regeneration process for the plant, the same way the blood does in the human body.

Chemically, essential oils are also very similar to the human body. The three primary elements in both human beings and essential oils are carbon, hydrogen, and oxygen. This shared chemistry makes essential oils one of the most compatible of all plant substances with human biochemistry.

This similarity goes deeper. Essential oils have a protein-like structure that is similar to that found in human cells and tissues. This makes essential oils compatible with human protein and enables them to be readily identified and accepted by the body.

Essential oils have a unique ability to penetrate cell membranes and diffuse throughout the blood and tissues. The unique, lipid-soluble structure of essential oils is very similar to the makeup of our cell membranes. The molecules of essential oils are also relatively small, giving them the ability to easily penetrate the cells. When topically applied to the feet or elsewhere, essential oils can travel throughout the body in a matter of minutes.

The ability of some essential oils to decrease the viscosity or thickness of the blood can enhance circulation and immune function. Adequate circulation is vital to good health, since it affects the function of every cell and organ, including the brain.

Research indicates that when essential oils are diffused, they can increase atmospheric oxygen and provide negative ions, which can inhibit bacterial growth. This suggests that essential oils could play an important role in air purification and neutralizing odors. Because of their ionizing action, essential oils have the ability to break down and render potentially harmful chemicals nontoxic.

In the human body, essential oils stimulate the secretion of antibodies, neurotransmitters, endorphins, hormones, and enzymes. Oils containing limonene have been shown to be antiviral. Other oils, like lavender, have been shown to promote the growth of hair and increase the rate of wound healing. Essential oils also act as pro-vitamins, assisting in the conversion of vitamins. They increase the uptake of oxygen and ATP (adenosine triphosphate), the fuel for individual cells.

European scientists have studied the ability of essential oils to work as natural chelators, binding with heavy metals and petrochemicals and ferrying them out of the body.

Today about 200 types of oils are distilled, with several thousand chemical constituents and aromatic molecules identified and registered. The quantity, quality, and type of these aromatic compounds will vary depending on climate, temperature, and distillation factors. Today, 98 percent of essential oils are used in the perfume and cosmetic industry. Only about 2 percent are produced for therapeutic and medicinal applications.

Because essential oils are composites of hundreds of different chemicals, they can exert many different effects on the body. For example, clove oil can be simultaneously antiseptic and anaesthetic when applied topically. It can also be antitumoral. Lavender oil has been used for burns, insect bites, headaches, PMS, insomnia, stress, and hair growth.

Moreover, because of their complexity, essential oils do not disturb the body's natural balance or homeostasis: If one constituent exerts too strong an effect, another constituent may block or counteract it. Synthetic chemicals, in contrast, usually have only one action and often disrupt the body's natural balance or homeostasis.

Using European AFNOR/ISO Standards to Identify Therapeutic-Grade Oils

One of the most reliable indicators of essential oil quality is whether the oil is AFNOR or ISO certified. This standard differentiates true therapeutic-grade essential oils from similar Grade A essential oils with inferior chemistry.

The AFNOR standard (Association French Normalization Organization Regulation) was written by a botanical chemist, Hervi Casabianca, Ph.D., while working with different analytical laboratories throughout France. He recognized that the constituents within an essential oil had to occur in certain percentages in order for the oil to be considered therapeutic. He combined his studies with research conducted by other scientists and doctors. The Central Service Analysis Laboratory is certified by the French government for essential oil analysis.

As a result, many oils that are listed as therapeutic-grade, such as frankincense, can be checked to see if they meet AFNOR standards. If some constituents are too high or too low, they cannot be AFNOR or ISO certified.

For example, the AFNOR standard for *Lavendula angustiofolia* (true lavender) dictates that the level of linalool should range from 30 to 34 percent and linalyl acetate range between 26-30 percent. As long as these marker compounds are within a specific parameter, they are recognized as therapeutic-grade essential oils.

As a general rule, if two or more marker compounds in an essential oil fall outside of their proper percentages, the oil may not be able to meet the AFNOR standard. It cannot be recognized as therapeutic-grade essential oil, even though it is still Grade A and of high quality.

What distinguishes a therapeutic-grade essential oil from a Grade A essential oil that is not therapeutic-grade or AFNOR-certified? A lavender oil produced in one region of France might have a slightly different chemistry than that grown in another region and as a result may not meet the standard. It may have excessive camphor levels (1.0 instead of 0.5), a condition that might be caused by distilling lavender that was too green. Or the levels of lavendulol may be too low due to certain weather conditions at the time of harvest.

By comparing the chemistry of lavender essential oil with the AFNOR standard, you may also distinguish true lavender from various species of hybrid lavender (lavendin). Usually lavendin has high camphor levels and almost no lavendulol and is easily identified. However, Tasmania produces a lavendin that yields an essential oil with naturally low camphor levels that mimics the chemistry of true lavender. Only by analyzing the chemical fingerprint of this Tasmanian lavendin using high resolution gas chromatography and comparing it with the AFNOR standard for genuine lavender can this hybrid lavender be identified.

Currently, there is no agency responsible for certifying that essential oil is therapeutic grade. The only indication that an oil is therapeutic grade is if it meets ISO or AFNOR standards. (ISO is the International Standards Organization which has set standards for therapeutic-grade essential oils adopted from AFNOR.) The oils used in the product discussed in this book has been and are constantly analyzed and graded according to the AFNOR standards.

To our knowledge, there is only one essential oil producer in North America who has been collaborating with government-certified analytical chemists in Europe to ensure that their essential oils meet AFNOR standards.

In the United States, few companies use the proper analytical equipment and methods to properly analyze essential oils. Most labs use equipment best-suited for synthetic chemicals—not for essential oil analysis. We know of only two firms that use the proper machinery and test-standards—Flora Research and Young Living Essential Oils. Both of these companies have made serious efforts to adopt the European testing standards, widely regarded as the gold standard for testing essential oils. In addition to operating its analytical equipment on the same standard as the European-certified laboratories, Young Living is also in the process of expanding its analytical library of chemicals in order to perform more thorough chemical analysis.

Properly analyzing an essential oil by gas chromatography is a complex undertaking. Your injection mixture, film thickness, column diameter and length, and oven temperature must fall within certain parameters.

Your column length should be at least 50 or 60 meters. However, almost all labs in the United States use a 30-meter column that is not long enough to achieve separation of all the essential oil constituents. While 30-meter columns are adequate for analyzing synthetic chemicals and marker compounds in vitamins, minerals, and herbal extracts, they are far too short to properly analyze the complex mosaic of natural chemicals found in an essential oil.

A longer column also enables double-phased ramping to be conducted, which enables constituents that occur in small percentages to be identified by increasing the separation of compounds. Without a longer column, it would be extremely difficult to identify these molecules, especially if they are chemically similar to each other or the marker compound.

While gas chromatography is an excellent tool for dissecting the anatomy of an essential oil, it does have limitations. Dr. Brian Lawrence, one of the foremost experts on essential oil chemistry, has commented that it is very difficult to distinguish between natural and synthetic compounds using GC analysis. If synthetic linalyl acetate was added to pure lavender, a GC cannot tell whether that compound is synthetic or natural, only that it is linalyl acetate.

This is why oils must be analyzed by a technician specially trained on the interpretation of a gas chromatograph (GC) chart. He examines the entire chemical fingerprint of the oil to determine its purity and potency, measuring how various compounds in the oil occur in relation to each other. If some chemicals occur in higher quantities than others, these provide important clues to determine if the oil is adulterated or pure.

Adulteration of essential oils will become more and more common as the supply of top-quality essential oils dwindles and demand explodes. These adulterated essential oils will jeopardize the integrity of aromatherapy in the United States and may put many people at risk.

(See AFNOR/ISO Standard charts in Appendix.)

Adulterated Oils and Their Dangers

Today most of the lavender oil sold in America is a hybrid called lavandin, grown and distilled in China, Russia, France, and Tasmania. They bring it into France, cut it with synthetic linolyl acetate to improve the fragrance, add propylene glycol or SD 40, DEP, and DOP, which are solvents that have no smell and increase the volume, and then sell it in the United States as lavender oil. Oftentimes lavandin is heated to evaporate off (flash off) the camphor and then is adulterated with synthetic linelyl acetate so that it appears as lavender. We don't know the difference, and we are happy to buy and sell it for $5 to $7 per half ounce in health food stores, beauty salons, grocery and department stores, and through mail order.

Frankincense is another example of an adulterated oil. The frankincense resin that is sold in Somalia costs between $30,000 and $35,000 per ton. The essential oil requires 12 hours to be steam distilled from the resin and is very expensive. Frankincense oil that sells for $25 per ounce or less is invariably distilled with alcohol or other solvents. When these cut, synthetic, and adulterated oils cause rashes, burns, or other irritations, we wonder why we do not get the benefit we were expecting and conclude that essential oils do not have much value.

Statistics show that one company—Proctor & Gamble—uses twice as much essential oil as is produced in the entire world. From where are these "essential" oils coming?

In France, production of true lavender oil (*Lavandula angustifolia*) dropped from 87 tons in 1967 to only 12 tons in 1998. During this same period the demand for lavender oil has grown over 100 times. So where do essential oil marketers

obtain enough lavender to meet demand? They use a combination of synthetic and adulterated oils. There are huge chemical houses on the East Coast that specialize in the duplication of every essential oil that exists. For every kilo of pure essential oil that is produced, there are between 10 and 100 kilos of synthetic oil created.

Adulterated and mislabeled essential oils present dangers for consumers. One woman who had heard of the ability of lavender oil to heal burns used lavender oil from a local health food store when she spilled boiling water on her arm. When the pain intensified and the burn worsened, she later complained that lavender oil was worthless for healing burns. When her "lavender" oil was later analyzed, it turned out to be lavandin, a hybrid lavender that is chemically very different from pure *Lavandula angustifolia*. Lavandin contains high levels of camphor (12-18 percent) and will burn the skin. In contrast, true lavender contains virtually no camphor and has burn-healing agents not found in lavandin.

Adulterated oils that are cut with synthetic extenders can be very detrimental, causing rashes, burning, and skin irritations. Petrochemical solvents, such dipropylene glycol and diethylphthalate, can all cause allergic reactions, besides being devoid of any therapeutic effects.

Some people assume that because an essential oil is 100 percent pure it will not burn their skin. This is not true. Pure essential oils may cause skin irritation if applied undiluted. If you apply straight oregano oil to the skin, it may cause severe reddening and burning. Citrus and spice oils, like cinnamon and orange, may also produce rashes. Even the terpenes in conifer oils, like pine, may cause skin irritation on sensitive people.

Some writers have claimed that a few compounds when isolated from the essential oil and tested in the lab can exert toxic effects. Even some nature-identical essential oils (a structured essential oil that has been chemically duplicated from 5 to 15 synthetic compounds) can produce unwanted side effects or toxicities. However, even though isolated compounds may be toxic, pure essential oils, in most cases, are not. This is because natural essential oils contain hundreds of different compounds, some of which balance and counteract each other, acting as buffers and balancers for the compounds that can be toxic.

Many tourists in Egypt are eager to buy local essential oils, especially lotus oil. Venders convince them that the oils are 100 percent pure, even going so far as to touch a lighted match to the neck of the oil container to show that the oil is not diluted with alcohol or other petrochemical solvents. However, this test provides no reliable indicator of purity. Many synthetic marker compounds can be added to an essential oil that are not flammable. Moreover, flammable solvents that are added to a vegetable oil base will have a hard time catching fire. Even more confusing is the fact that some natural essential oils high in terpenes can be flammable.

Facts or Fiction: Myths and Misinformation

Much currently available information on essential oils should be regarded with caution. Many aromatherapy books are merely compilations of two or three other books. The content is similar, only phrased and worded differently. Because the information has been copied from sources that have never been documented, the same misinformation repeatedly resurfaces.

Many aromatherapy books claim that essential oils, like clary sage, fennel, sage, and bergamot, can trigger an abortion. In fact several years ago a rumor circulated about a laboratory research project in which the uterus of a rat was turned inside out and a cold drop of clary sage oil was applied to the exposed uterine wall. When this caused a contraction of the muscle, clary sage was labeled as abortion causing. One must ask, what would have happened if cold water had been dropped on the exposed uterus? Would not the uterine wall have contracted also? Following this reasoning, water could be labeled as abortion causing as well.

The truth is that to our knowledge there has never been a single documented case that any of these essential oils have caused an abortion. Moreover, many people mistakenly assume that the sclareol in clary sage acts like estrogen, even though it does not. Sclareol is not an estrogen, although it can mimic estrogen if there is an estrogen deficiency. If there is not an estrogen deficiency, sclareol will not create more estrogen in the body. As a rule, essential oils bring balance to the human body.

The belief that pure essential oils will not leave a stain when poured on a tissue is unfounded. Any essential oil high in waxes will leave stains. Oils like frankincense, cedarwood, ylang ylang, or German chamomile will also leave a noticeable residue. However, an essential oil spiked with synthetic dilutents or solvent may not leave a stain.

It is frustrating to watch people who were totally unfamiliar with essential oils three years ago now authoring books and billing themselves as authorities. Yet when questioned, these "experts" cannot distinguish between a phenol, cineol, or aldehyde.

The Powerful Influence of Aromas on Both Mind and Body

What is the mechanism by which the fragrance of an essential oil can directly affect everything from your emotional state to your lifespan?

When a fragrance is inhaled, the odor molecules travel up the nose where they are trapped by olfactory membranes well protected by the lining inside the nose. Each odor molecule fits like a little puzzle piece into specific receptor cells lining a membrane known as the olfactory epithelium. Each one of these hundreds of millions of nerve cells is replaced every 28 days. When stimulated by odor molecules, this lining of nerve cells triggers electrical impulses to the olfactory bulb, which then transmits the impulses to the gustatory center (where the sensation of taste is perceived), the amygdala (where emotional memories are stored), and other parts of the limbic system of the brain. Because the limbic system is directly connected to those parts of the brain that control heart rate, blood pressure, breathing, memory, stress levels, and hormone balance, essential oils can have some very profound physiological and psychological effects.

The sense of smell is the only one of the five senses directly linked to the limbic lobe of the brain, the emotional control center. Anxiety, depression, fear, anger, and joy all emanate from this region. This is why the scent of a special fragrance can evoke memories and emotions before we are even consciously aware of it. Where smells are concerned, we react first and think later. In contrast, all other senses (touch, taste, hearing, and sight) are routed through the thalamus, which acts as the switchboard for the brain, passing stimuli onto the cerebral cortex and other parts of the brain.

The limbic lobe (a group of brain structures that include the hippocampus and amygdala that is located below the cerebral cortex) can also directly activate the hypothalamus. The hypothalamus is one of the most important parts of the brain, acting as our hormonal control center. It releases chemical messengers that can affect everything from our sex drive to energy levels. The production of growth hormones, sex hormones, thyroid hormones, and neurotransmitters, like serotonin, are all governed by the hypothalamus. This is why the hypothalamus is referred to as the "master gland."

Essential oils—through their fragrance and unique molecular structure—can directly stimulate both the limbic lobe and the hypothalamus. In this way, essential oils can exert a profound effect on body and mind. Not only can inhalation of essential oils be used to combat stress and emotional trauma, but they can also stimulate the production of hormones from the hypothalamus that can result in increased thyroid hormone (our energy hormone) and growth hormone (our youth and longevity hormone).

Essential oils may also be used to reduce appetite and produce dramatic reductions in weight because of their ability to stimulate the ventromedial nucleus of the hypothalamus, a section of the brain that governs our feeling of satiety or fullness following meals. In one large clinical study, Alan Hirsch, M.D., used fragrances, including peppermint, to trigger significant weight losses in a large group of patients who had previously been unsuccessful in any type of weight management program. During the course of the six-month study involving over 3,000 people, the average weight loss exceeded five pounds a month. According to Dr. Hirsch, some patients actually had to be dropped from the study to avoid becoming underweight.

Another double-blind, randomized study by Hirsch documents the ability of aroma to enhance libido and sexual arousal. When 31 male volunteers were subjected to the aromas of 30 different essential oils, each one exhibited a marked increase in arousal, based on measurements of brachial penile index and the measurement of both penile and brachial blood pressures. Among the scents that produced the most sexual excitement was a combination of lavender and pumpkin.

Fragrances enhance sexual desire through their stimulation of the amygdala, which is the emotional center of the brain.

In 1989, Dr. Joseph Ledoux, of the New York Medical University discovered that the amygdala plays a major role in storing and releasing emotional trauma and that aroma may exert a profound effect in triggering a response from this gland.

In studies conducted at Vienna and Berlin Universities, researchers found that sesquiterpenes in the essential oils of sandalwood and frankincense can increase levels of oxygen in the brain by up to 28%. Such an increase in brain oxygen may lead to a heightened level of activity in the hypothalamus and limbic systems of the brain, which can have dramatic effects not only on emotions, learning, and attitude, but also on many physical processes of the body, such as immune function, hormone balance, and energy levels. High levels of sesquiterpenes also occur in melissa, myrrh, and clove oil.

People who have undergone nose surgery or suffer olfactory impairment may find it difficult or impossible to detect a complete odor. The same is true of people who heavily use makeup, perfume, cologne, hair sprays, hair colorings, perms, or other products with synthetic odors. These types of people may not derive the full physiological and emotional benefits of essential oils and their fragrances.

Proper stimulation of the olfactory nerves may present an entirely new—and powerful—form of therapy that may be used as an adjunct against many forms of illness. Essential oils, through inhalation, may occupy a key position in this relatively unexplored frontier in medicine.

Chemical Sensitivities and Allergies

Occasionally, individuals beginning to use essential oils will suffer rashes or allergic reactions. This may be due to using an undiluted spice, conifer, or citrus oil, or it may be caused by an interaction of the oil with residues of synthetic, petroleum-based personal care products that have leached into the skin.

When using essential oils on a daily basis, it is imperative to avoid personal care products containing ammonium or hydrocarbon-based chemicals. These include quaternary compounds, such as quarternarium 1-29 and polyquarternarium 1-14. These compounds are found ubiquitously in a variety of handcreams, mouthwashes, shampoos, antiperspirants, after-shave lotions, and hair-care products. These chemicals can be fatal when ingested, especially benzalkonium chloride, which is the most popular. In small concentrations they can be toxic and present the possibility of reacting with essential oils and producing chemical byproducts of unknown toxicity.

Other compounds that present concerns are sodium lauryl sulfate, propylene glycol, and the aluminum salts found in many deodorants.

Of particular concern are the potentially-hazardous preservatives and synthetic fragrances that abound in virtually all modern personal-care products. Some of these include methylene chloride, methyl isobutyl ketone, and methyl ethyl ketone. These are not only toxic in their own right but can react with some compounds in natural essential oils. The result can be a severe case of dermatitis or even septicemia (blood poisoning).

A classic case of a synthetic fragrance causing widespread damage occurred in the 1970s. AETT (acetylethyltetramethyltetralin) appeared in numerous brands of personal care products throughout the United States. Even after a series of animal studies revealed that it caused significant brain and spinal cord damage, the FDA refused to ban the chemical. Finally, the cosmetic industry voluntarily withdrew it after allowing it to be distributed for years. How many more other toxins masquerading as preservatives or fragrances are currently being used in personal care products?

Even worse, many chemicals are easily absorbed through the skin due to its permeability. One study found that 13 percent of BHT (butylated hydroxytoluene) and 49% of DDT (a carcinogenic pesticide) are absorbed into the skin (Steinman 1997). Once absorbed they can become trapped in the fatty subdermal layers where they can leach into the blood stream. Sometimes these chemicals can remain trapped in fatty tissues underneath the skin for months or even years, where they harbor the potential of reacting with essential oils that may be topically applied later on. The user may mistakenly assume that the threat of an interaction between oils and synthetic cosmetics used months before is small. However, a case of dermatitis is an ever-present possibility nevertheless.

Producing Therapeutic-Grade Essential Oils

Organic Herb Farming

The key to producing oils that are of genuine therapeutic quality starts with the proper cultivation of the herbs in the field.

- Plants should be grown on virgin land uncontaminated by chemical fertilizers, pesticides, fungicides, or herbicides.

- Because robust, healthy plants produce higher quality essential oils, the soil should be nourished with enzymes, minerals, and organic biosolids. The mineral content of the soil is crucial to the proper development of the plant, and soils that lack minerals result in plants that produce inferior oils.

- Land should be watered with reservoir or watershed water. Mountain stream water is best because of its purity and high mineral content. Municipally-treated water or secondary run-off water from residential and commercial areas can introduce undesirable chemicals and residues into the plant and the essential oil.

- Different species of plants produce different qualities of oils. Only those cultivars that produce the highest quality essential oil should be selected.

- The timing of the harvest is one of the most important factors in the production of therapeutic-grade oils. If the plant is harvested at the wrong time of the season or even at the improper time of day, it can produce a substandard essential oil. In some instances, changing harvest time by even a few hours can make a huge difference. For example, German chamomile harvested in the morning will produce an oil with far more azulene (a powerful anti-inflammatory compound) than chamomile harvested in the late afternoon. Other factors that should be taken into consideration during the harvest include the amount of dew on the leaves, the percentage of plant in bloom, and weather conditions during the two weeks prior to harvest.

- To prevent herbs from drying out prior to being distilled, the distillers should be located as close to the field as possible. Transporting herbs to distillers hundreds or thousands of miles away heightens the risk of exposure to pollutants, dust, and petrochemical residues.

Steam Distillation

Essential oils can be extracted from the plant by a variety of methods, including solvent-extraction, carbon dioxide extraction, and steam distillation. Steam distillation is one of the most common and has several advantages over other methods.

Steam distillation involves creating steam and sending it into a cooking chamber that holds the raw plant material. As the steam rises, it ruptures the oil membranes in the plant and releases the essential oil. The steam carries the oil to the condenser, where the oil-water mixture reliquefies. It is then sent to a separator where the oil is separated from the water. The run-off water is called "floral water."

Distillation

Distillation can determine or destroy the value of the oil. Essential oil distilling is not just a job, it is an art. The operator of the distiller must have a full understanding of the value of essential oils in order to produce quality oils. If the pressure is too high, or if the temperature is too high, it may change the molecular structure of the fragrance molecule, altering the chemical constituents. As an example, the distilling process for lavender should not exceed three pounds of pressure, and temperatures should not exceed 245 degrees.

However, there are many variants of steam distillation. Subtle differences in distillation equipment and processing conditions can translate into huge differences in essential oil quality. The size of cooking chamber, the type of condenser and separator, and the degree of temperature and pressure can all have a huge impact on the oil. In many respects the way essential oils are steam-distilled can enhance or destroy them. Distillation is more than a science; it is an art. If the pressure or temperature is too high, or if the cooking chambers are constructed from reactive metals, the oil may not be therapeutic-grade, even though it still may technically be "Grade A."

Vertical steam distillation gives us the greatest potential for protecting the therapeutic benefits and quality of essential oils. In ancient distillation, low pressure (5 pounds and under) and low temperature were extremely important to produce the therapeutic benefits. Marcel Espieu, president of the Lavender Growers Association for 21 years in southern France, has long maintained that the best oil quality can only be produced when the pressure was zero pounds during distillation.

Temperature also has a distinct effect. At certain temperatures, the oil fragrance, as well as the chemical constituents, may be altered. High pressures and high temperatures seem to cause a harshness in the oil. Even the oil pH and the electrical polarity are greatly affected.

For example, cypress requires a maximum of 24 hours of distillation at 265 degrees and 5 pounds of pressure to extract most of the therapeutically active constituents. If distillation time is cut by only two hours, 18 to 20 constituents will be missing from the oil. However, most cypress is distilled for only 2 hours and 15 minutes. The short distillation times allow the producer to cut costs and produce a cheaper oil, since money is saved on fuel to generate the steam. It also mean less wear and tear on equipment.

In France, lavender produced commercially is often distilled for only 15 to 20 minutes at 155 lbs. of pressure with a steam temperature approaching 350 degrees F. Although this oil costs less and is easily marketed, it is of poor quality. It retains few, if any, of the therapeutic properties of the high grade lavender distilled at 0 lbs. of pressure for two hours.

In many large commercial fields during distillation, essential oil growers and distillers are introducing chemicals into the steam distillation process to increase the volume of oil produced. Chemical trucks can now pump solvents directly into the boiler water. This expands oil production by as much as 18 percent. However, these chemicals inevitably leach into the distilling water and mix

Essential Oil	Starting Material	Oil Production	Optical Rotation	Pressure in lbs	Distilling Temp.	Distilling Time
Cypress	2000 lb	1 lb	24	0	220	24 hrs.
Pine	1000 lb	1 lb	2	0	180	8 hrs.
Myrtle	500 kl	1 kl	22	1-2	200	7-9 hrs.
Palmarosa	600 kl	1 kl	6	2	200	4 hrs.
Lemongrass	650 kl	17.5 kl	0	5	230	2.75 hrs.
Citronella	150 lb	1 lb	0	5	225	4.5 hrs.
Rosewood	500 kl	1 kl	-4	30	287	3 hrs.
Cinnamon	1300 lb	5 oz	0	5	225-235	9-24 hrs.
Clove	450 kl	5 lit	0	10	229	18 hrs.
Eucalyptus	250 lb	1 lb	5	5	225	3-18 hrs.
Melaleuca	1000 lb	10-15 lb	3	3	218	2-3 hrs.
Geranium	500 lb	6 lb	-8	1.2	200	1-3 hrs.

with the essential oil, fracturing the molecular structure of the oil and altering both its fragrance and therapeutic value. Moreover, these chemicals remain with oil after it is sold because it is almost impossible to completely separate them out of the oil.

Other ways that essential oil producers can increase the quantity of oil extracted is through redistillation. This refers to the repeated distillation of the plant material to maximize the volume of oil by using second, third, and fourth stages of steam distillation, with each distillation generating successively weaker and less potent essential oils. Such essential oils are also degraded due to their prolonged exposure to water used in the redistillation; this water can hydrolize or oxidize the oil and begin to chemically break down the constituents responsible for its aroma and therapeutic properties.

Combining Traditional Steam Distillation with Modern Technology

Few people appreciate how chemically complex essential oils are. They are rich tapestries of literally hundreds of chemical components, some of which—even in small quantities—contribute important therapeutic benefits. The key to preserving as many as possible of these delicate aromatic constituents is to steam distill plant material in small batches using low pressure and low heat. This is the traditional method of distillation that has been used for centuries in Europe but is being abandoned in favor of high-volume pressure cookers designed to operate at over 400 degrees F. and 50 pounds of pressure.

Even more important, the cooking chamber where the plants are distilled should be constructed of a non-reactive metal, like stainless steel, to reduce the possibility of the essential oil being chemically altered by the more reactive metals, such as steel or copper.

No solvents or synthetic chemicals should be used or added to the water used to generate steam because they might jeopardize the integrity of the essential oil. Even the addition of chemicals to water used in the closed-loop heat-exchange systems of the condenser can be dangerous, since there is no guarantee that they can be completely isolated from the essential oil. It is unfortunate that many essential oils distilled commercially are

Different Types of Oil Production

Expressed oils are pressed from the rind of fruits, such as grapefruit, lemon, orange, and tangerine. Rich in terpene alcohols, expressed oils technically are not "essential oils," even though they are highly regarded for their therapeutic properties. Expressed oils should only be obtained from organically grown crops, since pesticide residues can become highly concentrated in the oil.

Steam distillation is the oldest and most traditional method of extraction. Plant material is inserted into a cooking chamber, and steam is passed through it. After the steam is collected and condensed, it is run through a separator to collect the oil.

Solvent-extraction involves the use of oil-soluble solvents, such as hexane, dimethylenechloride, and acetone. Because there can be no guarantee that solvent residues will not be found in the finished product, none of Young Living's essential oils are processed using solvent extraction.

Absolutes are technically not "essential oils" but are "essences." They are obtained from the grain alcohol extraction of a concrete, which is the solid waxy residue that is derived from the extraction of plant materials, usually flower petals. This method of extraction is used primarily for botanicals where the fragrance and therapeutic parts of the plant can only be unlocked using solvents. Jasmine and neroli are extracted this way.

processed using boiler water laden with chemicals and descaling agents.

Absolutely no pesticides, herbicides, fungicides, or agricultural chemicals of any kind should be used in the cultivation of herbs earmarked for distillation. These chemicals—even in minute quantities—can react with the essential oil and degrade its purity and quality and render it less therapeutically effective. Of even graver concern, some pesticides can intermix with the essential oil in the cultivation of our crops.

Essential Oil Production

Producing pure essential oils is very costly. It often requires several hundred or even thousands of pounds of raw plant material to produce a single pound of essential oil. For example, it takes three tons of melissa to produce one pound of oil. Its extremely low yield explains why it sells for $9,000 to $15,000 a kilo. It takes 5,000 pounds of rose petals to produce one pound of rose oil. It is not difficult to understand why these oils are so expensive.

The vast majority of oils are produced for the perfume industry, which is only interested in their aromatic qualities. High pressure, high temperatures, and the use of chemical solvents are used in this distillation process to produce greater quantity of oil at a faster rate. To many people, these oils smell exquisite but lack true therapeutic properties. Many of the important chemical constituents necessary to produce therapeutic results are either flashed off with the high heat or do not have enough time to be released from the plant material.

The Benefits of Therapeutic-Grade Essential Oils

1. Essential oils are so small in molecular size that they can quickly penetrate the tissues of the skin.

2. Essential oils are lipid solubles and are capable of penetrating cell walls, even if they have hardened because of an oxygen deficiency. In fact, essential oils can affect every cell of the body within 20 minutes and are then metabolized like other nutrients.

3. Essential oils contain oxygen molecules which help to transport nutrients to starving human cells. Because a nutritional deficiency is an oxygen deficiency, disease begins when the cells lack the oxygen for proper nutrient assimilation. By providing the needed oxygen, essential oils also work to stimulate the immune system.

4. Essential oils are very powerful antioxidants that create an unfriendly environment for damaging free radicals. They prevent all mutations, work as free-radical scavengers, prevent fungus, and prevent oxidation in the cells.

5. Essential oils are antibacterial, anticancerous, antifungal, anti-infectious, antimicrobial, anti-tumoral, antiparasitic, antiviral, and antiseptic. Essential oils have been shown to destroy all tested bacteria and viruses while simultaneously restoring physiological balance to the body.

6. Essential oils may detoxify the cells and blood in the body.

7. Essential oils containing sesquiterpenes have the ability to pass the blood-brain barrier.

8. Essential oils are aromatic and when diffused may provide air purification by:

    A. Removing metallic particles and toxins from the air;

    B. Increasing atmospheric oxygen;

    C. Increasing ozone and negative ions in the area, which inhibit bacterial growth;

    D. Eliminating odors from mold, cigarettes, and animals; and

    E. Filling the air with a fresh, aromatic scent.

9. Essential oils promote emotional, physical, and spiritual well being.

10. Essential oils have a bio-electrical frequency that is several times greater than the frequency of herbs, food, and even the human body. Clinical research has shown that essential oils can quickly raise the frequency of the human body, restoring it to its normal, healthy level.

How to Identify Disease Using Essential Oils

Frequency is a measurable rate of electrical energy that is constant between any two points. Every living thing has an electrical frequency. Research on human frequency is fascinating.

- Robert O. Becker, M.D., documents the electrical frequency of the human body in his book, *The Body Electric.*

- A "frequency generator" was developed in the early 1920s by Royal Raymond Rife, M.D. He found that by using certain frequencies he could destroy a cancer cell or virus. He found that these frequencies could prevent the development of disease, and others would destroy disease.

- Nikola Tesla said that if you could eliminate certain outside frequencies that interfered with our own electrical frequencies, we would have greater disease resistance.

- Bjorn Nordenstrom is a radiologist from Stockholm, Sweden, who wrote the book *Biologically Closed Circuits.* He discovered in the 1980s that by putting an electrode inside a tumor and running a milliamp D.C. (Direct Current) through the electrode, he could dissolve the cancer tumor and stop its growth. He found electropositive and electronegative energy fields in the human body.

- Bruce Tainio of Tainio Technology in Cheney, Washington, developed new equipment to measure the bio-frequency of humans and foods. He used this biofrequency monitor to determine the relationship between frequency and disease.

Measuring in hertz, it was found that processed/canned food had a zero MHz frequency; fresh produce measured up to 15 MHz; dry herbs from 12-22 MHz; and fresh herbs from 20-27 MHz. Essential oils started at 52 MHz and went as high as 320 MHz, which is the frequency of rose oil. A healthy body typically has a frequency ranging from 62 to 78 MHz, while disease begins at 58 MHz.

Clinical research shows that with essential oils having the highest frequency of any natural substance known to man, they create an environment in which microbes cannot live. Truly, the chemistry and frequencies of essential oils have the ability to help man maintain an optimal health frequency.

It is wonderful to discover that essential oil frequencies are several times greater than frequencies of herbs and foods.

For years research has been conducted on the use of electrical energy to reverse disease. Scientists in the field of natural healing have believed there has to be a more natural way to increase the body's electrical frequency. This led to the research and subsequent discovery of electrical frequencies in essential oils.

Patients felt better emotionally when oils were diffused in their rooms. It seemed that, within seconds, their heads would clear through simple inhalation. Certain oils acted within 1-3 minutes; others acted within seconds. It is fascinating to think that an oil applied to the bottom of the feet could travel to the head and take effect within one minute. The more results that have been seen, the more research has been initiated.

Unhealthy Substances Cause Frequency Changes

$$CH_2 = C - CH_2 - CH_2$$
with C

19

PEOPLE'S DESK REFERENCE FOR ESSENTIAL OILS

In one test, the frequency of two individuals – the first a 26 yr. old male and the second a 24 yr. old male – was measured at 66 MHz each. The first individual held a cup of coffee (without drinking any), and his frequency dropped to 58 MHz in 3 seconds. He put the coffee down and inhaled an aroma of essential oils. Within 21 seconds, his frequency had returned to 66 MHz. The second individual took a sip of coffee and his frequency dropped to 52 MHz in the same 3 seconds. However, no essential oils were used during the recovery time, and it took 3 days for his frequency to return to its initial 66 MHz.

One surprising aspect of this study measured the influence that thoughts have on the body's electrical frequency. Negative thoughts lowered the measured frequency by 12 MHz and positive thoughts raised the measured frequency by 10 MHz. It was also found that prayer and meditation increased the measured frequency levels by 15 MHz.

The Chemistry of Essential Oils

Essential Oil Constiuents

Essential Oil
Aromatic Ring Structure
CAMPHOR

CH₃
      C
H   C   C
H   C   C
H₃C   CH₃
H   C   C
H   C   C
H   H
      C
   H   H

Unlike synthetic chemicals, essential oil chemicals are diverse in their effects. No two oils are alike. Some constituents, such as aldehydes found in lavender and chamomile, are antimicrobial and calming. Eugenol, found in cinnamon and clove, is antiseptic and stimulating. Ketones, found in lavender, hyssop, and patchouly, stimulate cell regeneration and liquefy mucous. Phenols, found in oregano and thyme oil, are highly antimicrobial. Sesquiterpenes, predominant in sandalwood and frankincense, are soothing to inflamed tissue and produce profound effects on emotions and hormonal balance.

The complex chemistry of essential oils makes them ideal to kill and prevent the spread of bacteria, since microorganisms have a hard time mutating in the presence of so many different antiseptic compounds. In 1985, Dr. Jean C. Lapraz said that he could not find any microbe that could live in the presence of the essential oils of cinnamon or oregano. This is significant as we face life-threatening, drug-resistant viruses and bacteria. Today, we see microbial mutations that are starting to create panic in many parts of the world.

The essential oils of ravensara, oregano, mountain savory, clove, black cumin, cistus, Idaho tansy, hyssop, and frankincense are highly antibacterial and immune supportive properties that have been documented by many researchers, such as Daniel Pénoël, M.D. and Pierre Franchomme, Ph.D. These oils are found in varying amounts in the blends of ImmuPower, Thieves, and Exodus II.

Constituents	Essential Oil	Property	Effect
Ketones	Sage	neurotoxic	mucolytic
Aldehydes	Lemongrass	irritant	calming
Esters	Lavender	soothing	balancing
Ethers	Tarragon	soothing	balancing
Alcohols	Ravensara	energizing	toning
Phenols	Savory	hepatotoxic	stimulant
Terpenes	Pine	skin irritant	stimulant

Understanding Essential Oil Chemistry

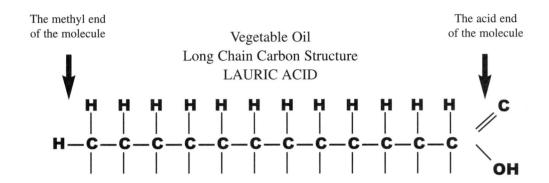

The methyl end of the molecule

The acid end of the molecule

Vegetable Oil
Long Chain Carbon Structure
LAURIC ACID

Basic Chemical Structure

The aromatic constituents of essential oils (ie., terpenes, monoterpenes, phenols, aldehydes, etc.) are constructed from long chains of carbon and hydrogen atoms, which have a predominantly ring-like chemical structure. Links of carbon atoms form the backbone of these chains, with oxygen, nitrogen, sulfur, and other carbon atoms that are attached at various points of the chain.

Essential oils are chemically different from fatty oils (also known as fatty acids). In contrast to the simple linear carbon-hydrogen structure of fatty oils, essential oils have a far more complex aromatic-ring structure and contain sulfur and nitrogen atoms that fatty oils do not have.

The terpenoids found in many essential oils are actually constructed out of the same basic building block—a five-carbon molecule known as isoprene.

When two isoprene units link together, they create a monoterpene; when three join, they create a sesquiterpene; and so on. Some of largest molecules found in essential oils are triterpenoids, which consist of 30 carbon atoms or six isoprene units linked together. Carotenoids, which consist of 40 carbons and eight isprene units, only occur in essential oils in tiny quantities because they are too heavy to be extracted via steam distillation.

Different molecules in an essential oil can exert different effects. For example, German chamomile *(Matricaria recutita)* contains azulene, a dark blue compound that has powerful anti-inflammatory compounds. German chamomile also contains bisobolol, a compound studied for its sedative and mood-balancing properties. There are other compounds in German chamomile that perform different functions, like speeding the regeneration of tissue.

Chemotypes

A single species of plant can have several different chemotypes (or cultivares) based its chemical composition. This means that basil *(Ocimum basilicum)* grown in one area might produce an essential oil with a completely different chemistry than that from a basil grown in another location. The plant's growing environment, such as soil pH and mineral content, can dramatically affect the plant's chemistry as well.

Chemotypes of *Ocimum basilicum*

Ocimum basilicum Linalol Fenchol CT (Germany)
• antiseptic

Ocimum basilicum Methyl Chavicol CT (Reunion, Comoro, or Egypt)
• anti-inflammatory

Ocimum basilicum Eugenol CT (Madagascar)
• anti-inflammatory, pain-relieving

Another species of plant that occurs in a variety of different chemotypes is rosemary (*Rosmarinus officinalis*).

Rosmarinus officinalis CT Camphor is high in camphor. Camphor serves best as a general stimulant and works synergistically with other oils, such as black pepper, and can be a powerful energy stimulant.

Rosmarinus officinalis CT Cineol is rich in 1,8 cineol, which is used in other countries for pulmonary congestion and to help with the elimination of toxins from the liver and kidneys.

Rosmarinus officinalis CT Verbenon is high in verbenon and is the most gentle of the rosemary chemotypes. It offers powerful regenerative properties and has outstanding benefits for skin care.

Thyme (*Thymus vulgaris*) also has several different chemotypes. Some of these include:

Thymus vulgaris CT Carvacrol is germicidal and anti-inflammatory.

Thymus vulgaris CT Linalool is anti-infectious (skin).

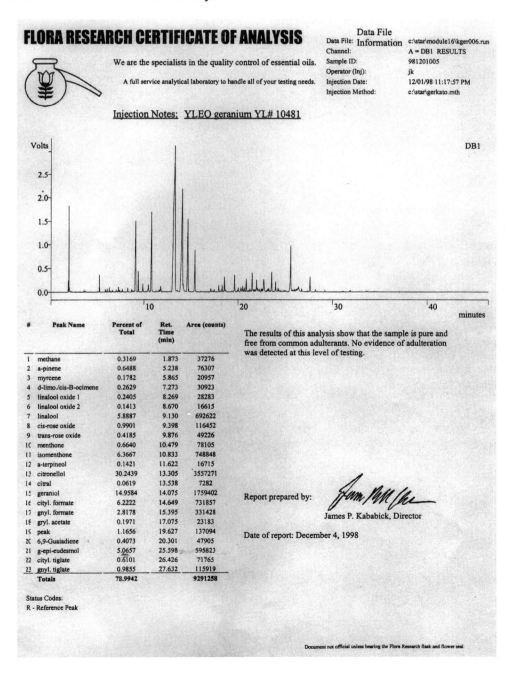

FLORA RESEARCH CERTIFICATE OF ANALYSIS

We are the specialists in the quality control of essential oils.

A full service analytical laboratory to handle all of your testing needs.

Data File Information

Data File:	c:\star\module16\kger006.run
Channel:	A = DB1 RESULTS
Sample ID:	981201005
Operator (Inj):	jk
Injection Date:	12/01/98 11:17:57 PM
Injection Method:	c:\star\gerkato.mth

Injection Notes: YLEO geranium YL# 10481

The results of this analysis show that the sample is pure and free from common adulterants. No evidence of adulteration was detected at this level of testing.

#	Peak Name	Percent of Total	Ret. Time (min)	Area (counts)
1	methane	0.3169	1.873	37276
2	a-pinene	0.6488	5.238	76307
3	myrcene	0.1782	5.865	20957
4	d-limo./cis-B-ocimene	0.2629	7.273	30923
5	linalool oxide 1	0.2405	8.269	28283
6	linalool oxide 2	0.1413	8.670	16615
7	linalool	5.8887	9.130	692622
8	cis-rose oxide	0.9901	9.398	116452
9	trans-rose oxide	0.4185	9.876	49226
10	menthone	0.6640	10.479	78105
11	isomenthone	6.3667	10.833	748848
12	a-terpineol	0.1421	11.622	16715
13	citronellol	30.2439	13.305	3557271
14	citral	0.0619	13.538	7282
15	geraniol	14.9584	14.075	1759402
16	cityl. formate	6.2222	14.649	731857
17	gnyl. formate	2.8178	15.395	331428
18	gryl. acetate	0.1971	17.075	23183
19	peak	1.1656	19.627	137094
20	6,9-Guaiadiene	0.4073	20.301	47905
21	g-epi-eudesmol	5.0657	25.598	595823
22	cityl. tiglate	0.6101	26.426	71765
23	gnyl. tiglate	0.9855	27.632	115919
	Totals	**78.9942**		**9291258**

Status Codes:
R - Reference Peak

Report prepared by:

James P. Kababick, Director

Date of report: December 4, 1998

Document not official unless bearing the Flora Research flask and flower seal.

Classification of Essential Oil Constituents

Carbohydrates
  Monosaccharides
  Oligosaccharides
  Sugar Alcohols & Cyclitols

Lipids
  Organic Acids
  Fatty Acids
  Lipids

Hydrocarbons & Derivatives
  Acetylenes
  Thiophenes

Nitrogen-containing constituents
  Amino Acids
  Amines
  Cyanogenic Glucosides
  Glucosinates
  Purines
  Pyrinidines
  Proteins
  Peptides
  Alkaloids
  Amaryllidaceae Alkaloids
  Betain Alkalydes
  Di-Terpinoid Alkalides

Indul Alkaloids
  Monoterpene Alkaloids
  Sesquiterpene Alkaloids
  Peptide Alkalides
  Phenolics
  Anthoycylines
  Benzofurans
  Chromones
  Coumarins
  Flavonoids
  Flavonones
  Isoflavonoids
  Neoflavonoids
  Phenolics
    Phenolic Acids
    Phenolic Ketones
    Phenolproponoids
Terpenoids
  Monoterpenoids
  Sesquiterpenoids
  Sesquiterpene Lactones
  Di-terpenoids
  Triterpenoids
  Saponin
  Steroid Saponins
  Phytosterols
  Carotenoids

Scientific Research: Essential Oils

Scientific Research List

1. "Effect of a Diffused Essential Oil Blend on Bacterial Bioaerosols"

2. "Antibacterial Properties of Plant Essential Oils"

3. "Influence of Some Spice Essential Oils on *Aspergillus parasiticus* Growth and Production of Aflatoxins in a Synthetic Medium"

4. "Antioxidant Activity of Some Spice Essential Oils on Linoleic Acid Oxidation in Aqueous Media"

5. "Antimicrobial Activity of Some Egyptian Spice Essential Oils"

6. "Antimicrobial Properties of Spices and Their Essential Oils"

7. "The Antimicrobial Activity of Essential Oils and Essential Oil Components Towards Oral Bacteria"

8. "Anticarcinogenic Effects of the Essential Oils From Cumin, Poppy and Basil"

9. "Effects of Essential Oil on Lipid Peroxidation and Lipid Metabolism in Patients with Chronic Bronchitis"

10. "Effect of Essential Oils on the Course of Experimental Atherosclerosis"

11. "Inhibition of Growth and Aflatoxin Production in *Aspergillus parasiticus* by Essential Oils of Selected Plant Materials"

12. "Odors and Learning"

13. "Weight Reduction through Inhalation of Odorants"

14. "Anti-inflammatory Activity of *Passiflora incarnata* L. in Rats"

15. "Medroxyprogesterone Interferes with Ovarian Steroid Protection Against Coronary Vasospasm"

16. "Methyl-Sulfonyl-Methane (M.S.M.): A Double-Blind Study of Its Use in Degenerative Arthritis"

17. "Chemopreventive Effect of Perillyl Alcohol on 4-(methylnitrosamino)-1-(3-pyridyl)-1-butanone Induced Tumorigenesis in (C3H/HeJ X A/J)F1 Mouse Lung"

18. "Chemoprevention of Colon Carcinogenesis by Dietary Perillyl Alcohol"

1. Effect of a Diffused Essential Oil Blend on Bacterial Bioaerosols

Author: S. C. Chao, D. G. Young, and C. J. Oberg

Journal: Journal of Essential Oil Research 10, 517-523 (Sept/Oct 1998)

Location: Weber State University, Ogden, UT

Conclusion: Diffusion of the oil blend, Thieves, can significantly reduce the number of aerosol-borne bacteria.

Abstract: A proprietary blend of oils (named Thieves) containing cinnamon, rosemary, clove, eucalyptus, and lemon was tested for its antibacterial activity against airborne *Micrococcus luteus*, *Pseudomonas aeruginosa,* and *Staphylococcus aureus*. The bacteria cultures were sprayed in an enclosed area, and Thieves was diffused for a given amount of time. There was an 82 percent reduction in *M. luteus* bioaerosol, a 96 percent reduction in the *P. aeruginosa* bioaerosol, and a 44 percent reduction in the *S. aureus* bioaerosol following 10 minutes of exposure.

2. Antibacterial properties of plant essential oils

Author: S. G. Deans, G. Ritchie

Journal: International Journal of Food Microbiology 5, 165-180 (1987)

Location: Scotland Agricultural College

Conclusion: Many essential oils have antibacterial properties.

Abstract: Fifty plant essential oils were tested in different concentrations for antibacterial activity against 25 genera of bacteria. The ten most antibacterial oils were: angelica, bay, cinnamon, clove, thyme, almond, marjoram, pimento, geranium, and lovage.

3. Influence of Some Spice Essential Oils on Aspergillus parasiticus Growth and Production of Aflatoxins in a Synthetic Medium

Author: R. S. Farag, Z. Y. Daw, S. H. Abo-Raya

Journal: Journal of Food Science, Vol 54, No. 1, 74-76 (1989)

Location: Cairo University, Giza, Egypt

Conclusion: Essential oils of thyme, cumin, clove, caraway, rosemary, and sage all possess antifungal properties.

Abstract: The essential oils of thyme, cumin, clove, caraway, rosemary, and sage were tested for antifungal properties. The essential oils completely inhibited growth of fungal mycelium and aflatoxin production. The oils from most effective to least effective were: thyme > cumin > clove > caraway > rosemary > sage. The basic components of these oils were determined by gas-liquid chromatography to be: thyme—thymol, cumin—cumin aldehyde, clove—eugenol, caraway—carvone, rosemary—borneol, and sage—thujone.

4. Antioxidant Activity of Some Spice Essential Oils on Linoleic Acid Oxidation in Aqueous Media

Author: R. S. Farag, A.Z.M.A. Badei, F. M. Hewedi, G.S.A. El-Baroty

Journal: JAOCS, Vol. 66, No. 6 (June 1989)

Location: Cairo University, Giza, Egypt

Conclusion: Essential oils of caraway, clove, cumin, rosemary, sage, thyme possess antioxidant activity on linoleic acid oxidation.

Abstract: Essential oils of caraway, clove, cumin, rosemary, sage and thyme were examined for antioxidant activity in linoleic acid. These oils were all found to have an antioxidant effect which increased when their concentrations were increased. The effectiveness of these essential oils on linoleic acid oxidation was in the following order: caraway, sage, cumin, rosemary, thyme, clove.

5. Antimicrobial Activity of Some Egyptian Spice Essential Oils

Author: R.S. Farag, Z. Y. Daw, F. M. Hewedi, G.S.A. El-Baroty

Journal: Journal of Food Protection, Vol. 52 (September 1989)

Location: Cairo University, Giza, Egypt

Conclusion: Essential oils of sage, rosemary, caraway, cumin, clove, and thyme were shown to have antimicrobial properties.

Abstract: Essential oils of sage, rosemary, caraway, cumin, clove, and thyme were studied for their antibacterial effects. The minimum inhibitory concentration for each essential oil was also determined. Various essential oils were inhibitory at extremely low concentrations (0.25-12 mg/ml). Gram-positive bacteria were shown to be more sensitive to the essential oils than were gram-negative. Thyme and cumin oils had stronger antimicrobial activity than the other oils. The chemical structures of compounds in the essential oils were related to the antimicrobial activity.

6. Antimicrobial Properties of Spices and Their Essential Oils

Author: L. R. Beuchat

Journal: Nat. Antimicrob. Syst. Food Preserv. 167-79 (1994)

Location: University of Georgia, Griffin, Georgia

Conclusion: Many spices and herbs possess antimicrobial properties against various bacteria, yeasts, and molds.

Abstract: Many spices and herbs possess antimicrobial actions. These include plants of the genus *Allium*, such as onions and garlic; spices such as thyme, oregano, savory, sage, cinnamon, clove, vanilla, and others. Microbes inhibited by these herbs and spices include gram-positive and gram-negative bacteria, yeasts, and molds.

7. The Antimicrobial Activity of Essential Oils and Essential Oil Components Towards Oral Bacteria

Author: S. Shapiro, A. Meier, B. Guggenheim

Journal: Oral Microbiology and Immunology 1994: 202-208 (Copyright Munksgaard 1994)

Location: University of Zurich, Switzerland

Conclusion: Essential oils of tea tree, peppermint, and sage showed potent antimicrobial action against anaerobic oral activity.

Abstract: Antimicrobial activity of some essential oils on anaerobic oral bacteria was analyzed. The most potent essential oils tested were Australian tea tree oil, peppermint oil, and sage oil. Thymol and eugenol were the most potent oil components.

8. Anticarcinogenic Effects of the Essential Oils From Cumin, Poppy and Basil

Author: K. Aruna, V. M. Sivaramakrishnan

Journal: Phytotherapy Research, Vol. 10, 577-580 (1996)

Location: Cancer Institute (W.I.A.) Adyar Madras, India

Conclusion: Essential oils of cumin, poppy, and basil all possess potent anticarcinogenic properties.

Abstract: Essential oils of cumin, poppy, and basil were assessed for anticarcinogenic properties. The activity of glutathione-S-transferase, a carcinogen-detoxifying enzyme, was increased by over 78 percent in the stomach, liver, and esophagus of Swiss mice when they were treated with cumin, poppy, and basil essential oils.

9. Effects of Essential Oil on Lipid Peroxidation and Lipid Metabolism in Patients with Chronic Bronchitis

Author: S. A. Siurin

Journal: Klinicheskaia Meditsina, 75(10):43-5 (1997)

Location: Scientific Group NII of Pulmonology, Monchegorsk, Russia.

Conclusion: Lavender essential oil aids in normalizing lipid levels.

Abstract: Essential oils were tested in 150 patients with chronic bronchitis for their effects on lipid peroxidation and lipid metabolism. Essential oils of rosemary, basil, fir, eucalyptus, and lavender were found to have antioxidant effect and lavender was found to normalize lipid levels.

10. Effect of Essential Oils on the Course of Experimental Atherosclerosis

Author: V. V. Nikolaevskii, N. S. Kononova, A. I. Pertsoviskii, I.F. Shinkarchuk

Journal: Patologicheskaia Fiziologiia i Eksperimentalnaia Terapiia (5):52-3 (Sep-Oct 1990)

Conclusion: Inhalation of lavender and monarda essential oils reduces cholesterol content in the aorta of rabbits, providing an angioprotective effect.

Abstract: Lavender, monarda, and basil essential oils were tested in rabbits for their effect on atherosclerosis. When inhaled, lavender and monarda essential oils did not affect blood cholesterol content, but reduced cholesterol content in the aorta. These oils provide a heart-protective effect.

11. Inhibition of Growth and Aflatoxin Production in Aspergillus parasiticus by Essential Oils of Selected Plant Materials

Author: A. Tantaoui-Elaraki, L. Beraoud

Journal: Journal of Environmental Pathology, Toxicology and Oncology;13(1):67-72 (1994)

Location: Hassan II Institute for Agriculture and Veterinary Medicine, Rabat-Instituts, Morocco

Conclusion: Several essential oils (cinnamon, thyme, oregano, and cumin) were shown to have strong antifungal properties.

Abstract: Essential oils of cinnamon, thyme, oregano, cumin, curcumin, ginger, lemon, and orange were tested on *Aspergillus parasiticus* for antifungal properties. The most inhibitory essential oils were cinnamon, thyme, oregano, and cumin.

12. Odors and Learning

Author: A. R. Hirsch, M.D., L. H. Johnston, M.D.

Journal: J. Neurol Orthop Med Surg 17:119-126 (1996)

Location: Smell & Taste Research Foundation, Chicago, Illinois, USA

Conclusion: Pleasant odors increased performance of individuals on cognitive tasks.

Abstract: This study assessed the effects of hedonically positive odors on performance of cognitive tasks. Results indicate that normally performing subjects completed a cognitive task an average 17 percent faster on subsequent trials when a pleasing odor was present. Further studies are desirable to determine if odors would be useful in general education and education of those with learning disabilities.

13. Weight Reduction through Inhalation of Odorants

Author: A. R. Hirsch, M.D., R. Gomez

Journal: Annals of Clinical and Laboratory Science (Official Journal of the Association of Clinical Scientists) Volume 24 September-October Number 5

Location: Smell & Taste Research Foundation, Chicago, Illinois, USA

Conclusion: Use of aroma inhalers aided study volunteers in weight loss over a 6-month period.

Abstract: To measure the role of olfaction in weight loss, odorant inhalers were given to 3,193 overweight volunteers. Study participants were instructed to inhale odorants 3 times in each nostril whenever hunger occurred. Average weight loss was 2.1 percent body weight per month. These results suggest inhalation of odorants may induce sustained weight loss over a 6-month period.

14. Anti-inflammatory Activity of Passiflora incarnata L. in Rats

Author: F. Borrelli, L. Pinto, A. A. Izzo, N. Mascolo, F. Capasso, V. Mercati, E. Toja, G. Autore

Journal: Phytotherapy Research, Vol. 10, S104-S106 (1996)

Location: University of Naples, Naples, Italy

Conclusion: *Passiflora incarnata* extract was found to have anti-inflammatory activity in rats.

Abstract: Ethanolic extract of *Passiflora incarnata* (passion flower) was tested for anti-inflammatory activity in rats. The extract significantly inhibited swelling and inflammation.

15. Medroxyprogesterone Interferes with Ovarian Steroid Protection Against Coronary Vasospasm

Author: K. Miyagawa, J. Rosch, F. Stanczyk, K. Hermsmeyer

Journal: Nature Medicine, Vol. 3 (3); (March 1997)

Location: Oregon Health Sciences University, Beaverton, Oregon

Conclusion: Progesterone was found to cause less risk of cardiovascular disease than medroxyprogesterone, a synthetic progesterone.

Abstract: Progesterone and medroxyprogesterone, a synthetic progesterone, were tested on rhesus monkeys. Medroxyprogesterone was found to cause an increased risk of cardiovascular disease compared to progesterone.

16. Methyl-Sulfonyl-Methane (M.S.M.) A Double-Blind Study of Its Use in Degenerative Arthritis

Author: R. M. Lawrence

Journal: Preliminary correspondence, not yet published

Location: UCLA School of Medicine, Los Angeles, CA

Conclusion: MSM helps patients with degenerative arthritis in pain management.

Abstract: A double-blind study was conducted on patients suffering from degenerative joint disease. After 6 weeks, patients given MSM showed an 82 percent improvement in pain on average. MSM is a safe, non-toxic method of managing pain.

17. Chemopreventive Effect of Perillyl Alcohol on 4-(methylnitrosamino)-1-(3-pyridyl)-1-butanone Induced Tumorigenesis in (C3H/HeJ X A/J)F1 Mouse Lung

Author: L. E. Lantry, Z. Zhang, F. Gao, K. A. Crist, Y. Wang, G. J. Kelloff, R. A. Lubet, M. You

Journal: Journal of Cellular Biochemistry Supplement; 27:20-5 (1997)

Location: Medical College of Ohio, Toledo, OH.

Conclusion: Perillyl alcohol possesses chemopreventive effects in a mouse lung tumor experiment.

Abstract: Perillyl alcohol, a naturally occurring monoterpene found in lavender, cherries, and mint was given to laboratory mice which were then exposed to carcinogens. Perillyl-treated mice had a 22 percent reduction in tumor incidence compared to non-treated mice. Perillyl alcohol is an effective chemopreventive compound in mouse lung tumors.

18. Chemoprevention of Colon Carcinogenesis by Dietary Perillyl Alcohol

Author: B. S. Reddy, C. X. Wang, H. Samaha, R. Lubet, V. E. Steele, G. J. Kelloff, C. V. Rao

Journal: Cancer Research 1;57(3): 420-5 (1997 Feb)

Location: American Health Foundation, Valhalla, NY

Conclusion: Perillyl alcohol is shown to have chemopreventive activity in colon cancer in lab rats.

Abstract: Perillyl alcohol, a monoterpene found in lavender, was administered to rats which were then given azoxymethane (AOM), an agent causing colon carcinogenesis. Perillyl alcohol inhibited the incidence of adenocarcinomas of the colon and small intestine as compared to the control.

Everyday Use of Essential Oils

Safety

There are a few guidelines to keep in mind when using essential oils, especially if you are new to this practice. They are listed below and will be elaborated on throughout the chapter. However, no list of "do's and don'ts" could ever replace common sense. It is foolish to dive headlong into a pond when you don't know the depth of the water. Start gradually, and find what works best for you and your family.

Guidelines for Safe Use

- Always keep a bottle of a pure vegetable or carrier oil handy when using essential oils. Vegetable oils dilute essential oils if they cause discomfort or skin irritation.

- Keep bottles of essential oils tightly closed and store in a cool location away from light. If stored properly, essential oils will maintain their potency for many years.

- Keep essential oils out of reach of children. Treat them as you would any product for therapeutic use.

- Essential oils rich in menthol (such as peppermint) should not be used on the throat or neck area of children under 30 months of age.

- Direct sunlight and essential oils. Lemon, bergamot, orange, grapefruit, tangerine, angelica, and other citrus oils may cause a rash or darker pigmentation if applied to skin exposed to direct sunlight or UV rays within 3 to 4 days.

- Keep essential oils away from eye area and do not put into ears. Do not handle contact lenses or rub eyes with essential oils on your fingers. Oils with high phenol content—oregano, cinnamon, thyme, clove, lemongrass, and bergamot—may damage contacts and irritate eyes.

- Pregnant women may want to consult a health care professional when starting any type of health program.

- Epileptics and those with high blood pressure should consult their health care professional before using essential oils. Use caution with hyssop, fennel, and Idaho tansy oils.

- People with allergies should test a small amount of oil on a small area of sensitive skin, such as the inside of the arm, before applying the oil on other areas. The bottom of the feet is one of the safest, most effective places to use essential oils.

- Before taking GRAS (Generally regarded as Safe-FDA approved) essential oils internally, use a spray applicator or dilute with an oil-soluble liquid like honey, olive oil, or soy milk.

- Do not add undiluted essential oils directly to bathwater. Use Bath Gel Base as a dispersing agent for all oils applied to your bath.

Because essential oils are soluble with the lipid membranes of cells, they have an unmatched ability to disperse within minutes throughout the body. Consider how nicotine skin patches and hormone skin patches rely on transdermal absorption to deliver drugs into the bloodstream.

Before you start...

- Always skin test an essential oil before using it. Each person's body is different, so apply oils to a small area first.

- Apply one oil or blend at a time. When layering oils that are new to you, allow enough time (3 to 5 min.) for the body to respond before applying a second oil.

Exercise caution when applying essential oils to skin that has been exposed to cosmetics, personal care products, soaps, and cleansers containing synthetic chemicals. Some of them—especially petroleum-based chemicals—can penetrate and remain in the skin and fatty tissues for days or even weeks. Essential oils may react with such chemicals and cause skin irritation, nausea, headaches or other uncomfortable effects.

Essential oils can react with toxins built up in the body from chemicals in food, water and work environment. If you experience a reaction to essential oils, it may be wise to temporarily discontinue their use and start an internal cleansing program before resuming regular use of essential oils. Always double your water intake when using essential oils.

You may also want to try the following alternative to a detoxification program to determine the root of the problem:

- Dilute the oils—1 to 3 drops of oil to 1/2 tsp. massage oil, V-6 Mixing Oil, or any pure vegetable oil, such as jojoba or olive. More dilution may be needed.

- Reduce the number of oils used at one time.

- Use single oils or oil blends one at a time.

- Reduce the amount of oil used.

- Reduce the frequency of application.

- Drink more purified or distilled water.

- Ask your health professional to monitor detoxification.

- Skin-test the diluted essential oil on a small patch of skin. If any redness or irritation results, cleanse skin thoroughly and reapply.

- If skin irritation or other uncomfortable side effects persist, discontinue use.

You may also want to avoid using products that contain the following ingredients to eliminate potential problems.

- Cosmetics, deodorants, and skin care products containing aluminum, petrochemicals, or other synthetic ingredients.

- Synthetic chemicals in perms, hair coloring, and hair sprays. Avoid shampoos and soaps containing chemicals, such as sodium lauryl sulfate and lead acetate.

- Garden sprays, paints, detergents, and cleansers containing toxic chemicals and solvents.

You can use essential oils anywhere except on your eyes and ears. Caution: Essential oils may sting if applied in or around the eyes. Some oils may be painful on mucous membranes unless diluted properly. Immediate dilution is strongly recommended if skin becomes painfully irritated or if oil accidentally gets into eyes. Flushing the area with a vegetable oils should minimize discomfort almost immediately. DO NOT flush with water. Essential oils are oil soluble, not water soluble. Water will only spread the oils over a larger surface, possibly exacerbating the problem.

Keep all essential oils out of reach of children and only apply to children under skilled supervision. If a child or infant swallows an essential oil:

- Administer a mixture of milk, cream, yogurt, or another safe, oil-soluble liquid.

- Call your poison control center or seek immediate emergency medical attention if necessary.

Topical Application

Topical application means to apply the oils locally on the skin. Lavender is safe to use on children without dilution. However, you must be sure it is not lavandin that is labeled as lavender or is a genetically-engineered lavender. When applying most other oils on children, dilute the essential oil with a carrier oil. For dilution, add 15 to 30 drops of essential oil to one ounce of a quality carrier oil.

Carrier oils extend essential oils—making them last longer and giving you more efficient use. When massaging, the carrier oil helps lubricate the skin. Some excellent carrier oils include cold-pressed grapeseed, olive, wheat germ, jojoba, and sweet almond oils, or a blend of these.

When starting an essential oil application, always apply the oil first to the bottom of the feet. This allows the body to become acclimated to the oil, minimizing the chance of a reaction. The Vita

Flex foot charts identify areas for best application. Start by applying 3 to 6 drops of a single or blended oil, spreading it over the bottom of each foot.

When applying the oils to another person, place the oil or mixture in the palm of your left hand and mix clockwise with the fingers of your right hand, before applying. This will increase the frequency of the oil. When applying the oils to yourself, use 1 to 2 drops of oil on 2 to 3 locations 2 times a day. Increase to 4 times a day if needed. Rub the oil on briefly and allow it to absorb for 2 to 3 minutes to avoid staining your clothing.

As a general rule, when applying oils to yourself or another for the first time, do not apply more than 2 singles or blends at one time.

When mixing carrier oil with essential oils, it is best to use containers made of glass or earthenware, rather than plastic because plastic particles can leach into the oil and then into the skin once it is applied.

Massage

Start by putting 2 drops of a single oil or blend on location and massaging in. If working on a larger area, such as the back, mix 20 to 30 drops of the selected oil into carrier oil.

Acupuncture

Licensed doctors can dramatically increase the effectiveness of acupuncture by using essential oils. To start, place several drops of essential oil into the palm of your hand. Dip the needle tip into the oil and spin clockwise 3 times before inserting the needle so that the electrical charge of the needle matches the frequency of the oil. You can pre-mix several oils in your hand if you wish to use more than one oil.

Acupressure

When performing acupressure treatment, apply 1 to 3 drops of essential oil to the acupressure point. When stimulating acupressure points, apply oils with the finger. Using an auricular probe that dispenses oil can enhance the application, with the slender point of the probe further increasing the effectiveness of the application. Start be pressing firmly and releasing. Avoid applying pressure to any particular pressure point too long. You may continue along the acupressure points and meridians or use the reflexology or Vita Flex points as well. Once you have completed the small point stimulation, massage the general area with the oil.

Hot Packs

For deeper penetration of an essential oil, use hot packs. Start by dipping a cloth in comfortably hot water. Wring the cloth out and place it on location. After allowing it to cool, wrap it loosely with another dry towel or blanket to seal in the heat. Use this technique 1-3 times daily as needed.

Cold Packs

Apply essential oils on location, followed by cold water or ice packs when treating inflamed or swollen tissues. Frozen packages of peas or corn make excellent ice packs that will mold to the contours of the body part and will not leak. Keep the cold pack on until the swelling diminishes. For neurological problems, always use cold packs, never hot.

Layering

This technique consists of applying oils one at a time. For example, place marjoram over a sore muscle, massage into the tissue gently until the area is dry, then apply the next oil until the oil is absorbed and skin is dry. Then layer on the third oil.

Creating a Compress

- Rub 1-3 drops on location, diluted or neat, depending on the oil and the skin sensitivity at that location.

- Cover with a hot, damp towel.

- Cover the moist towel with a dry towel for 10-60 minutes.

As the oil penetrates, you may experience a warming or even a burning sensation, especially in areas where the greatest benefits occur. If burning becomes uncomfortable, apply massage oil, V-6 Mixing Oil, or any pure vegetable oil to the location.

A second type of application is very mild and is even suitable for infants, children, or those with sensitive skin.

- Place 5 to 15 drops of essential oil into a basin filled with warm water.

- Vigorously agitate the water and let it stand for 1 minute.

- Water temperature should be about 100°F (38°C), unless the patient suffers neurological conditions; in this case, use cool water.

- Place a dry face cloth on top of the water to soak up oils that have floated to the surface.

- Wring out the water and apply the cloth on the location. To seal in warmth, cover with a thick towel for no more than 1 hour.

Bath

Adding essential oils to bathwater is challenging because oil does not mix with water. For even dispersion, drop in the oils while running the bath, or add 2 to 3 drops of oil to a cup of Epsom salts or bath gel base and pass this mixture under the faucet. Either method will help the oils disperse evenly and prevent stronger oils from stinging sensitive areas.

You can also use premixed bath gels containing essential oils as a liquid soap in the shower or bath. Lather down with the bath gel, let it soak in, and then rinse. To maximize benefits, leave them on the skin or scalp for several minutes to allow the essential oils to penetrate. You can create your own aromatic bath gels by placing 5 to 15 drops of essential oil in 1/2 ounce of unscented bath gel base.

Shower

Essential oils may be added to bath salts (such as epsom salts) and used in the shower. The RainSpa shower head contains a special attached receptacle that may be loaded with essential oil salts. This allows essential oils to not only make contact with the skin but also diffuses the fragrance of the oils in the air. The shower head receptacle can hold approximately 1/4 to 1/2 cup of bath salts.

Start by adding several drops of essential oil to 1/4 cup of bath salt and loading the shower head receptacle. This should provide enough material for about two to three showers. The shower head has a bypass feature that allows the user to switch from bath salt water to regular tap water.

How to Enhance the Benefits of Topical Application

The longer essential oils stay in contact with the skin, the more likely they are to be absorbed. Rose Ointment or AromaSilk Body Lotion may be layered on top of the essential oils to reduce evaporation of the oils and enhance penetration. It also helps seal and protect cuts and wounds.

Other Uses

Inhalation

Direct

- Place two or more drops into the palm of the left hand, and rub clockwise with the right hand.

- Cup hands together over the nose and mouth and breathe deeply.

OR

- Add several drops of an essential oil to a bowl of hot (not boiling) water

- Inhale the vapors that rise from the bowl.

- To increase the intensity of the oil vapors inhaled, place a towel over the head

OR

- Apply oils to a cotton ball, tissue, or handkerchief (do not use synthetic fiber or fabric)

- Inhale directly

Indirect or Subtle Inhalation (Wearing as a perfume or cologne)

- Rub 2 or more drops of oil on your chest, neck, upper sternum, wrists, or under nose and ears

- Breathe in the fragrance throughout the day.

Diffusing

A cold-air diffuser is designed to atomize a microfine mist of essential oils into the air, where they can remain suspended for up to several hours. Unlike aromalamps or candles, it disperses oils without the heating or burning that can render the oil therapeutically less beneficial and even create toxic compounds. Research shows that cold air diffusing certain oils may:

- Reduce bacteria, fungus, mold, and unpleasant odors.

- Relax, relieve tension, and clear the mind.

- Help in weight management.

- Improve concentration, alertness, and mental clarity.

- Stimulate neurotransmitters.

- Stimulate secretion of endorphins.

- May stimulate growth hormone production and receptivity.

- Digests petrochemicals on the receptor sites.

- Improve the secretion of IgA antibodies that fight candida.

- Improve digestive function.

- Improve hormonal balance.

- Relieve tension and headaches

- Dispel odors

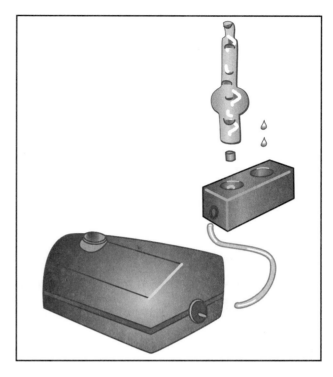

Start by diffusing oils for 15-30 minutes a day. As you become accustomed to the oils and recognize their effects, increase the diffusing time to 1-2 hours.

By connecting your diffuser to a timer, you can gain better control over the length and duration of diffusing. For some respiratory conditions, you can diffuse the oils during the night.

If you don't have a diffuser, add several drops of essential oil to a spray bottle, add water, and shake. You can use this to mist your entire house.

OTHER EASY WAYS TO DIFFUSE OILS

- Add essential oils to cedar chips to make your own potpourri.

- Put scented cedar chips in closets or drawers to deodorize.

- Drop any conifer essential oil onto each log in the fireplace. As they burn, they will disperse a lovely smell. There is little therapeutic benefit.

- Place a bowl of water with a few drops of oil on a wood stove.

- Dampen a cloth, apply essential oils to it, and place it near the intake duct of your heating and cooling system.

Humidifier and Vaporizer

Essential oils, like peppermint, lemon, or frankincense, make ideal additions to humidifiers or vaporizers.

Vaginal Retention Implant

- Place 10-20 drop of essential oil into a tablespoon of carrier oil.

- Use a small syringe to implant the mixture into the vagina and retain it overnight.

- If a capsule is used, it must be implanted immediately after the oils are added.

- A pad or tampon may need to be used to aid in the retention of the essential oil solution.

Rectal Implant and Retention Enema

This method is effective for getting to the urinary tract, the reproductive organs, and the lungs. Always use sterile applicator.

- Mix 20 to 35 drops of essential oil in a teaspoon of carrier oil.

- Place mixture in a small syringe and inject into the rectum.

- Retain mixture through the night (or longer for best results) .

- Clean and disinfect applicator after each use.

Water Distillers and Filters

You can apply oils, like peppermint, lemon, clove, and cinnamon, to the post-filter side of your water purifier. This will help purify the water.

Dishwashing Soap

You can purchase affordable, effective dishwashing soap through a natural products catalog. To add fragrance or antiseptic action to your soap, add several drops of essential oils, like lavender, lemon, bergamot, and oranges.

Cleaning and Disinfecting

A few drops of oil may be added to the washing machine or the dishwasher to help disinfect and purify. Some popular oils are lemon and peppermint, although any antibacterial oil would work well.

Painting

When painting, add a 5 ml. bottle of your favorite essential oil to 1 gallon of paint. The oil will counteract the unpleasant smell of paint. Because essential oils are not fatty oils, they will leave no oil spots on the walls.

Laundry

Essential oils may be used to enhance the cleanliness and fragrance of your laundry. As unpleasant as it seems, mites live in your bedding, feeding from the dead skin cells you constantly shed. Recent research has shown that eucalyptus oil kills dust mites. To achieve effective dust mite control, add 25 drops of eucalyptus to each washload, or approximately 1/2 ounce to a jug of laundry detergent.

Instead of using toxic and irritating softening agents in the dryer, toss in a dampened washcloth loaded with 10 drops of lavender, lemon, melaleuca, bergamot, or other oils. While the oils will not reduce static cling, they will impart a distinctive fragrance to the clothes.

In addition, because clothing (like everything else) has a frequency, consider moving toward natural fabrics instead of synthetics. Cotton, linen, silk, and wool possess energy frequencies harmonious to the human body.

Surface Cleansers: Counters, Furniture, etc.

In addition to purchasing products free of toxicity, for a nominal price you can create many household products on your own. Instead of purchasing standard household cleaners for surfaces, you can create your own version by filling a plastic spray bottle with water and a squirt of dishwashing soap. Add 3 to 5 drops each of lavender, lemon, and pine essential oils. Shake, and your homemade cleaner is ready to spray. This simple solution is extremely economical, yet it cleans and disinfects as well as any commercial cleaner. Furthermore, it smells delicious.

Additional antibacterial and antiviral oils that are excellent for cleansing include cinnamon, clove, eucalyptus, thyme, spruce, lemongrass, and grapefruit.

Floors and Carpet

By combining essential oils with common household detergents, you create your own nontoxic aromatic floor and carpet cleaners.

To clean hard floors, add 1/4 cup of white vinegar to a bucket of water. Then add 5-10 drops of lemon oil or another suitable oil. If the floor is especially dirty, add several drops of dishwashing soap. This will clean even the dirtiest floor.

To make a carpet freshener, add 16 drops of essential oils to a cup of baking soda or borax powder. Mix well and place in a covered container overnight so that the oil can be absorbed. Sprinkle over your carpet and then vacuum.

You can also saturate a cloth with several drops of essential oil and deposit it into the collecting bag of your vacuum. This will diffuse a pleasant odor as you clean. If you have a vacuum that collects dirt into water, simply add a few drops into the water reservoir before cleaning. This refreshes both the carpet and the room.

Insecticide and Repellent: Dust Mites, Fleas, Tics, Ants, Spiders, etc.

Many of us use chemicals to deal with insects. Essential oils, like lavender, lemon, peppermint, lemongrass, eucalyptus, cinnamon, thyme, basil, and citronella, effectively repel many types of insects including mites, lice, and fleas. Peppermint put on the doorsill prevents ants from entering.

If you need moth repellents for your linens and woolens, don't use commercial mothballs. These are toxic. Natural essential oils, like camphor, citronella, lavender, lemongrass, or rosemary, can just as effectively repel them. You can make a

sachet by placing several drops of essential oil on a cotton ball. Then wrap and tie it into a small handkerchief or square of cotton. Hang this cloth in storage areas or add it to your chest of linens. Refresh as often as necessary.

You can put this sachet in your bureau drawers to keep your clothes freshly scented. Lavender and rose make classic scents. For children's sleepwear, Roman chamomile is especially fragrant and relaxing. To scent stationery, stretch out a scented cotton ball and place in an envelope.

Hot Tubs and Saunas

Hot tubs, jacuzzis, and saunas act as reservoirs for germs, especially if you entertain frequently. Lavender, cinnamon, clove, eucalyptus, thyme, lemon, or grapefruit can be used to disinfect and fragrance the water. Use 3 drops per person. For saunas, add several drops of rosemary, thyme, pine, or lavender to a spray bottle with water and then spray down the surfaces. You can also use the scented water to splash on the hot sauna stones.

Deodorizing - Kitchens, Bathrooms, etc.

(See chapter for EVERYDAY USES.)

The kitchen and bathroom are often a source of odors and bacteria.

Single oils:

• Rosemary with lemon, eucalyptus, and lavender.

Use: Add 1-3 drops to the corresponding single oils above (according to your sensitivity).

Blends:

• Lavender with Purification.

Use: Add 1-3 drops of each single oil to the corresponding blend above (according to your sensitivity).

Mix:
• 2 drops rosemary
• 4 drops lemon
• 3 drops eucalyptus
• 4 drops lavender in 1 quart water.

Shake well and put in a spray bottle.

Mix:

- 3 to 4 drops lavender
- 5 to 6 drops Purification in 1 quart water.

Shake well and put in a spray bottle.

Use to freshen, deodorize, and disinfect the air, work areas, cupboards, sinks, tiles, woodwork, carpets, etc. These blends are safe for the family and the environment.

Since the oils separate easily from water, always shake well and keep on shaking as you use these mixtures. They will deodorize and clean the air, instead of covering the odors.

Cooking

Many essential oils make excellent food flavorings. Only 1-2 drops of an essential oil is equivalent to a full bottle of dried herbs.

They are so concentrated that they work well for flavoring.

Single oils: Basil, cinnamon, clove, fennel, ginger, lemon, lavender, marjoram, mountain savory, nutmeg, oregano, peppermint, rosemary, sage, spearmint, tarragon, and thyme.

You'll have to experiment with the blends.

For a recipe that serves 4 to 6 people, add 1 to 2 drops of an oil and stir in after cooking, just before serving so the oil does not evaporate.

Cooking uses:

- Salad dressings or salad oil: Lemon, lavender, rosemary, clove, or peppermint in V-6 Mixing Oil.
- Cakes, frostings, puddings, fruit pies: Lavender, lemon, clove, or peppermint.
- Pie Crusts: V-6 Mixing Oil has been reported to produce very flaky crusts.
- Herbal teas: Lavender, lemon, peppermint, Melissa, and Stevia.

- Cool refreshing drink: Lemon or peppermint added to a pitcher of cold water.
- Flavored honey: warm until it becomes a thin liquid, stir in favorite oil.

Internal and Oral Use as a Dietary Supplement

All essential oils that are Generally Regarded As Safe (GRAS) or certified as Food Additives (FA) by the FDA may be safely taken internally as a dietary supplement. In fact, some oils (valerian, lemon, grapefruit, orange, and tangerine) are more effective taken orally.

Essential oils should be diluted in vegetable oil, honey, soy milk, or rice milk prior to ingestion. More or less dilution may be required, depending on how strong (hot) the oil is. More potent oils, like cinnamon, oregano, lemongrass, and thyme, will require far more dilution than relatively mild oils, like lavender or rose (which may not need any dilution at all). As a general rule, dilute 1 drop of essential oil in 1 teaspoon of honey or in 4 ounces of a beverage like soy milk or rice milk.

Usually no more than 2 or 3 drops should be ingested at one time (during any 4 to 8 hour period). Because essential oils are so concentrated, 1 to 2 drops is often sufficient to achieve significant benefits.

Essential oils should not be given as dietary supplements to children under six years of age. Parents should exercise caution before orally administering essential oils to any child, and oils should always be diluted prior to ingestion.

Essential oils are extremely concentrated, so they should be kept out of reach of infants and children. If a large quantity of oil is ingested at one time (more than 5 drops), please contact your physician or poison control center immediately.

List of Oils Certified as GRAS or Food Additives by the FDA

Angelica		GRAS	FA	Grapefruit		GRAS	FA	Peppermint		GRAS	FA
Basil		GRAS	FA	Helichrysum			FA	Petitgrain		GRAS	FA
Bergamot		GRAS	FA	Hyssop		GRAS	FA	Pine	(FL)	GRAS	FA
Celery Seed		GRAS	FA	Juniper		GRAS	FA	Rosemary		GRAS	FA
Cedarwood			FA	Jasmine		GRAS	FA	Rose		GRAS	FA
Chamomile, Roman	GRAS	FA	Laurus nobilis		GRAS	FA	Rosewood			FA
Chamomile, German	GRAS	FA	Lavendin		GRAS	FA	Savory		GRAS	FA
Cinnamon Bark		GRAS	FA	Lavender		GRAS	FA	Sage		GRAS	FA
Cistus			FA	Lemon		GRAS	FA	Sandalwood	(FL)	GRAS	FA
Citrus rinds (all)		GRAS	FA	Lemongrass		GRAS	FA	Spearmint		GRAS	FA
Citronella		GRAS	FA	Lime		GRAS	FA	Spikenard			FA
Clary Sage		GRAS	FA	Melaleuca alternifolia			FA	Spruce	(FL)	GRAS	FA
Clove		GRAS	FA	Melissa (lemonbalm)	GRAS	FA	Tarragon		GRAS	FA
Coriander		GRAS	FA	Manderin		GRAS	FA	Tangerine		GRAS	FA
Cumin		GRAS	FA	Marjoram		GRAS	FA	Thyme		GRAS	FA
Dill		GRAS	FA	Myrrh	(FL)	GRAS	FA	Valerian	(FL)	GRAS	FA
Eucalyptus	(FL)	GRAS	FA	Myrtle		GRAS	FA	Vetiver		GRAS	FA
Elemi			FA	Neroli		GRAS	FA	Ylang ylang		GRAS	FA
Fennel			FA	Nutmeg		GRAS	FA				
Fir			FA	Orange		GRAS	FA				
Frankincense	(FL)	GRAS	FA	Oregano		GRAS	FA				
Galbanum	(FL)	GRAS	FA	Palmarosa		GRAS	FA				
Geranium		GRAS	FA	Patchouly	(FL)	GRAS	FA				
Ginger		GRAS	FA	Pepper		GRAS	FA				

Code

FA = FDA-approved food additive
(FL) = Flavoring agent
GRAS = Generally regarded as safe

Vita Flex Therapy

Vita Flex Therapy means "vitality through the reflexes." It is a specialized form of hand and foot massage that is exceptionally effective in delivering the benefits of essential oils throughout the body. It is said to have originated in Tibet thousands of years ago, long before acupuncture was developed, and is based on a complete system of internal body controls. Oils are applied to contact points, and energy is released through electrical impulses created by contact between the fingertips and reflex points. This electrical charge follows the nerve pathways to a break in the electrical circuit caused by toxins, damaged tissues, or loss of oxygen. There are more than 1,400 Vita Flex points throughout the human body, encompassing the entire realm of body and mind, that are capable of releasing many kinds of tension, congestion, and imbalances.

In contrast to the steady stimulation of Reflexology, Vita Flex uses a rolling and releasing motion that involves placing all four fingers flat on the skin, rolling onto the fingertips, and continuing over onto the fingernail. Use medium pressure. Move ahead about half the width of the finger and repeat until the Vita Flex point, or area, is covered. Repeat this movement over the area three times.

Combine this technique with 1-2 drops of essential oil to those areas of the feet that correspond to the system of the body you wish to support (SEE DIAGRAM). The Vita Flex (VF) numbers correspond to locations on the feet and are noted on the foot chart. Rapid and extraordinary results are experienced when combining essential oils with Vita Flex stimulation, as it increases the effect of both. Vita Flex and Raindrop Therapy are both demonstrated and explained on the "Science and Application" video available from Essential Science Publishing.

The following diagram on page 42 shows the nervous system connection for the electrical points throughout the body.

VitaFlex Points

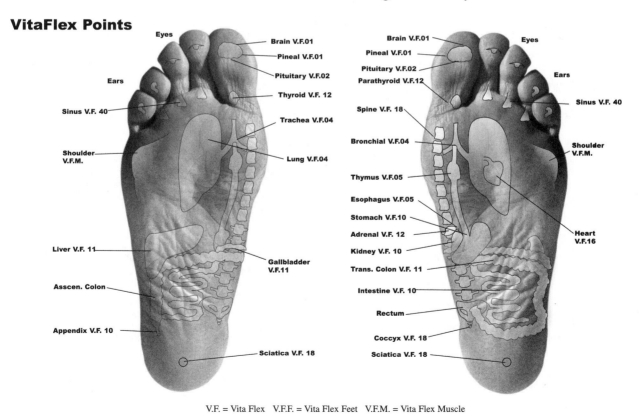

V.F. = Vita Flex	V.F.F. = Vita Flex Feet		V.F.M. = Vita Flex Muscle	
V.F. 1 Clarity	V.F. 1 My-Grain	V.F. 4 R.C.	V.F. 4 Raven	V.F. 5 Immupower
V.F. 10 Di-Tone	V.F. 11 Juva Flex	V.F.F. 11 Thieves	V.F. 12 EndoFlex	V.F. 16 Aroma Life
V.F. Pane Away	V.F. 22 Dragon Time	V.F. 22 Mister	V.F.F. Valor	V.F.M. Aroma Siez

Nervous System Connection Points

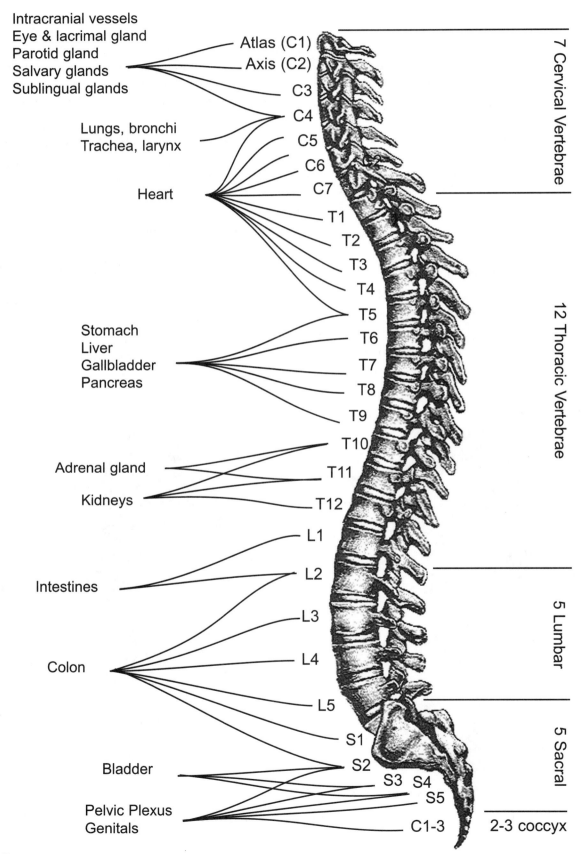

Intracranial vessels
Eye & lacrimal gland
Parotid gland
Salvary glands
Sublingual glands

Atlas (C1)
Axis (C2)
C3
C4
C5
C6
C7
T1
T2
T3
T4
T5
T6
T7
T8
T9
T10
T11
T12
L1
L2
L3
L4
L5
S1
S2
S3 S4
S5
C1-3

Lungs, bronchi
Trachea, larynx

Heart

Stomach
Liver
Gallbladder
Pancreas

Adrenal gland

Kidneys

Intestines

Colon

Bladder

Pelvic Plexus
Genitals

7 Cervical Vertebrae

12 Thoracic Vertebrae

5 Lumbar

5 Sacral

2-3 coccyx

Raindrop Therapy

Raindrop Therapy is a powerful, non-invasive tool for helping to correct defects in the curvature of the spine. During the years that it has been practiced, it has resolved numerous cases of scoliosis and kyphosis and eliminated the need for back surgery for thousands of people.

Raindrop Therapy originated from the research of D. Gary Young and a Lakota medicine man almost two decades ago. It integrates Vita Flex and massage therapy with essential oils to bring the body into structural and electrical alignment.

Raindrop Therapy is based on the theory that many types of scoliosis and spinal misalignments are caused by viruses or bacteria that lie dormant along the spine. These pathogens create inflammation, which, in turn, contorts and disfigures the spinal column.

Raindrop Therapy uses a sequence of highly antimicrobial essential oils designed to simultaneously reduce inflammation and kill the viral agents responsible for it. The principle oils used are: thyme (*Thymus vulgaris*), oregano (*Origanum compactum*), birch (*Betula alleghaniensis*), cypress (*Cupressus sempervirens*), peppermint (*Mentha piperita*), basil (*Ocimum basilicum*), and marjoram (*Origanum majorana*). The oils are dispensed like little drops of rain from a height of about six inches and massaged alongside the vertebrae. Although the entire process takes about 40 minutes to complete, the oils will continue to work in the body for 5 to 7 days following treatment, with continued re-alignment taking place during this time.

The Raindrop Therapy is not a cure-all or a magic bullet. A healthy body is the result of a well-rounded program of exercise and proper diet. Health is everything we do, say, hear, see, and eat. The Raindrop Therapy is only one tool to help restore a balance of good health.

Although this therapy is explained as simply as possible, it is recommended that you view the "Science and Application" video from Essential Science Publishing so that you can see this therapy demonstrated firsthand. Viewing this video, combined with the outline presented here, will make this revolutionary therapy relatively easy to understand and put into practice.

Order in Which to Apply Essential Oils

STEP 1—**Valor** is the most important oil used in this applications, because it works on both physical and emotional levels, supporting the electrical and energy alignment of the body. The key to using this blend of oils is patience. Once the frequencies begin to balance in these areas, a structural alignment can then occur.

STEP 2—**Thyme** is documented to be highly antimicrobial. Thyme acts directly on the viral or bacterial activity responsible. The essential oil easily penetrates the skin and travels throughout the body.

STEP 3—**Oregano** has an antimicrobial action even more aggressive than thyme. It also has anti-inflammatory properties.

STEP 4—**Basil** has antispasmodic activity that relaxes muscles. It is also antimicrobial.

STEP 5—**Marjoram** is antispasmodic and may help relax the muscles.

STEP 6—**Birch** is anti-inflammatory and analgesic and relieves pain. It is excellent for bone since its primary constituent, methyl salicylate, has a cortisone-like activity.

STEP 7—**Cypress** improves circulation and relieves spasms and swelling.

STEP 8—**Peppermint** has pain-killing properties. It is also antimicrobial, working synergistically with the other oils to enhance their activity.

STEP 9—**Ortho Ease Massage Oil** is a blend of vegetable and essential oils with many of the same properties as those just listed.

V-6 Mixing Oil or any massage oil is required to dilute essential oils high in phenols that may produce an excess warming or reddening to the skin, a problem that occurs often with fair- and light-skinned people. Following the application of thyme and oregano, it may be necessary to apply 2-3 drops of massage oil over areas with excess warming or reddening.

Ortho Ease is to be applied over the entire area after you have finished with the Raindrop Therapy. This blend has been reported to be beneficial for stress, muscle cramps, arthritic pain, and tension.

Preparation

- Remove all jewelry. This includes watches, pendants, rings, bracelets, earrings, etc. These could interfere with the electrical frequencies and the flow of energy.

- Remove all tight-fitting clothing.

- When giving the therapy, you should have your fingernails clipped and filed down as short as possible. This will avoid your unintentionally scratching your patient.

- When needing to drop the oils into your hand, put them into the non-dominant hand. Then use the dominant hand to rub them three times clockwise to stir the oils. This will increase their frequency.

- You will need three medium-size towels, hot water, and a sheet or blanket to protect the modesty of the individual while they move around.

To begin:

- The patient should lie face down on the massage table with the head slightly lower than the rest of the body, preferably resting in the face cradle.

- The patient should lie as straight as possible with the hips flat on the table. The arms can be resting alongside the body.

Step 1: Application of Valor. This procedure forms the foundation of everything that follows.

- Place 6 drops of Valor in each hand.

- Apply oil to the bottom of the feet: right hand holding right foot and left hand holding left foot. The facilitator may kneel or sit while touching the feet.

- The palm of the hand should be flat against the bottom of the feet, with as much hand-to-foot contact as possible.

- Apply 3 drops on each shoulder: right hand placed on right shoulder and left hand placed on left shoulder. There must be as much hand to shoulder contact as possible. It works best if there are two people to apply Valor. One to apply oils to the feet, the other to apply oils to the shoulders. However, if you are working by yourself, the application works well just holding the feet, which is the most important.

- Let your mind be free and peaceful. Encourage the recipient to take deep breaths. Have them inhale and exhale deeply and slowly, allowing them to engage in their own healing. You may feel an energy flowing up through the patient into your body. The receiver may feel a little heat or tingling on the feet, or an energy working up through the legs to the back, even as high as the head. With some individuals, the giver may feel the hands become cold. Many times you may feel a pulsating feeling.

- Do not break contact with the individual. Hold your position for 5-10 minutes.

In most cases, you will see some realignment of the spine. The vertebrae can move under the skin with just this small amount of application. The results will depend largely on the frequency of the person holding the feet. If there are people present with negative attitudes, or if the person applying the oils lacks a high enough frequency to block out the negative interference, the results may be less than optimal. One should not touch another person if they are feeling angry, negative, or sick.

Step 2: Application of oregano and thyme.

- Hold the bottle six inches above the skin and evenly space 5 drops of each oil along the spine from bottom to top (sacrum to atlas).

- Apply one oil, layering it on along the curvature of the spine. Apply the second oil the same way. It does not matter which oil is applied first.

- You don't need large drops; more is not better. If there is a burning sensation, apply massage oil.

- With 4-inch brush-like strokes using the nail side of your fingertips, lightly feather up the spine. Repeat this action two more times, always starting at the sacrum.

- With 4-inch brush-like strokes, flare your fingertips out to the side as your feather up the spine. The right hand will move to the right and the left hand to the left. Repeat motion two more times.

- Starting at the sacrum, stroke up **8 inches** before flaring out again. Repeat two more times.

- Starting at the sacrum, stroke up **12 inches** before flaring out again. Repeat two more times.

- Continue this therapy until your strokes feather up the full length of the spine up to the atlas. Flare your fingertips out over the shoulders when you reach the top. Repeat two more times.

- Repeat this whole sequence three times.

Step 3: Application of basil, birch, cypress, marjoram, and peppermint.

- Apply 4- 5 drops of basil along the length of the spine. Layer it in by evenly spreading it with your fingertips.

- Repeat, using the other 4 oils in sequence.

- Starting on one side of the spine, gently massage the oils in along the spine. **Do not work directly on the spine. Do not force it or apply direct pressure.** Start at the sacrum and use the fingertips of both hands placed side by side.

- In a circular clockwise motion, work up the side of the spine to the atlas, pushing or pulling the tissue in the direction you want the spine to move.

- After finishing one side of the spine, start on the other side. Repeat this procedure two or more times.

- Using the index and middle finger of either hand, place the fingers so that they straddle the spine. Start at the coccyx (bottom of spine) and move to the top. Always work directionally toward the brain. With mild pressure and the fingers on either side of the spine, place one hand over the top of the fingers. Then, in a gentle see-sawing motion, rock the fingers back and forth while moving gently down the spine to the sacrum. Repeat this procedure two more times.

- Beginning at the sacrum, with your thumbs on either side of the spine, you will use the Vita Flex therapy working up the spine approximately a thumb's width apart with each move up to the atlas. With the thumbs on each side of the spine, nail side up and slightly angled out, rock the thumbs so they point upward with the joints slightly bent. Then, apply a mild pressure straight down. Continue to roll your thumbs slightly over onto the nails, and then release. Move your thumbs up about 1/2-a-thumb's width and apply the same therapy. Do this all the way to the atlas. Repeat two more times.

Step 4: Back massage with massage oil.

Apply 20-25 drops of Ortho Ease to each side of the spine, (not on the spine) into the muscle tissue of the back. Work the oils in all over the back, using a gentle massage for a few minutes. After the oils have been massaged in, rest for five minutes. Then apply Ortho Ease over the entire back and legs.

Step 5: Towel placement.

- Place a dry towel over the back. Then lay a hand towel (soaked in hot water and folded in thirds) along the entire length of the spine.

- Place another dry towel (folded in half) over the wet towel.

- Pay close attention because the back can become very hot. The heat will generally build slowly and peak in 5-8 minutes before cooling down to the point where it feels pleasant. The greater the inflammation and viral infection along the spine, the hotter the area along the spine will become.

Some will experience no heat, while others will find it mild and pleasant. Still others may find it uncomfortably hot. Pay attention to your patient. Ask questions. If the heat becomes too uncomfortable, remove the towels and apply massage oil on the back. Then work it in. This will usually remove the heat within minutes.

After placing the towels, wait several minutes to gauge the individual's response. If the back does not become very hot, have the individual roll over on his/her back. This usually creates more heat.

Step 6: Leg massage with birch, basil, cypress, and peppermint.

- Apply 5-6 drops each of birch, basil, cypress, and peppermint along the inside of the lower legs. Start at the top of the knee and follow the shin bone down to the heel and sideways to the big toe on each foot. Apply one oil at a time, in order, massaging each oil in before applying the next oil.

- Place the fingers of one hand along the inside of the shinbone just below the knee. Work the fingers down to the ankle and then along the foot up to the top of the big toe using the Vita Flex therapy. Roll your fingers up and then over onto the nails of the fingers, applying slightly more pressure at the top of the roll and releasing as you come over onto the nails. The person on whom you are working would appreciate short nails. Repeat this procedure three times on each leg.

Step 7: Stretching.

- This next step works best with two people. With the individual on his/her back, have your assistant hold each leg tightly, just above the ankles, while you cradle the individual's head under your right hand. Then place your left hand around the chin and gently pull to create slight tension.

- Hold this traction for several minutes. Do not pull hard. The person holding the feet will act as the anchor, while you begin a mild rocking motion, repeatedly pulling and releasing. Continue the rocking motion from 4-8 minutes.

Step 8: Checking results.

- With the individual lying face down, with his/her head snug in the head-cradle of the massage table, make sure the person is lying straight. Remove the towels and then check the spine. Corrections may or may not be visible. At this point you may need to add another therapy. Occasionally results take several days to take effect.

COMMENTARY:

This is the basic Raindrop Therapy, although there are several variations. However, these are not easy to explain and require class instruction and demonstration. Every person is different, and what works for one may not work for another. Different body types respond to the applications in ways you may not expect. Learn to be sensitive to the person on whom you are working so that you can respond to his or her needs.

The question is often asked, "How long does this application last?" Again, each person responds differently. Generally speaking, the level of health and proper diet are key factors, as are exercise and attitude. One application may last four months for one person, but then for another it may be necessary to have the application repeated every week until the body begins to respond. The key is to retrain the body. In some cases, you will have to develop a new memory in the tissue in order for the body to stay where it should be. This may take a few weeks or even a full year.

Spinal alignment may have a completely different look when the individual is lying down, rather than sitting. There is more torque on the spine in a sitting or standing position, so these are the positions in which X-rays are usually taken. There may appear to be a total correction when the individual is lying down and then appear to be crooked when they are in a sitting position. This variance is normal and may be apparent until a total retraining of the tissue can occur. The object is to achieve straightening in all positions.

The Raindrop Therapy is a powerful tool that not only can assist therapists but help everyone achieve a balance in the body.

Emotional Response with Essential Oils

Today, we live in a society of emotional turmoil. There is more focus on emotional behavior and psychological conditions of the body now than at any time in our history. Many doctors are recognizing that a number of diseases are caused by emotional problems that link back to infancy or even to problems that occurred during conception or while in the womb. These emotional problems may have compromised the immune system or genetic structuring, causing children to become allergic to something that the mother was eating or drinking while pregnant.

Essential oils play an important role in assisting people in getting beyond these emotional barriers. The aldehydes and esters of certain essential oils are very calming and sedating to the central nervous system (which consists of both the sympathetic and parasympathetic systems). These substances allow us to relax instead of letting anxiety build up in our body. Anxiety creates an acidic condition that activates the transcript enzyme that transcribes that emotion on the RNA template and stores it in the DNA. That emotion then becomes a predominant factor in our lives from that moment on.

When we have an emotional situation come up, instead of being overwhelmed by it, we can diffuse the oils, put them in our bath, or wear them as cologne. The oil molecules will absorb into the bloodstream, go into the limbic system to the nasal and boucle cavity. They will activate the amygdala (which is the memory center for fear and trauma) and sedate and relax the sympathetic/para-sympathetic system. The oils help support the body in minimizing the acid that is created so that it does not create a reaction to the transcript enzyme.

Essential oils can help us cope with day-to-day problems. When you apply the essential oils, they will help you balance so that you can methodically work through the situation.

Essential oils also help us stay centered in our goals. People have great difficulty staying focused in today's fast-paced world. For example, if you are struggling to retain or remember information, breathing the essential oils of peppermint, cardamom, or rosemary helps the brain filter out any outside interference and allows you to lock in on what is most critical. Someone who is focusing on creating a business but finds other problems that interfere with that focus, could breathe the essential oils of galbanum, frankincense, sandalwood and melissa. These oils are extremely beneficial in enabling a person to bring his or her mind into a center of focus. The blend Gathering will also bring focus to people's minds.

For emotional clearing and release, the essential oil blend Trauma Life is especially helpful.

Oils For Emotional Application

Abuse

Blends: SARA, Hope, Joy, Peace & Calming, Inner Child, Grounding, Trauma Life.

Single oils: Geranium, ylang ylang, sandalwood.

Agitation

Blends: Peace & Calming, Joy Valor, Harmony, Forgiveness

Single Oils: Bergamot, cedarwood, clary sage, frankincense, geranium, juniper berry, lavender, myrrh, marjoram, rosewood, rose, ylang ylang, sandalwood.

Anger

Blends: Release, Valor, Sacred Mountain, Joy, Harmony, Hope, Forgiveness, Present Time, Trauma Life, Surrender.

Single Oils: Bergamot, cedarwood, Roman chamomile, frankincense, lavender, lemon, marjoram, myrrh, orange, rose, sandalwood, ylang ylang.

Anxiety

Blends: Valor, Hope, Peace & Calming, Present Time, Joy.

Single Oils: Orange, Roman chamomile, ylang ylang, lavender.

Apathy

Blends: Joy, Harmony, Valor, 3 Wise Men, Hope, White Angelica, Motivation, Passion.

Single Oils: Frankincense, geranium, marjoram, jasmine, orange, peppermint, rosewood, rose, sandalwood, thyme, ylang ylang.

Argumentative

Blends: Peace & Calming, Joy, Harmony, Hope, Valor, Acceptance, Humility, Surrender, Release.

Single Oils: Cedarwood, Roman chamomile, eucalyptus, frankincense, jasmine, orange, thyme, ylang ylang.

Boredom

Blends: Dream Catcher, Motivation, Valor, Awaken, Passion, Gathering.

Single Oils: Cedarwood, spruce, Roman chamomile, cypress, frankincense, juniper berry, lavender, fir, rosemary, sandalwood, thyme, ylang ylang, black pepper.

Concentration

Blends: Clarity, Awaken, Gathering, Dream Catcher, Magnify Your Purpose, Brain Power.

Single Oils: Cedarwood, cypress, eucalyptus, juniper berry, lavender, lemon, basil, helichrysum, myrrh, orange, peppermint, rosemary, sandalwood, ylang ylang.

Confusion

Blends: Clarity, Harmony, Valor, Present Time, Awaken, Brain Power, Gathering.

Single Oils: Cedarwood, spruce, fir, cypress, peppermint, frankincense, geranium, ginger, juniper berry, marjoram, jasmine, rose, rosewood, rosemary, basil, sandalwood, thyme, ylang ylang.

Day Dreaming

Blends: Sacred Mountain, Gathering, Valor, Harmony, Present Time, Dream Catcher, 3 Wise Men, Magnify Your Purpose, Envision, Brain Power.

Single Oils: Eucalyptus, ginger, spruce, lavender, helichrysum, lemon, myrrh, peppermint, rosewood, rose, rosemary, sandalwood, thyme, ylang ylang.

Depression

Blends: Valor, Motivation, Passion, Hope, Joy, Brain Power, Present Time, Envision, Sacred Mountain, Harmony.

Single Oils: Frankincense, sandalwood, geranium, lavender, angelica, orange, grapefruit, ylang ylang.

Despair

Blends: Joy, Valor, Harmony, Hope, Gathering, Grounding, Forgiveness, Motivation.

Single Oils: Cedarwood, spruce, fir, clary sage, frankincense, lavender, geranium, lemon, orange, lemongrass, peppermint, spearmint, rosemary, sandalwood, thyme, ylang ylang.

Despondency

Blends: Peace & Calming, Inspiration, Harmony, Valor, Hope, Joy, Present Time, Gathering, Inner Child, Trauma Life, Envision.

Single Oils: Bergamot, clary sage, cypress, geranium, ginger, orange, rose, rosewood, sandalwood, ylang ylang.

Disappointment

Blends: Hope, Joy, Valor, Present Time, Harmony, Dream Catcher, Gathering, Magnify Your Purpose, Passion, Motivation.

Single Oils: Clary sage, eucalyptus, frankincense, geranium, ginger, juniper berry, lavender, spruce, fir, orange, thyme, ylang ylang.

Discouragement

Blends: Valor, Sacred Mountain, Hope, Joy Dream Catcher, Into the Future, Magnify Your Purpose, Envision.

Single Oils: Bergamot, cedarwood, frankincense, geranium, juniper berry, lavender, lemon, orange, spruce, rosewood, sandalwood.

Fear

Blends: Valor, Present Time, Hope, White Angelica, Trauma Life.

Single Oils: Bergamot, clary sage, Roman chamomile, cypress, geranium, juniper berry, marjoram, myrrh, spruce, fir, orange, sandalwood, rose, ylang ylang.

Forgetfulness

Blends: Clarity, Valor, Present Time, Gathering, 3 Wise Men, Dream Catcher, Acceptance, Brain Power.

Single Oils: Cedarwood, Roman chamomile, eucalyptus, frankincense, rosemary, basil, sandalwood, peppermint, thyme, ylang ylang.

Frustration

Blends: Valor, Hope, Present Time, Sacred Mountain, 3 Wise Men, Humility, Peace & Calming, Surrender, Passion.

Single Oils: Roman chamomile, clary sage, frankincense, ginger, juniper berry, lavender, lemon, orange, peppermint, thyme, ylang ylang, spruce.

Grief/Sorrow

Blends: Forgiveness, Valor, Joy, Hope, Present Time, White Angelica, Release, Trauma Life.

Single Oils: Bergamot, Roman chamomile, clary sage, eucalyptus, juniper berry, lavender.

Guilt

Blends: Valor, Release, Inspiration, Inner Child, Gathering, Harmony, Present Time, Magnify Your Purpose.

Single Oils: Roman chamomile, cypress, juniper berry, lemon, marjoram, geranium, frankincense, sandalwood, spruce, rose, thyme.

Irritability

Blends: Valor, Hope, Peace & Calming, Surrender, Forgiveness, Present Time, Inspiration.

Single Oils: All oils except eucalyptus, peppermint, black pepper.

Jealousy

Blends: Valor, Sacred Mountain, White Angelica, Joy, Harmony, Humility, Forgiveness, Valor, Surrender, Release.

Single Oils: Bergamot, eucalyptus, frankincense, lemon, marjoram, orange, rose, rosemary, thyme.

Mood Swings

Blends, Peace & Calming, Gathering, Valor, Dragon Time, Mister, Harmony, Joy, Present Time, Envision, Magnify Your Purpose, Brain Power.

Single Oils: Bergamot, clary sage, sage, geranium, juniper berry, fennel, lavender, peppermint, rose, jasmine, rosemary, lemon, sandalwood, spruce, yarrow, ylang ylang.

Obsessiveness

Blends: Sacred Mountain, Valor, Forgiveness, Acceptance, Humility, Inner Child, Present Time, Awaken, Motivation, Surrender, Passion.

Single Oils: Clary sage, cypress, geranium, lavender, marjoram, rose, sandalwood, ylang ylang, helichrysum.

Panic

Blends: Harmony, Valor, Gathering, White Angelica, Peace & Calming, Trauma Life, Awaken, Grounding.

Single Oils: Bergamot, Roman chamomile, frankincense, lavender, marjoram, birch, myrrh, rosemary, sandalwood, thyme, ylang ylang, spruce, fir.

Resentment

Blends: Forgiveness, Harmony, Humility, White Angelica, Surrender, Joy.

Single Oils: Jasmine, rose, tansy.

Restlessness

Blends: Peace & Calming, Sacred Mountain, Gathering, Valor, Harmony, Inspiration, Acceptance, Surrender.

Single Oils: Angelica, bergamot, cedarwood, basil, frankincense, geranium, lavender, orange, rose, rosewood, ylang ylang, spruce.

Shock

Blends: Clarity, Valor, Inspiration, Joy, Grounding, Trauma Life, Brain Power.

Single Oils: Helichrysum, basil, roman chamomile, myrrh, ylang ylang, rosemary.

Auricular Therapy

Auricular aromatherapy, the integration of essential oils with standard auricular therapy, was developed by D. Gary Young after using essential oils in an acupuncture application in his clinic. He found that using essential oils in conjunction with acupuncture was extremely beneficial. He could localize and identify different functions and conditions that the body would respond to through direct acupuncture stimulation with essential oils than through acupuncture or oil application by themselves.

Acupuncture with essential oils seems to enhance benefits substantially. As he left his clinical practice and retired to researching, farming, and teaching, he could not continue the practice of acupuncture, so he started developing techniques that everyone could use. That was the technique of

Physical Ear Chart

M - Mouth
E - Esophagus
CO - Cardiac Orifice
St - Stomach
SI - Small Intestine
LI - Large Intestine
Pr - Prostate
Bl - Bladder
Ur - Ureter
Kid - Kidney
Pan - Pancreas,
    Gall Bladder
Liv - Liver
Spl - Spleen
H - Heart
W - Windpipe,
    Trachea
Tri - Triple Warmer

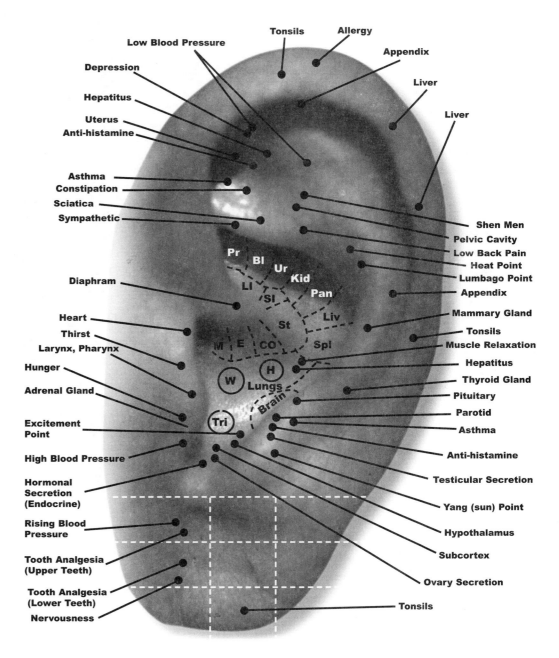

Low Blood Pressure
Tonsils
Allergy
Appendix
Depression
Liver
Hepatitus
Liver
Uterus
Anti-histamine
Asthma
Constipation
Sciatica
Sympathetic
Shen Men
Pelvic Cavity
Low Back Pain
Heat Point
Lumbago Point
Appendix
Diaphram
Mammary Gland
Heart
Tonsils
Thirst
Muscle Relaxation
Larynx, Pharynx
Hepatitus
Hunger
Thyroid Gland
Adrenal Gland
Pituitary
Parotid
Excitement Point
Asthma
High Blood Pressure
Anti-histamine
Hormonal Secretion (Endocrine)
Testicular Secretion
Rising Blood Pressure
Yang (sun) Point
Tooth Analgesia (Upper Teeth)
Hypothalamus
Subcortex
Tooth Analgesia (Lower Teeth)
Ovary Secretion
Nervousness
Tonsils

Pr Bl Ur Kid
LI SI Pan
St Liv
M E CO Spl
W Lungs H
Tri Brain

auricular probe therapy, using a small, pen-like instrument with a rounded end to apply the oils to the acupuncture meridians or Vita Flex points. This concept can be used in the emotional and physical realm by applying oils to the acupressure points of the ears.

For working the spine and dealing with neurological problems that exist because of spinal cord injury, it was found to be extremely beneficial to deliver the oils to the exact location of the neurological damage.

Auricular probe therapy is a program that Gary has been researching, developing, and teaching doctors that has a tremendous value and will grow to be a well-known modality of therapy in the future.

Emotional Ear Chart

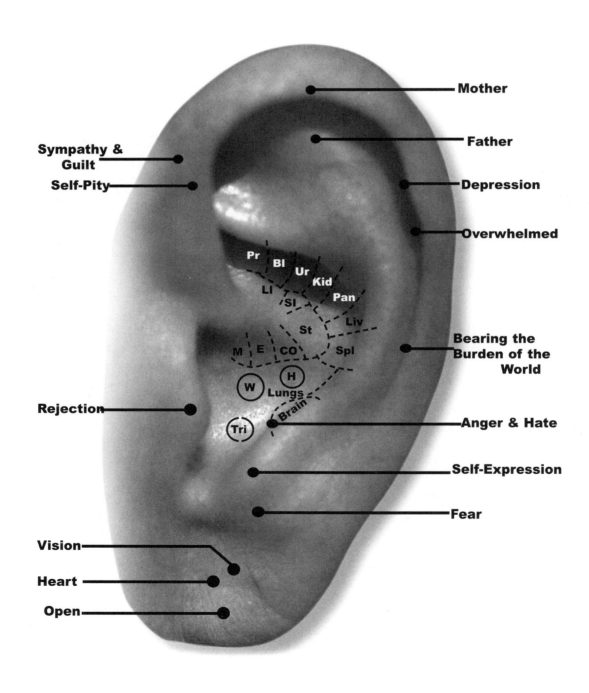

How to be Sure Your Essential Oils Are Therapeutic Grade

Are the fragrances subtle, rich, organic, and delicate? Do they "feel" natural?

Do the fragrances of your oils vary from batch to batch as an indication that they are pure and painstakingly distilled in small batches rather than industrially processed on a large scale?

Does your supplier send each batch of essential oils it receives through up to five different chemical analyses before it is released?

Are these tests performed by independent labs?

Does your supplier grow and distill its own organically grown herbs?

Are the distillation facilities part of the farm where the herbs are grown so they are freshly distilled, or do the herbs lose their potency as they wait for days to be processed?

Does your supplier use low pressure and low temperature to distill essential oils and preserve all of their fragile chemical constituents? Are the distillation cookers fabricated from costly stainless steel alloys to reduce the likelihood of the oils chemically reacting with metal?

Does your supplier have representatives traveling worldwide to personally inspect the fields and distilleries where the herbs are grown and distilled?

Do they scrutinize the facilities to check that no synthetic chemicals are being used in any of these processes?

How many years has your supplier been doing all of this?

How To Maximize the Shelf Life of Your Essential Oils

The highest quality essential oils are bottled in dark glass. The reason for this is two-fold: Glass is more stable than plastic and does not "breathe" the same way plastic does. Moreover, the darkness of the glass protects the oil from light that may chemically alter or degrade it over time.

After using, keep the lid tightly sealed. Bottles that are improperly sealed can result in the loss of some of the lighter, lower-molecular-weight parts of the oil, especially the monoterpenes and sesquiterpenes. In addition, over time the oxygen in the air may react with and oxidize the essential oil.

Store out of light, especially sunlight. Ultraviolet rays may chemically alter and damage the fragile components of the essential oils. While the brown glass of the oil bottles does afford some protection against visible light, the darker the storage conditions the longer your oil will last.

Store in a cool location. Excessive heat can derange the molecular structure of the oil the same way ultraviolet light can. This can lead to changes in the fragrance of the essential oil.

Single Oils

Angelica (*Angelica archangelica*)

Botanical Family: Apiaceae or Umbelliferae (parsley)

Plant Origin: France, Belgium

Extraction Method: Steam distilled from root.

Chemical Constituents: Monoterpenes (73%): phellandrene, α and β-pinenes, limonene (13%); Esters; Terpene alkaloids; Coumarins: bergoptene.

Action: It is anticoagulant and sedating to the nervous system. It reduces inflammation of the intestinal wall. Emotionally, it is calming, assisting in the release and dissociation of negative feelings.

Found In: Awaken, Forgiveness, Grounding, Harmony, Passion, and Surrender.

Traditional Uses: Known as the "holy spirit root" or the "oil of angels by the Europeans, it had healing powers so strong that it was believed to be of divine origin. From the time of Paracelsus, it was credited with the ability to protect from the plague. The stems were chewed during the plague of 1660 to prevent infection. When burned, the seeds and roots were thought to purify the air.

Indications: Angelica may help with bruises, colic, coughs, respiratory infections, indigestion, menopause, pre-menstrual tension, loss of appetite, and rheumatic conditions.

Application: Apply to Vita Flex points on bottom of feet or diffuse.

Fragrant Influence: It brings memories back to the point of origin before trauma or anger was experienced, helping us to release and let go of negative feelings. It is soothing and calming.

Safety Data: If pregnant or under a doctor's care, consult your physician. Avoid if diabetic. Avoid direct sunlight after use.

Companion Oils: Patchouly, vetiver, clary sage, and most citrus oils.

Frequency: Physical and emotional; approximately 85 Mhz.

NOTE: Because angelica contains bergopten, it may be photo-sensitizing and should not be applied to skin that will be exposed to direct sunlight or ultraviolet light within 72 hours.

Basil (*Ocimum basilicum*)

Botanical Family: Lamiaceae or Labiatae (mint)

Plant Origin: Egypt, India, Utah, France

Extraction Method: Steam distilled from leaves, stems, and flowers.

Chemical Constituents: Methyl chavicol (70-75%), 12-14% linalol; Terpene alcohols: linalol, citronnellol; Terpene esters: fenchyle acetate, linalyl acetate: Phenols: eugenol: Phenols methl-ethers (90%): methyl chavicol (85-88%), methal eugenol: Ketones: camphor; Oxides: 1,8 ceneol.

Historical Use: Used extensively in traditional Asian Indian medicine, basil's name is derived from "basileum," the Greek name for king. In the 16th century, the powdered leaves were inhaled to treat migraines and chest infections.

Action: Powerful antispasmodic, anti-infectious, antiviral, anti-inflammatory, decongestant (veins, arteries of the lungs, prostate), antibacterial.

Found In: Aroma Siez, Clarity, and M-Grain

Traditional Uses: The Hindu people put basil sprigs on the chests of the dead to protect them from evil spirits. Italian women wore basil to attract possible suitors.

Indications: Migraines, mental fatigue, menstrual periods (scanty).

Other Uses: Relaxing to both striated and smooth muscles, soothes insect bites, stimulates the sense of smell. May help bronchitis and chest infections.

Application: Apply to tip of nose, on temples, and on location of stings and bites. For mental fatigue, inhale first, then apply to crown of head, forehead, heart, and navel. May be added to food or water as a dietary supplement.

Fragrant Influence: Helps with mental fatigue.

Safety Data: If pregnant or under a doctor's care, consult your physician. Do not use if epileptic. Skin test for sensitivity.

Companion Oils: Bergamot, cypress, birch, geranium, lemongrass, lavender, and marjoram.

Frequency: Low (Physical); approximately 52 MHz.

Selected Research:

Fyfe L, et al. "Inhibition of Listeria monocytogenes and Salmonella enteriditis by combinations of plant oils and derivatives of benzoic acid: the development of synergistic antimicrobial combinations." *Int J Antimicrob Agents.* 1997;9(3):195-9.

Wan J, et al. "The effect of essential oils of basil on the growth of Aeromonas hydrophila and Pseudomonas fluorescens." *J Appl Microbiol.* 1998;84(2):152-8.

Lachowicz KJ, et al. "The synergistic preservative effects of the essential oils of sweet basil (Ocimum basilicum L.) against acid-tolerant food microflora." *Lett Appl Microbiol.* 1998;26(3):209-14.

Bergamot *(Citrus bergamia)*

Botanical Family: Rutaceae (citrus)

Plant Origin: Italy, Ivory Coast

Extraction Method: Pressed from the rind or peel. Rectified and void of terpenes. Produced by solvent extraction or vacuum distilled.

Chemical Constituents: Monoterpenes, a-pinene, Aldehydes: citrals (45%); Furocoumarins.

Action: Calming, antiseptic, anti-infectious, anti-inflammatory, hormonal support, antibacterial, strep, staph.

Found In: Dream Catcher, Joy, and White Angelica.

Traditional Uses: It is believed that Christopher Columbus brought bergamot to Bergamo in Northern Italy from the Canary Islands. A mainstay in traditional Italian medicine, bergamot has been used in the Middle East for hundreds of years for skin conditions associated with an oily complexion. Bergamot is responsible for the distinctive flavor of the renowned Earl Grey Tea, and was used in the first genuine eau de cologne.

Indications: Stress, appetite (loss of), indigestion, agitation, depression, infection, inflammation, intestinal parasites, rheumatism, insomnia, insect repellent, and vaginal candida.

Other Uses: This oil may help bronchitis, cold sores, oily complexion, anxiety, nervous tension, coughs, cystitis, urinary tract infections, respiratory infection, sore throat, thrush, and tonsillitis. Jean Valnet, M.D. recommends it as an antidepressant and to regulate appetite.

Application: Diffuse, apply to forehead, on temples, and on location of stings and bites. Apply where you would a deodorant. May be added to food or water as a dietary supplement.

Fragrant Influence: It may help to relieve anxiety, stress, and tension. It has about 300 chemical constituents contributing refreshing, mood-lifting qualities.

Safety Data: If pregnant or under a doctor's care, consult your physician. *Citrus aurantium spp. bergamia* is very photo-sensitizing and should NOT be applied to skin that will be exposed to direct sunlight or ultraviolet light within 72 hours.

Birch *(Betula alleghaniensis)*

Botanical Family: Betulaceae

Plant Origin: Canada, Scandinavia

Extraction Method: Steam distilled from wood

Chemical Constituents: Esters: methyl salicylate (89%)

Action: Analgesic, antispasmodic, anti-inflammatory, liver stimulant, supports bone function.

Found In: PanAway and Raven

Traditional Uses: The American Indians and early European settlers flavored their tea with birch bark. Birch's main constituent, methyl salicylate, is also found in willow trees and is similar to the salicylic acid used as aspirin.

Indications: Arthritis, rheumatism, inflammation, muscular pain, tendonitis, hypertension, cramps. Contains an active principle similar to cortisone and is beneficial for bone, muscle, and joint discomfort.

Other Uses: This oil may be beneficial for cystitis, acne, bladder infection, gout, gallstones, edema, eczema, osteoporosis, skin diseases, ulcers, and urinary tract disorders.

Application: It is safest to apply after diluting with massage oil or V-6 Mixing Oil, It also may be applied neat to the bottom of the feet. For baths, add 3 to 5 drops to bath water with 1/2 oz. of Bath Gel Base.

Fragrant Influence: It stimulates and increases awareness in all levels of the sensory system.

Safety Data: If pregnant or under a doctor's care, consult your physician. Do not use if epileptic. Skin test for allergies.

Companion Oils: Basil, Roman chamomile, cypress, geranium, juniper, lavender, lemongrass, marjoram, and peppermint.

Black Cumin *(Cuminum cyminum)*

Botanical Family: Apiaceae or Umbelliferae (parsley)

Plant Origin: Egypt

Extraction Method: Steam distilled from seeds.

Chemical Constituents: Monoterpenes (30-60%): pinene (13-22%), paracymene (3-9%), terpinene (12-32%); Coumarins.

Action: Antiviral, stomatic, digestive and liver regulator.

Found In: ImmuPower, ParaFree, and Protec

Traditional Uses: Cumin seeds have been retrieved from the tombs of the pharoahs of Egypt. The Hebrews used cumin as an antiseptic for circumcision.

Indications: Immune stimulant, antiviral. This oil may help with poor circulation, indigestion, digestive spasms, headaches, and migraines.

Other Uses: *Cuminum cyminum* is rarer and more expensive than the commonly used white cumin found in supermarkets. It is antiseptic, calming, and a powerful support to the immune system.

Application: Diffuse or apply topically.

Fragrant Influence: Stimulates appetite.

Safety Data: If pregnant or under a doctor's care, consult your physician. Avoid direct sunlight for up to 12 hours after use.

Companion Oils: Cinnamon, patchouly, jasmine, ylang ylang, rose, and sandalwood.

Cajeput *(Melaleuca leucadendra)*

Botanical Family: Myrtaceae (myrtle)

Chemical Constituents: Cineol (45-70%); Aldehydes: benzoic, butyric, valeric; Monoterpenes: pinene; Terpene Alcohols: terpineol.

Action: Antimicrobial, analgesic (mild), antispasmodic, antineuralgic, antiseptic (pulmonary, urinary, and intestinal), insecticidal, and expectorant.

Traditional Uses: In Malaysia and other Indonesian islands, cajeput was used for respiratory infections, headaches, rheumatism, toothache, skin conditions, throat infections, and sore muscles. Cajeput derives its name from the Malayasian word for white tree.

Indications: Cajeput may help with arthritis, acne, respiratory infections, asthma, bronchitis, urinary complaints, coughs, cystitis, stiff joints, toothache, hay fever, bursitis, headaches, insect bites, intestinal problems, laryngitis, dysentery, psoriasis, rheumatism, sinusitis, skin (oily and spots), sore throat, and viral infections.

Application: Diffuse or rub on bottom of feet.

Safety Data: If pregnant or under a doctor's care, consult your physician. Use with caution. Do not use synthetic cajeput, it could cause further blistering and skin eruption. Skin test for sensitivity.

Companion Oils: Eucalyptus, peppermint, juniper, and birch.

Cardamon *(Elettaria cardamomum)*

Botanical Family: Zingiberaceae (ginger)

Chemical Constituents: Monoterpenes: sabinene, mycene, limonene; monoterpenols; linalol, terpinene; Esters (40%); linalyle acetate (3.4%), terpenal acetate (30-45%); Terpene oxides (45%): 1.9 ceneole (40-45%).

Action: Antispasmodic (neuro muscular), anti-bacterial, expectorant, anti-infectious, and combats worms.

Found In: Clarity

Traditional Uses: Cardamom has been used for paralysis, rheumatism, cardiac disorders, epilepsy, spasms, pulmonary disease, digestive, intestinal, and urinary complaints.

Indications: Cardamom may help with indigestion, appetite (loss of), coughs, debility, halitosis, mental fatigue, headaches, heartburn, nausea, and sciatica. It may also alleviate menstrual problems and irregularities.

Application: Diffuse, rub on bottom of feet, stomach, solar plexus, and thighs.

Fragrant Influence: Uplifting, refreshing, and invigorating.

Safety Data: If pregnant or under a doctor's care, consult physician.

Companion Oils: Bergamot, neroli, clove, rose, cedarwood, orange, cinnamon, cistus, and ylang ylang.

Canadian Red Cedar *(Thuja plicata)*

Botanical Family: Cupressaceae (Cypress)

Plant Origin: Canada

Extraction Method: Steam distilled from bark and sawdust.

Chemical Constituents: Thujle acid methyl ester, Terpinen-4-ol, Sesquiterpene: β–caryophylline; Monoterpene ester: Linalyl acetate.

Action: Antifungal, antibacterial, hair follicle stimulator, antiparasitic, insect repellent.

Traditional Uses: It was used traditionally by the Canadian Native American Indians to help them enter a higher spiritual realm. They used it to stimulate the scalp and as an anti-microbial and antiseptic agent.

Application: Diffuse. Apply on crown of head or on location.

Safety Data: If pregnant or under a doctor's care, consult physician.

Cedarwood *(Cedrus atlantica)*

Botanical Family: Pinaceae (pine)

Plant Origin: Morocco, USA. *Cedrus atlantica* is the species most closely related to the biblical Cedar of Lebanon.

Extraction Method: Steam distilled from bark.

Chemical Constituents: Sesquiterpenes (50%): Sesquiterpenols (30%); Sesquiterpenones (20%).

Action: Mildly antiseptic, it may be effective against hair loss (alopecia areata), tuberculosis, bronchitis, gonorrhea, and skin disorders such as acne and psoriasis. It can reduce hardening of artery walls. It is high in sesquiterpenes which can stimulate the limbic region of the brain (the center of our emotions). It also may help stimulate the pineal gland, which releases melatonin, an antioxidant hormone associated with deep sleep.

Found In: Brain Power, Grounding, Inspiration, Into The Future, Passion, Sacred Mountain, SARA.

Traditional Uses: Throughout antiquity, cedarwood used in medicines and cosmetics. The Egyptians used it for embalming the dead. It was used as both a traditional medicine and incense in Tibet. It is recognized for its calming, purifying properties and is used to benefit the skin and underlying tissues.

Indications: Bronchitis, anger (calming effect), hair loss, arteriosclerosis, diuretic, tuberculosis, calming, nervous tension, and urinary infections.

Other Uses: It may help with acne, anxiety, arthritis, congestion, coughs, cystitis, dandruff, psoriasis, purification, respiratory system, sinusitis, skin diseases, and fluid retention. It may help open the pineal gland. It also helps to reduce oily secretions.

Application: Diffuse or apply topically on location.

Safety Data: If pregnant or under a doctor's care, consult physician.

Companion Oils: Bergamot, cypress, eucalyptus, juniper, and rosemary.

Bible References:

Leviticus 14:4— "Then shall the priest command to take for him that is to be cleansed two birds alive [and] clean, and cedar wood, and scarlet, and hyssop:"

Leviticus 14:6— "As for the living bird, he shall take it, and the cedar wood, and the scarlet, and the hyssop, and shall dip them and the living bird in the blood of the bird [that was] killed over the running water:"

Leviticus 14:49— "And he shall take to cleanse the house two birds, and cedar wood, and scarlet, and hyssop:"

Leviticus 14:51— "And he shall take the cedar wood, and the hyssop, and the scarlet, and the living bird, and dip them in the blood of the slain bird, and in the running water, and sprinkle the house seven times:"

Leviticus 14:52— "And he shall cleanse the house with the blood of the bird, and with the running water, and with the living bird, and with the cedar wood, and with the hyssop, and with the scarlet."

Numbers 19:6— "And the priest shall take cedar wood, and hyssop, and scarlet, and cast [it] into the midst of the burning of the heifer."

Numbers 24:6— "As the valleys are they spread forth, as gardens by the river's side, as the trees of lign aloes which the Lord hath planted, [and] as cedar trees beside the waters."

2 Samuel 5:11— "And Hiram king of Tyre sent messengers to David, and cedar trees, and carpenters, and masons: and they built David an house."

2 Samuel 7:2— "That the king said unto Nathan the prophet, See now, I dwell in an house of cedar, but the ark of God dwelleth within curtains."

2 Samuel 7:7— "In all [the places] wherein I have walked with all the children of Israel spake I a word with any of the tribes of Israel, whom I commanded to feed my people Israel, saying, Why build ye not me an house of cedar?"

1 Kings 4:33— "And he spake of trees, from the cedar tree that [is] in Lebanon even unto the hyssop that springeth out of the wall: he spake also of beasts, and of fowl, and of creeping things, and of fishes."

1 Kings 5:6— "Now therefore command thou that they hew me cedar trees out of Lebanon; and my servants shall be with thy servants: and unto thee will I give hire for thy servants according to all that thou shalt appoint: for thou knowest that [there is] not among us any that can skill to hew timber like unto the Sidonians."

1 Kings 5:8— "And Hiram sent to Solomon, saying, I have considered the things which thou sentest to me for: [and] I will do all thy desire concerning timber of cedar, and concerning timber of fir."

1 Kings 5:10— "So Hiram gave Solomon cedar trees and fir trees [according to] all his desire."

1 Kings 6:9— "So he built the house, and finished it; and covered the house with beams and boards of cedar."

1 Kings 9:11— "([Now] Hiram the king of Tyre had furnished Solomon with cedar trees and fir trees, and with gold, according to all his desire,) that then king Solomon gave Hiram twenty cities in the land of Galilee."

2 Kings 19:23— "By thy messengers thou hast reproached the Lord, and hast said, With the multitude of my chariots I am come up to the height of the mountains, to the sides of Lebanon, and will cut down the tall cedar trees thereof, [and] the choice fir trees thereof: and I will enter into the lodgings of his borders, [and into] the forest of his Carmel."

1 Chronicles 22:4— "Also cedar trees in abundance: for the Zidonians and they of Tyre brought much cedar wood to David."

2 Chronicles 1:15— "And the king made silver and gold at Jerusalem [as plenteous] as stones, and cedar trees made he as the sycomore trees that [are] in the vale for abundance."

2 Chronicles 2:8— "Send me also cedar trees, fir trees, and algum trees, out of Lebanon: for I know that thy servants can skill to cut timber in Lebanon; and, behold, my servants [shall be] with thy servants,"

2 Chronicles 9:27— "And the king made silver in Jerusalem as stones, and cedar trees made he as the sycomore trees that [are] in the low plains in abundance."

Ezra 3:7— "They gave money also unto the masons, and to the carpenters; and meat, and drink, and oil, unto them of Zidon, and to them of Tyre, to bring cedar trees from Lebanon to the sea of Joppa, according to the grant that they had of Cyrus king of Persia."

Isaiah 41:19— "I will plant in the wilderness the cedar, the shittah tree, and the myrtle, and the oil tree; I will set in the desert the fir tree, [and] the pine, and the box tree together:"

Ezekiel 17:3— "And say, Thus saith the Lord God; A great eagle with great wings, longwinged, full of feathers, which had divers colours, came unto Lebanon, and took the highest branch of the cedar:"

Ezekiel 17:22— "Thus saith the Lord God; I will also take of the highest branch of the high cedar, and will set [it]; I will crop off from the top of his young twigs a tender one, and will plant [it] upon an high mountain and eminent:"

Ezekiel 17:23— "In the mountain of the height of Israel will I plant it: and it shall bring forth boughs, and bear fruit, and be a goodly cedar: and under it shall dwell all fowl of every wing; in the shadow of the branches thereof shall they dwell."

Zechariah 11:2— "Howl, fir tree; for the cedar is fallen; because the mighty are spoiled: howl, O ye oaks of Bashan; for the forest of the vintage is come down."

Selected Research:

Hay IC, et al. "Randomized trial of aromatherapy. Successful treatment for alopecia areata." *Arch Dermatol.* 1998;134(11):1349-52.

Chamomile (German) *(Matricaria recutita)*

Botanical Family: Asteraceae or Compositae (daisy)

Plant Origin: Utah, Egypt, Hungary

Extraction Method: Steam distilled from flowers.

Chemical Constituents: Sesquiterpenes: chamazulene; Sesquiterpenols: α bisabolol, farnesol; Sesquiterpene oxides; Sesquiterpenes lactones; Coumarins; Ethers.

Action: Sedating, calming, anti-inflammatory, antispasmodic, decongestant. It supports digestive, liver and gallblader function, reduces scarring, and relieves allergies.

Found In: EndoFlex and Surrender.

Traditional Uses: Has been highly esteemed for over 3,000 years and has been used for many types skin conditions and stress-related complaints.

Indications: Insomnia, nervous tension, stress, bursitis, tendonitis, inflammation, carpel tunnel syndrome, headaches, acne, liver and gallbladder disease, parasites, and ulcers.

Other Uses: It is a cleanser of the blood, helps increase liver function and secretion, and supports the pancreas. German chamomile promotes the regeneration of skin and can be used for abscesses, burns, rashes, cuts, dermatitis, teething pains, acne, eczema, chronic gastritis, infected nails, cystitis, inflamed joints, menopausal problems, sores, skin disorders, stress-related complaints, toothaches, ulcers, and wounds.

Application: Diffuse, add to food or water as a dietary supplement. or apply topically on location. Among the gentlest oils used in aromatherapy, all of the chamomiles are suitable for use on children.

Fragrant Influence: Dispels anger, stabilizes the emotions, and helps to release emotions linked to the past. It may also be used to soothe and clear the mind.

Safety Data: If pregnant or under a doctor's care, consult physician.

Companion Oils: Birch, fir, lavender, geranium, helichrysum, spearmint, hyssop, lemongrass, marjoram, sandalwood, spruce, and melaleuca.

Frequency: Emotional; approximately 105 Mhz.

Chamomile (Roman) *(Chamaemelum nobile)*

Botanical Family: Asteraceae or Compositae (daisy)

Plant Origin: Utah, Egypt

Extraction Method: Steam distilled from flowers.

Chemical Constituents: Alcohols terpenes; Esters (75-80%); acetates, isobutyrate d'isobutyle; Terpene ketones; pinocarvone (13%); Lactones sesquiterpenes.

Action: Calming for preanesthesia and tension, antispasmodic, anti-inflammatory, antiparasitic, skin regeneration.

Found In: Gentle Baby, JuvaFlex, Motivation, M-Grain, and Surrender

Traditional Uses: It is used extensively in Europe for the skin. For centuries, mothers have used chamomile to calm crying children, ease earaches, reduce fevers, soothe stomachaches and indigestion, and relieve toothaches and teething pain.

Indications: It may help calm and relieve restlessness and tension. Its anti-infectious properties benefit cuts, scrapes, and bruises.

Other Uses: Roman chamomile neutralizes allergies and increases the ability of the skin to regenerate. It is a cleanser of the blood and also helps the liver to reject poisons and to discharge them. This oil may help with allergies, bruises, cuts, depression, insomnia, muscle tension, nerves (calming and promoting nerve health), restless legs, and skin conditions, such as, acne, dermatitis, eczema, rashes, and sensitive skin. It can effectively minimize irritability and nervousness in hyperactive children.

Application: Diffuse, apply topically on bottom of feet, ankles, wrists or on location. Add to food or water as a dietary supplement. Among the gentlest oils used in aromatherapy, all of the chamomiles are suitable for use on children.

Fragrant Influence: Because it is calming and relaxing, it can combat depression, insomnia, and stress. It minimizes anxiety, irritability, and nervousness. It may also dispel anger, stabilize the emotions, and help to release emotions that are linked to the past.

Safety Data: If pregnant or under a doctor's care, consult your physician. Test for skin sensitivity.

Companion Oils: Lavender, rose, geranium, or clary sage.

Cinnamon Bark (*Cinnamomum verum*)

Botanical Family: Lauraceae (laurel)

Plant Origin: Sri Lanka, Madagascar, India

Extraction Method: Steam distilled from bark

Chemical Constituents: Esters; Phenols; Aldehydes arom.: cinnamaldehyde (63-76%), hydroxycinnamald; Coumarins.

Action: Highly antimicrobial, anti-infectious, antibacterial for large spectrum of infection, antiviral, antifungal (candida), general tonic, sexual stimulant, increases blood flow when previously restricted, light anticoagulant.

Found In: Abundance, Christmas Spirit, Exodus II, Gathering, Magnify Your Purpose, and Thieves.

Traditional Uses: Cinnamon Bark is one of the most antimicrobial essential oils. It has been produced in Sri-Lanka for over 2,000 years. Researchers found that viruses cannot live in the presence of cinnamon oil.

Indications: Sexual stimulant, tropical infection, typhoid, vaginitis.

Other Uses: This oil may be beneficial for circulation, infections, coughs, exhaustion, respiratory infections, digestion, rheumatism, and warts. This oil also fights viral and infectious diseases.

Application: Diffuse, apply topically on bottom of feet, ankles, and wrists. May be added to food or water as a dietary supplement.

Fragrant Influence: Thought to attract wealth.

Safety Data: If pregnant or under a doctor's care, consult your physician. Repeated use can result in extreme contact sensitization. Skin test for sensitivity. Diffuse with caution; it may irritate the nasal membranes if it is inhaled directly from the diffuser.

Companion Oils: All citrus oils, frankincense, cypress, juniper, geranium, lavender, rosemary, and all spice oils.

Bible Reference:

Exodus 30:23— "Take thou also unto thee principal spices, of pure myrrh five hundred [shekels], and of sweet cinnamon half so much, [even] two hundred and fifty [shekels], and of sweet calamus two hundred and fifty [shekels]…"

Proverbs 7:17— "I have perfumed my bed with myrrh, aloes, and cinnamon."

Song of Solomon 4:14— "Spikenard and saffron; calamus and cinnamon, with all trees of frankincense; myrrh and aloes, with all the chief spices:"

Revelation 18:13— "And cinnamon, and odours, and ointments, and frankincense, and wine, and oil, and fine flour, and wheat, and beasts, and sheep, and horses, and chariots, and slaves, and souls of men."

Selected Research:

Tantaoui-Elaraki A, et al. "Inhibition of growth and aflatoxin production in Aspergillus parasiticus by essential oils of selected plant materials." *J Environ Pathol Toxicol Oncol.* 1994;13(1):67-72.

Cassia (*Cinnamomum cassia*)

Botanical Family: Lauraceae (laurel)

Chemical Constituents: t-cinnamaldehyde, Benzaldehyde, t-cinamyl acetate, t-cinnamic alcohol.

Plant Origin: China

Extraction Method: Steam distilled from bark.

Action: Antibacterial, antiviral, antifungal

Found In: Exodus II

Safety Data: If pregnant or under a doctor's care, consult physician.

NOTE: While the aroma is similar to cinnamon, cassia is chemically and physically quite different.

Cistus (*Cistus ladanifer*)

Botanical Family: Cistaceae

Plant Origin: France, Spain

Extraction Method: Steam distilled from branches.

Chemical Constituents: Monoterpenes; α pinene (50%), camphene (4%); Aldehydes; Centones.

Action: Anti-infectious, antiviral, antibacterial, powerful antihemorraging agent, helps reduce inflammation, neurotonic for the sympathetic nervous system.

Found In: ImmuPower

Traditional Uses: Known as the "rock rose" and has been studied for its effects on the regeneration of cells.

Indications: Bronchitis, respiratory infections, coughs, rhinitis, urinary infections, wounds, and wrinkles.

Other Uses: Cistus may strengthen and support the immune system (due to phenol action).

Application: Diffuse or apply topically mixed with massage oil.

Fragrant Influence: Calming to the nerves, elevates the emotions.

Safety Data: If pregnant or under a doctor's care, consult physician.

Companion Oils: Juniper, clary sage, lavender, lavandin, patchouly, pine, cypress, sandalwood, bergamot, and vetiver.

Citronella (*Cymbopogon nardus*)

Botanical Family: Poaceae or Gramineae (grasses)

Plant Origin: Sri Lanka, Philippines, Egypt

Extraction Method: Steam distilled from leaves.

Chemical Constituents: Terpene alcohols (35%): geraniol (18%), bomeol (6%), citronnellol (8%); Aldehydes (5-15%): citronnellal (5%); Esters (9%); Phenols (9%): methyl isoeugenol (7%).

Action: Antibacterial, insect-repellent, antifungal, anti-inflammatory, antiseptic, antispasmodic, deodorant, and insecticidal.

Found In: Purification

Traditional Uses: Various cultures have used this oil to treat intestinal parasites, digestive and menstrual problems, and as a stimulant.

Indications: This oil may alleviate headaches, respiratory infections, neuralgia, fatigue, oily skin, and headaches.

Other Uses: Can be used as an antiseptic to sanitize and deodorize surfaces. It makes an excellent insect repellent when combined with cedarwood.

Application: Diffuse or apply topically on bottom of feet or on location diluted with massage oil.

Fragrant Influence: Insecticidal and soothing to the tissues.

Safety Data: If pregnant or under a doctor's care, consult your physician. Repeated use can result in extreme contact sensitization. Skin test for sensitivity.

Companion Oils: Geranium, bergamot, lemon, cedarwood, orange, and pine.

Clary Sage (*Salvia sclarea*)

Botanical Family: Lamiaceae or Labiatae (mint)

Plant Origin: Utah, France

Extraction Method: Steam distilled from flowering plant.

Chemical Constituents: Contains over 250 constituents: Monoterpenes: α and β–pinenes, camphene, myrcene, limonene; Sesquiterpenes; Monoterpenols (15%): linalol (6-16%), terpinene; Sesquiterpenols; Diterpenols: sclareol; Terpene esters (75%): linalyle acetate (62-75%); Ethers; oxides: 1,8 cineol, linalol oxide; Ketones; Aldehydes; Coumarins.

Utah distilled clary sage contains 5-7% sclareol).

Action: Antidiabetic, helps reduce high cholesterol, estrogen-like, supports hormones, anti-infectious, antifungal, antispasmodic, relaxing, antibacterial, may help with epilepsy, menopause, PMS.

Found In: Dragon Time, Into the Future, and Passion

Traditional Uses: Nicknamed "clear eyes" during the Middle Ages for its ability to cure eye conditions.

Indications: Treats bronchitis, cholesterol, hemorrhoids, hormonal imbalance, insomnia, intestinal cramps, menstrual cramps, PMS, premenopause, and weak digestion.

Other Uses: This oil may be used for menstrual problems, depression, headaches, dandruff, insect bites, insomnia, kidney disorders, dry skin, throat reaction, ulcers, circulatory problems, and whooping cough.

Application: Diffuse, apply topically on bottom of feet, ankles, and wrists. May be added to food or water as a dietary supplement.

Fragrant Influence: Enhances one's ability to dream and is very calming and stress-relieving.

Safety Data: If pregnant or under a doctor's care, consult your physician. Use caution with infants and children.

Companion Oils: Cypress, bergamot, cedarwood, geranium, citrus oils, juniper, lavender, and sandalwood.

Clove (*Syzygium aromaticum*)

Botanical Family: Myrtaceae (myrtle)

Plant Origin: Madagascar, Spice Islands

Extraction Method: Steam distilled from bud and stem.

Chemical Constituents: Eugenol Acetate, β–Caryophyllene, α-Humelene

Action: Highly antimicrobial, antiseptic, analgesic, bactericidal, antioxidant, hemostatic (blood thinning), anti-inflammatory.

Found In: Abundance, En-R-Gee, ImmuPower, Melrose, PanAway, and Thieves

Traditional Uses: The people of Penang were free from epidemics until the sixteenth century, when Dutch conquerors destroyed the clove trees that flourished on the islands. Many of the islanders died from the epidemics that followed. Eugenol, its principal constituent, is used synthetically in the dental industry for the numbing of gums. Courmont et al., demonstrated that a solution of .05 percent eugenol from clove oil was sufficient to kill the tuberculosis bacillus.

Indications: Infectious diseases, intestinal parasites, tuberculosis, respiratory infections, pain, toothache, scabies, wounds (infected).

Other Uses: According to Jean Valnet, M.D., this oil can prevent contagious disease and may treat arthritis, bronchitis, cholera, cystitis, dental infection, amoebic dysentery, diarrhea, tuberculosis, acne, fatigue, thyroid dysfunction, halitosis, headaches, hypertension, insect bites, nausea, neuritis, dermatitis, rheumatism, sinusitis, skin cancer, chronic skin disease, bacterial colitis, sores (speeds healing of mouth and skin sores), viral hepatitis, warts, and lymphoma.

Application: Diffuse, apply topically diluted with massage oil, add 1 to 2 drops in 4 oz. of water and use as a gargle. May be applied neat on palms of hands, bottom of feet, and on gums and teeth. May be added to food or water as a dietary supplement. For oral hygiene, rub directly on the gums surrounding an infected tooth. To break tobacco addiction, place a drop on tongue with finger. For tickling cough, put a drop on back of tongue.

Fragrant Influence: It may influence healing, serve as a mental stimulant, encourage sleep, stimulate dreams, and create a sense of protection and courage.

Safety Data: If pregnant or under a doctor's care, consult your physician. Repeated use can result in contact sensitization. Skin test for sensitivity.

Companion Oils: Basil, bergamot, cinnamon bark, clary sage, clove, grapefruit, lavender, lemon, nutmeg, orange, peppermint, rose, rosemary, and ylang ylang.

Selected Clinical Studies:

Nishijima H, et al. "Mechanisms mediating the vasorelaxing action of eugenol, a pungent oil, on rabbit arterial tissue." *Jpn J Pharmacol.* 1999 Mar;79(3):327-34.

Jayashree T, et al. "Antiaflatoxigenic activity of eugenol is due to inhibition of lipid peroxidation." *Lett Appl Microbiol.* 1999; 28(3):179-83.

Wie MB, et al. "Eugenol protects neuronal cells from excitotoxic and oxidative injury in primary cortical cultures." *Neurosci Lett.* 1997: 4;225(2):93-6.

Rompelberg CJ, et al. "Effect of short-term dietary administration of eugenol in humans" *Hum Exp Toxicol.* 1996;15(2):129-35.

Reddy AC, et al. "Effect of curcumin and eugenol on iron-induced hepatic toxicity in rats." *Toxicology* 1996;107(1):39-45.

Nagababu E, et al. "The protective effects of eugenol on carbon tetrachloride induced hepatotoxicity in rats." *Free Radic Res.* 1995;23(6):617-27.

Naidu KA. "Eugenol--an inhibitor of lipoxygenase-dependent lipid peroxidation." *Prostaglandins Leukot Essent Fatty Acids.* 1995;53(5):381-3.

Nakamoto K, et al. "In vitro effectiveness of mouthrinses against candida albicans." *Int J Prosthodont.* 1995;8(5):486-9.

Rompelberg CJ, et al. "Antimutagenicity of eugenol in the rodent bone marrow micronucleus test." *Mutat Res.* 1995;346(2):69-75.

Azizan A, et al. "Mutagenicity and antimutagenicity testing of six chemicals associated with the pungent properties of specific spices as revealed by the Ames Salmonella/ microsomal assay." *Arch Environ Contam Toxicol.* 1995;28(2):248-58.

Sharma JN, et al. "Suppressive effects of eugenol and ginger oil on arthritic rats." *Pharmacology.* 1994;49(5):314-8.

Sukumaran K, et al. "Inhibition of tumour promotion in mice by eugenol." *Indian J Physiol Pharmacol.* 1994;38(4):306-8.

Shapiro S, et al. "The antimicrobial activity of essential oils and essential oil components towards oral bacteria." *Oral Microbiol Immunol.* 1994;9(4):202-8.

Didry N, et al. "Activity of thymol, carvacrol, cinnamaldehyde and eugenol on oral bacteria." *Pharm Acta Helv.* 1994;69(1):25-8.

Saeed SA, et al. "Antithrombotic activity of clove oil." *JPMA J Pak Med Assoc.* 1994;44(5):112-5.

Shirota S, et al. "Tyrosinase inhibitors from crude drugs." *Biol Pharm Bull.* 1994; 17(2):266-9.

Reddy AC, et al. "Studies on anti-inflammatory activity of spice principles and dietary n-3 polyunsaturated fatty acids on carrageenan-induced inflammation in rats." *Ann Nutr Metab.* 1994;38(6):349-58.

Hasan HA, et al. "Inhibitory effect of spice oils on lipase and mycotoxin production." *Zentralbl Mikrobiol.* 1993;148(8):543-8.

Srivastava KC. "Antiplatelet principles from a food spice clove." *Prostaglandins Leukot Essent Fatty Acids.* 1993;48(5):363-72.

Moleyar V, et al. "Antibacterial activity of essential oil components." *Int J Food Microbiol.* 1992;16(4):337-42.

Bilgrami KS, et al. "Inhibition of aflatoxin production & growth of Aspergillus flavus by eugenol & onion & garlic extracts." *Indian J Med Res.* 1992;96:171-5.

Coriander *(Coriandrum sativum)*

Botanical Family: Apiaceae or Umbelliferae (parsley)

Plant Origin: Russia, India

Extraction Method: Steam distilled seeds.

Chemical Constituents: Monoterpenes: Phellandrene; Aldehydes (85-95%); octanal, decanal, undecanal.

Action: Anti-inflammatory, sedative.

Traditional Uses: The seeds were found in the ancient Egyptian tomb of Ramses II. This oil has been researched at Cairo University for its effects in lowering glucose and insulin levels and supporting pancreatic function. It has been studied for its effects in strengthening the pancreas.

Indications: It also has soothing, calming properties.

Other Uses: Coriander may help with arthritis, diarrhea, respiratory infections, indigestion, digestive spasms, poor circulation, rheumatism, gout, infections (general), measles, headaches, nausea, muscular aches and pains, neuralgia, skin conditions (acne, psoriasis and dermatitis), and stress. It may also help during convalescence and after a difficult childbirth. Because of its estrogen content, it may regulate and help control pain-related to menstruation.

Application: Apply topically. May be added to food or water as a dietary supplement or flavoring.

Fragrant Influence: Soothing and calming.

Safety Data: If pregnant or under a doctor's care, consult your physician. Use sparingly, as coriander can be stupefying in large doses.

Companion Oils: Ginger, cinnamon, citronella, cypress, jasmine, neroli, petitgrain, bergamot, pine, clary sage, sandalwood, and other spice oils.

Cypress *(Cupressus sempervirens)*

Botanical Family: Cupressaceae (cypress)

Plant Origin: France, Spain

Extraction Method: Steam distilled from branches.

Chemical Constituents: Monoterpenes: α-pinene; Sesquiterpenes; Sesquiterpenols; Diterpenols.

Action: Improves circulation and supports the nerves and intestines. Anti-infectious, antibacterial, antimicrobial (causative agent of tuberculosis), strengthens blood capillaries. Acts as an insect repellent.

Found In: Aroma Life, Aroma Siez, and R.C.

Traditional Uses: It is one of the oils most used for the circulatory system.

Indications: Arthritis, bronchitis, circulation, cramps, hemorrhoids, insomnia, intestinal parasites, menopausal problems, menstrual pain, pancreas insufficiencies, pulmonary infections, rheumatism, spasms, throat problems, varicose veins, and fluid retention. Jean Valnet, M.D. suggests that it may be helpful for some cancers.

Other Uses: This oil may be beneficial for asthma, strengthening blood capillary walls, reducing cellulite, circulatory system, strengthening connective tissue, coughs, edema, improving energy, gallbladder, bleeding gums, hemorrhaging, laryngitis, liver disorders, muscular cramps, nervous tension, nose bleeds, ovarian cysts. It is outstanding when used in skin care, lessening scar tissue.

Application: Use topically with a massaging action toward the center of the body. Apply where you would wear a deodorant.

Fragrant Influence: It influences, strengthens, and helps ease the feeling of loss. It creates a feeling of security, grounding, and it helps to heal emotions.

Safety Data: If pregnant or under a doctor's care, consult physician.

Companion Oils: Bergamot, clary sage, juniper, lavender, lemon, orange, and sandalwood.

Bible Reference:

Isaiah 44:14—"He heweth him down cedars, and taketh the cypress and the oak, which he strengtheneth for himself among the trees of the forest: he planteth an ash, and the rain doth nourish [it]."

Davana *(Artemisia pallens)*

Botanical Family: Asteraceae or Compositae (daisy)

Action: Anti-infectious

Chemical Constituents: Davanone

Found In: Trauma Life

Indications: Stimulates the endocrine system, improves hormonal balance, and soothes rough, dry, and chapped skin.

Application: Diffuse or apply topically.

Safety Data: If pregnant or under a doctor's care, consult physician.

Dill *(Anethum graveolens)*

Botanical Family: Apiaceae or Umbelliferae (parsley)

Plant Origin: Austria, Hungary

Extraction Method: Steam distilled from whole plant.

Chemical Constituents: Carvone, Limonene, Phellandrene (depending on extraction method), eugenol, pinene, and others.

Action: Antispasmodic, antibacterial, expectorant, and stimulant.

Traditional Uses: The dill plant is mentioned in the Papyrus of Ebers from Egypt (1550 BC). Roman gladiators rubbed their skin with dill before each match. It is used in European hospitals.

Indications: It has been researched at Cairo University for its effects in glucose and insulin levels and supporting pancreatic function.

Other Uses: This oil may help bronchial, indigestion, constipation, headaches, indigestion, liver deficiencies, lower glucose levels, nervousness, normalize insulin levels, promote milk flow in nursing mothers, and support the pancreas function.

Application: Apply topically on abdomen and bottom of feet. May be added to food or water as a dietary supplement.

Fragrant Influence: It calms the autonomic nervous system and, when diffused with Roman chamomile, may help calm fidgety children.

Safety Data: If pregnant or under a doctor's care, consult your physician.

Companion Oils: Nutmeg and citrus oils.

Elemi *(Canarium luzonicum)*

Botanical Family: Burseraceae (frankincense)

Plant Origin: Philippines

Extraction Method: Steam distilled from the gum of the tree.

Chemical Constituents: Monoterpenes; Sesquiterpenes; Alcools sesquiterpenes: elemol.

Action: Antiseptic, antimicrobial

Traditional Uses: It has been used in Europe for hundreds of years in salves for skin and is included in the celebrated healing ointments, such as *baum paralytique*. Used by a 17th century physician, J. J. Wecker, on the battle wounds of soldiers, Elemi belongs to the same botanical family (Burseraceae) as frankincense (*Boswellia carteri*) and myrrh (*Commiphora myrrha*). The Egyptians used elemi for embalming, and subsequent cultures used it for skin care.

Indications: Glandular stimulant, helps reduce scarring, calming to the stomach, works against amoebic dysentery.

Other Uses: It is widely regarded today for soothing sore muscles, protecting and rejuvenating the skin, reducing wrinkles, and stimulating nerves. Its fragrance is very conducive toward meditation.

Application: Apply topically or diffuse. May be added to food or water as a dietary supplement. It is one of the gentlest oils in aromatherapy, and suitable for use on children.

Safety Data: If pregnant or under a doctor's care, consult physician.

Eucalyptus globulus

Botanical Family: Myrtaceae (myrtle)

Plant Origin: Australia, Brazil.

Extraction Method: Steam distilled from leaves.

Chemical Constituents: Monoterpenes: α-pinenes (10-12%); Sesquiterpenes: Sesquiterpenols; Terpene oxides: 1,8 cineole (70-75%).

Action: Expectorant, mucolytic, antimicrobial, antibacterial (staph, strep, pneumonia), antifungal (candida), antiviral, antiseptic, aids respiratory system.

Found In: R.C.

Traditional Uses: For centuries, Australian aborigines used the leaves as a disinfectant to cover wounds. Shown by laboratory tests to be a powerful antimicrobial agent, *E. globulus* contains a high percentage of eucalyptol (a key ingredient in many antiseptic mouth rinses). Often used for the respiratory system, eucalyptus has been investigated for its effect on insects in a study called, "Laboratory Evaluation of a Eucalyptus-based Repellent against Four Biting Arthopods" published by the *Phytotherapy Research*. Eucalyptus trees have been planted throughout parts of North Africa to successfully block the spread of malaria. According to Jean Valnet, M.D., a solution of 2 percent eucalyptus oil sprayed in the air will kill 70 percent of the airborne staph microorganisms. Some doctors still use solutions of eucalyptus oil in surgical dressings.

Indications: Asthma, candida, coughs, diabetes, herpes, hypoglycemia, lungs, measles, headaches, respiratory infections, sinusitis, shingles, and tuberculosis.

Other Uses: This oil may be used for aches/pains, acne, allergies, arthritis, bronchitis, burns, decongestant, respiratory infections, cystitis, endometriosis, increasing energy, gonorrhea, inflammation of the ear, eye, and sinus, malaria, rheumatism, respiratory infections, skin and throat infection/ sores, ulcers, vaginitis, and wounds.

Application: Apply topically, diffuse, or use in a humidifier. May be added to food or water as a dietary supplement.

Fragrant Influence: It promotes health, well-being, purification, and healing.

Safety Data: If pregnant or under a doctor's care, consult your physician. Do not take internally.

Companion Oils: Geranium, lavender, lemon, sandalwood, juniper, lemongrass, melissa, pine, and thyme.

Selected Research:

Tovey ER, et al. "A simple washing procedure with eucalyptus oil for controlling house dust mites and their allergens in clothing and bedding." *J Allergy Clin Immunol.* 1997; 100(4):464-6.

Weyers W, et al. "Skin absorption of volatile oils. Pharmacokinetics." *Pharm Unserer Zeit.* 1989;18(3):82-6.

Zanker KS, et al. "Evaluation of surfactant-like effects of commonly used remedies for colds." *Respiration.* 1980;39(3):150-7.

Modgil R, et al. "Efficacy of mint and eucalyptus leaves on the physicochemical characteristics of stored wheat against insect infestation." *Nahrung.* 1998;42(5):304-8.

Eucalyptus polybractea

Botanical Family: Myrtaceae (myrtle)

Plant Origin: Australia

Extraction Method: Steam distilled from leaves.

Chemical Constituents: Terpene oxides: 1,8 cineole (10%), Paracymene (30%), Sesquiterpenols.

Action: Anti-infectious, antiviral, antibacterial, anti-inflammatory, expectorant, mucolytic, insect repellent.

Indications: Acne, urinitis, cystitis.

Application: Diffuse or apply topically.

Safety Data: If pregnant or under a doctor's care, consult physician.

Eucalyptus citriodora

Botanical Family: Myrtaceae (myrtle)

Plant Origin: China

Extraction Method: Steam distilled from leaves.

Chemical Constituents: Monoterpene alcohols: citronnellol (15-20%), trans-pinocarveol, geraniol; Terpene Esters; Terpene aldehydes: citronnellal (40-80%).

Action: Analgesic, antiseptic, antiviral, antibacterial, antifungal, deodorant, expectorant, and insecticidal.

Found In: R.C.

Traditional Uses: *Eucalyptus citriodora* has been used to perfume the linen closet, and as an insect repellent, especially for cockroaches and silverfish.

Indications: Asthma, athlete's foot and other fungal infections, respiratory infections, cuts, dandruff, fevers, herpes, infectious skin conditions, laryngitis, scabs, shingles, sore throat, sores, and wounds.

Application: Diffuse or rub on bottom of feet or on location.

Safety Data: If pregnant or under a doctor's care, consult your physician. Do not take internally.

Eucalyptus radiata

Botanical Family: Myrtaceae (myrtle)

Plant Origin: Australia

Extraction Method: Steam distilled from leaves.

Chemical Constituents: Monoterpenes (8%); α-pinene; Monoterpenols (20%): linalol, borneal, geraniol, α-terpinol (14%); Monoterpenals: Terpene oxides: 1,8 cineole (62-72%).

Action: Anti-infectious, antibacterial, antiviral, expectorant, anti-inflammatory.

Found In: R.C., Raven, and Thieves

Traditional Uses: An antimicrobial oil studied for its action against viruses. This oil is used extensively for respiratory infections.

Indications: Conjunctivitis, vaginitis, acne, sinusitis, bronchitis.

Other Uses: This oil, when combined with bergamot, has been used effectively on herpes simplex. It may also help with acne, bronchitis, ear (inflammation), endometriosis, nasal and sinus congestion, sinusitis, and vaginitis.

Application: Diffuse or rub on bottom of feet or on location.

Safety Data: If pregnant or under a doctor's care, consult your physician. Do not take internally.

Fennel *(Foeniculum vulgare)*

Botanical Family: Apiaceae or Umbelliferae (parsley)

Plant Origin: Australia, Spain

Extraction Method: Steam distilled from the crushed seeds.

Chemical Constituents: Monoterpenes; α-pinene, limonene; Monoterpenols: fenchol; Phenols: methyl chavicol; Aldehydes; Ketones, camphor, Oxides: 1.9 cineol; Coumarins and furocoumarins.

Action: Stimulates estrogen production, facilitates birthing, increases lactation, promotes digestion, reduces indigestion, supports the heart and respiratory system, expels worms, stimulating to the circulatory and respiratory systems. It is antiseptic, antispasmodic, analgesic.

Found In: Di-Tone, Dragon Time, JuvaFlex, and Mister.

Traditional Uses: Fennel was believed to ward off evil spirits and to protect against spells cast by witches during medieval times. Sprigs were hung over doors to fend off evil spirits. For hundreds of years, fennel seeds have been used as a digestive aid to balance menstrual cycles. Recently it has been used mouthwashes and toothpastes.

Indications: Cystitis, sluggish digestion, fluid retention, gout, intestinal parasites, intestinal spasms, nausea, menopause and pre-menopause problems.

Other Uses: Fennel oil may be used for indigestion, stimulating the cardiovascular system, constipation, digestion, balancing hormones, supporting pancreatic function, PMS, and stimulating the respiratory system. It may break up fluids and toxins, and cleanse the tissues.

Application: Apply topically mixed with massage oil. Add to food or water as a dietary supplement or flavoring.

Safety Data: If pregnant or under a doctor's care, consult your physician. Use caution if epileptic.

Companion Oils: Basil, geranium, lavender, lemon, rosemary, and sandalwood.

Selected References:

Fyfe L, et al. "Inhibition of Listeria monocytogenes and Salmonella enteriditis by combinations of plant oils and derivatives of benzoic acid: the development of synergistic antimicrobial combinations." *Int J Antimicrob Agents.* 1997;9(3):195-9.

Fir *(Abies alba)*

Botanical Family: Pinaceae (pine)

Plant Origin: Balkans

Extraction Method: Steam distilled from needles.

Chemical Constituents: Monoterpenes (90-95%): alpina-Pinenes (24%), camphene (21%), limonene (34%).

Action: Antiseptic, anticatarrahal, stimulant

Found In: En-R-Gee, Grounding, Into The Future, Sacred Mountain.

Traditional Uses: Fir is used today as the traditional Christmas tree. Though highly regarded for its fragrant scent, the fir tree has been prized through the ages for its medicinal virtues in regards to respiratory conditions and muscular and rheumatic pain. It has been researched for its ability to kill airborne germs and bacteria.

Indications: Bronchitis, respiratory congestion, and fatigue.

Other Uses: It may be beneficial for discomfort from respiratory infections, fighting airborne germs/bacteria, treating arthritis, asthma, bronchial obstructions, coughs, rheumatism, sinusitis, and urinary tract infections.

Application: Diffuse or apply topically.

Aromatic Influence: Grounding, stimulating to the mind, relaxing to the body.

Safety Data: If pregnant or under a doctor's care, consult your physician. Skin test for sensitivity.

Companion Oils: Blue chamomile, cedarwood, frankincense, lavender, lemon, myrtle, and rosewood.

Bible Reference:

2 Samuel 6:5— "And David and all the house of Israel played before the Lord on all manner of [instruments made of] fir wood, even on harps, and on psalteries, and on timbrels, and on cornets, and on cymbals."

1 Kings 5:8— "And Hiram sent to Solomon, saying, I have considered the things which thou sentest to me for: [and] I will do all thy desire concerning timber of cedar, and concerning timber of fir."

1 Kings 5:10— "So Hiram gave Solomon cedar trees and fir trees [according to] all his desire."

1 Kings 6:15— "And he built the walls of the house within with boards of cedar, both the floor of the house, and the walls of the cieling: [and] he covered [them] on the inside with wood, and covered the floor of the house with planks of fir."

1 Kings 6:34— "And the two doors [were of] fir tree: the two leaves of the one door [were] folding, and the two leaves of the other door [were] folding."

1 Kings 9:11— "([Now] Hiram the king of Tyre had furnished Solomon with cedar trees and fir trees, and with gold, according to all his desire,) that then king Solomon gave Hiram twenty cities in the land of Galilee."

2 Kings 19:23— "By thy messengers thou hast reproached the Lord, and hast said, With the multitude of my chariots I am come up to the height of the mountains, to the sides of Lebanon, and will cut down the tall cedar trees thereof, [and] the choice fir trees thereof: and I will enter into the lodgings of his borders, [and into] the forest of his Carmel."

2 Chronicles 2:8— "Send me also cedar trees, fir trees, and algum trees, out of Lebanon: for I know that thy servants can skill to cut timber in Lebanon; and, behold, my servants [shall be] with thy servants."

2 Chronicles 3:5— "And the greater house he cieled with fir tree, which he overlaid with fine gold, and set thereon palm trees and chains."

Psalms 104:17— "Where the birds make their nests: [as for] the stork, the fir trees [are] her house."

Song Of Solomon 1:17— "The beams of our house [are] cedar, [and] our rafters of fir."

Isaiah 14:8— "Yea, the fir trees rejoice at thee, [and] the cedars of Lebanon, [saying], Since thou art laid down, no feller is come up against us."

Isaiah 37:24— "By thy servants hast thou reproached the Lord, and hast said, By the multitude of my chariots am I come up to the height of the mountains, to the sides of Lebanon; and I will cut down the tall cedars thereof, [and] the choice fir trees thereof: and I will enter into the height of his border, [and] the forest of his Carmel."

Isaiah 41:19— "I will plant in the wilderness the cedar, the shittah tree, and the myrtle, and the oil tree; I will set in the desert the fir tree, [and] the pine, and the box tree together:"

Isaiah 55:13— "Instead of the thorn shall come up the fir tree, and instead of the brier shall come up the myrtle tree: and it shall be to the Lord for a name, for an everlasting sign [that] shall not be cut off."

Isaiah 60:13— "The glory of Lebanon shall come unto thee, the fir tree, the pine tree, and the box together, to beautify the place of my sanctuary; and I will make the place of my feet glorious."

Ezekiel 27:5— "They have made all thy [ship] boards of fir trees of Senir: they have taken cedars from Lebanon to make masts for thee."

Ezekiel 31:8— "The cedars in the garden of God could not hide him: the fir trees were not like his boughs, and the chestnut trees were not like his branches; nor any tree in the garden of God was like unto him in his beauty."

Hosea 14:8— "Ephraim [shall say], What have I to do any more with idols? I have heard [him], and observed him: I [am] like a green fir tree. From me is thy fruit found."

Nahum 2:3— "The shield of his mighty men is made red, the valiant men [are] in scarlet: the chariots [shall be] with flaming torches in the day of his preparation, and the fir trees shall be terribly shaken."

Zechariah 11:2— "Howl, fir tree; for the cedar is fallen; because the mighty are spoiled: howl, O ye oaks of Bashan; for the forest of the vintage is come down."

Fleabane *(Conyza canadensis)*

Botanical Family: Asteraceae or Compositae (daisy)

Plant Origin: Canada

Extraction Method: Steam distilled from stems, leaves, and flowers.

Chemical Constituents: Monoterpenes; Sesquiterpenes: Terpene alcohols, Esters: lactones.

Action: Stimulates liver and pancreas, antirheumatic, antispasmodic, hormone-like, cardiovascular dilator. Daniel Penoël used it to treat children with retarded puberty.

Found In: Ultra Young

Safety Data: If pregnant or under a doctor's care, consult physician.

Note: This oil is still under study.

Frankincense *(Boswellia carteri)*

Botanical Family: Burseraceae (Frankincense)

Plant Origin: Somalia

Extraction Method: Steam distilled from gum/resin.

Chemical Constituents: Monoterpenes (40%); α pinene (43%), limonese; Sesquiterpenes; Alcools terpenes: borneol.

Action: Expectorant, antitumoral, immunostimulant, antidepressant.

Found In: Abundance, Acceptance, Brain Power, Exodus II, Forgiveness, Gathering, Harmony, Humility, ImmuPower, Inspiration, Into The Future, 3 Wise Men, Trauma Life, and Valor.

Traditional Uses: Also known as "olibanum," or "Oil from Lebenon" the name frankincense is derived from the Medieval French word for "real incense." Frankincense is considered the "holy anointing oil" in the Middle East and has been used in religious ceremonies for thousands of years. It was well known during the time of Christ for its anointing and healing powers and was one of the gifts given to Christ at His birth. "Used to treat every conceivable ill known to man," it was valued more than gold during ancient times, and only those with great wealth and abundance possessed. Researchers today have discovered that frankincense is high in sesquiterpenes, which helps stimulate the limbic system of the brain (the center of emotions) as well as the hypothalamus, pineal and pituitary glands. The hypothalamus is the master gland of the human body, controlling the release of many hormones including thyroid and growth hormone. Frankincense is now being researched and used therapeutically in European hospitals and is being investigating for its ability to improve human growth hormone production.

Indications: Asthma, depression, and ulcers. High in sesquiterpenes, it is stimulating and elevating to the mind and helps in overcoming stress and despair, as well as supporting the immune system.

Other Uses: This oil may help with allergies, bites (insect and snake), bronchitis, cancer, respiratory infections, diphtheria, headaches, hemorrhaging, herpes, high blood pressure, inflammation, stress, tonsillitis, typhoid, and warts. It contains sesquiterpenes, enabling it to go beyond the blood brain barrier. It increases the activity of leukocytes in defense of the body against infection.

Application: Diffuse or apply topically. May be added to food or water as a dietary supplement.

Fragrant Influence: It increases spiritual awareness and promotes meditation. Frankincense may also help improve attitude and uplift spirits, which may help to strengthen the immune system.

Safety Data: If pregnant or under a doctor's care, consult physician.

Companion Oils: All oils.

Bible Reference: There are over 52 references to frankincense (considering that "incense" is translated from the Hebrew/Greek "frankincense" and is referring to the same oil).

Exodus 30:34— "And the Lord said unto Moses, Take unto thee sweet spices, stacte, and onycha, and galbanum; [these] sweet spices with pure frankincense: of each shall there be a like [weight]:"

Leviticus 2:1— "And when any will offer a meat offering unto the Lord, his offering shall be [of] fine flour; and he shall pour oil upon it, and put frankincense thereon:"

Leviticus 2:2— "And he shall bring it to Aaron's sons the priests: and he shall take thereout his handful of the flour thereof, and of the oil thereof, with all the frankincense thereof; and the priest shall burn the memorial of it upon the altar, [to be] an offering made by fire, of a sweet savour unto the Lord:"

Leviticus 2:15— "And thou shalt put oil upon it, and lay frankincense thereon: it [is] a meat offering."

Leviticus 2:16— "And the priest shall burn the memorial of it, [part] of the beaten corn thereof, and [part] of the oil thereof, with all the frankincense thereof: [it is] an offering made by fire unto the Lord."

Leviticus 5:11— "But if he be not able to bring two turtledoves, or two young pigeons, then he that sinned shall bring for his offering the tenth part of an ephah of fine flour for a sin offering; he shall put no oil upon it, neither shall he put [any] frankincense thereon: for it [is] a sin offering"

Leviticus 6:15— "And he shall take of it his handful, of the flour of the meat offering, and of the oil thereof, and all the frankincense which [is] upon the meat offering, and shall burn [it] upon the altar [for] a sweet savour, [even] the memorial of it, unto the Lord."

Leviticus 24:7— "And thou shalt put pure frankincense upon [each] row, that it may be on the bread for a memorial, [even] an offering made by fire unto the Lord."

Numbers 5:15— "Then shall the man bring his wife unto the priest, and he shall bring her offering for her, the tenth [part] of an ephah of barley meal; he shall pour no oil upon it,

nor put frankincense thereon; for it [is] an offering of jealousy, an offering of memorial, bringing iniquity to remembrance."

1 Chronicles 9:29— "[Some] of them also [were] appointed to oversee the vessels, and all the instruments of the sanctuary, and the fine flour, and the wine, and the oil, and the frankincense, and the spices."

Nehemiah 13:5— "And he had prepared for him a great chamber, where aforetime they laid the meat offerings, the frankincense, and the vessels, and the tithes of the corn, the new wine, and the oil, which was commanded [to be given] to the Levites, and the singers, and the porters; and the offerings of the priests."

Nehemiah 13:9— "Then I commanded, and they cleansed the chambers: and thither brought I again the vessels of the house of God, with the meat offering and the frankincense."

Song Of Solomon 3:6— "Who [is] this that cometh out of the wilderness like pillars of smoke, perfumed with myrrh and frankincense, with all powders of the merchant?"

Song Of Solomon 4:6— "Until the day break, and the shadows flee away, I will get me to the mountain of myrrh, and to the hill of frankincense."

Song Of Solomon 4:14— "Spikenard and saffron; calamus and cinnamon, with all trees of frankincense; myrrh and aloes, with all the chief spices:"

Matthew 2:11— "And when they were come into the house, they saw the young child with Mary his mother, and fell down, and worshiped him: and when they had opened their treasures, they presented unto him gifts; gold, and frankincense, and myrrh."

Revelation 18:13— "And cinnamon, and odours, and ointments, and frankincense, and wine, and oil, and fine flour, and wheat, and beasts, and sheep, and horses, and chariots, and slaves, and souls of men."

Selected Research:

Michie, C.A., et al. "Frankincense and myrrh as remedies in children." *J R Soc Med.* 1991;84(10):602-5.

Wang, L.G., et al. "Determination of DNA topoisomerase II activity from L1210 cells--a target for screening antitumor agents." Chung Kuo Yao Li Hsueh Pao. 1991;12(2):108-14.

Galbanum *(Ferula gummosa)*

Botanical Family: Apiaceae or Umbelliferae (parsley)

Plant Origin: Iran

Extraction Method: Steam distilled from resin derive from stems and branches.

Chemical Constituents: Monoterpenes (65-85%), α-pinene (45-50%), camphene, limonene, myrcene, carvone; Sesquiterpenols; Esters; Coumarins.

Action: Anti-infectious, stimulant, supporting to the kidneys and genitals (menstruation), analgesic, light antispasmodic.

Found In: Exodus II and Gathering.

Traditional Uses: Mentioned in Egyptian papyri and the Old Testament (Exodus 30:34) it was esteemed for its medicinal and spiritual properties. Dioscorides, an ancient Roman historian, records that galbanum was used for its antispasmodic, diuretic, and pain-relieving properties.

Indications: Recognized for its antimicrobial and body supporting properties.

Other Uses: It may also help with abscesses, acne, asthma, bronchitis, chronic coughs, cramps, cuts, indigestion, inflammation, muscular aches and pains, nervous tension, poor circulation, rheumatism, scar tissue, stress, wrinkles, and wounds. Although it has a low frequency, when combined with other oils, such as frankincense or sandalwood, the frequency rises dramatically.

Application: Apply topically. May be added to food or water as a dietary supplement.

Fragrant Influence: Harmonic and balancing. It may help increase spiritual awareness and meditation.

Safety Data: If pregnant or under a doctor's care, consult physician.

Companion Oils: All oils.

Bible Reference:

Exodus 30:34—"And the Lord said unto Moses, Take unto thee sweet spices, stacte, and onycha, and galbanum; [these] sweet spices with pure frankincense: of each shall there be a like [weight]:"

Geranium *(Pelargonium graveolens)*

Botanical Family: Geraniaceae

Plant Origin: Egypt, India

Extraction Method: Steam distilled from the leaves.

Chemical Constituents: Monoterpenes; Sesquiterpenes; Monoterpene alcohols (60-68%): linalol, citronnellol (33%), geraniol (25%), nerol, menthol, Sesquiterpene alcohols; Terpene esters (20-33%); Oxides: 1,8 cineole: Aldehydes: neral, geranial (9.8%); Ketones.

Action: Antispasmodic, antitumoral, adrenal cortex stimulant, anti-inflammatory, astringent, hemostatic (stops bleeding) anti-infectious, antibacterial, antifungal, revitalizes skin tissue, dilates bile ducts for liver detoxification. Geranium balances the sebum, which is the fatty secretion in the sebaceous glands of the skin that keep the skin supple. Helps cleanse oily skin and restores and enlivens pale skin.

Found In: Acceptance, EndoFlex, Envision, Gathering, Gentle Baby, Harmony, Humility, JuvaFlex, Release, SARA, Trauma Life, and White Angelica.

Traditional Uses: Geranium has been used for centuries for skin care.

Indications: Skin conditions (dermatitis, eczema, psoriasis, vitiligo), herpes, shingles, bleeding, tumor growths, and hormone imbalances.

Other Uses: This oil may be used for acne, burns, circulatory problems (improves blood flow), depression, gingivitis, liver problems, sterility, digestion, eczema, insomnia, menstrual problems, neuralgia (severe pain along the nerve), regenerating tissue and nerves, pancreas imbalances, ringworm, shingles, sore throats, and wounds. Jean Valnet, M.D., recommends it for liver disorders and hepatitis.

Application: Diffuse and apply topically. May be added to food or water as a dietary supplement. Apply where you would use a deodorant.

Fragrant Influence: It may help to release negative memories. It may also help ease nervous tension and stress, balance the emotions, lift the spirit, and foster peace, well-being, and hope.

Safety Data: If pregnant or under a doctor's care, consult physician.

Companion Oils: All oils.

Selected Research:

Lis-Balchin, M., et al. "Antimicrobial activity of Pelargonium essential oils added to a quiche filling as a model food system." *Lett Appl Microbiol.* 1998;27(4):207-10.

Lis-Balchin, M., et al. "Comparative antibacterial effects of novel Pelargonium essential oils and solvent extracts." *Lett Appl Microbiol.* 1998;27(3):135-41.

Fang, H.J., et al. "Studies on the chemical components and anti-tumour action of the volatile oils from Pelargonium graveoleus." *Yao Hsueh Hsueh Pao.* 1989;24(5):366-71.

Ginger *(Zingiber officinale)*

Botanical Family: Zingiberaceae (ginger)

Plant Origin: China

Extraction Method: Steam distilled from root.

Chemical Constituents: Monoterpenes: α pinene, camphene, β–pinene, myrcene, limonene; Sesquiterpenes: zingiberene (30%); Hydrocarbons: Monoterpene alcohols: Sesquiterpene alcohols; Aldehydes; Ketones.

Action: Digestive tonic, relieves sexual tonic, reduces pain, expectorant.

Found In: Abundance, Di-Tone, Magnify Your Purpose, and Passion.

Traditional Uses: Ginger is used to combat the effects of motion sickness and has been studied for its gentle, simulating effects. Women in the country of Senegal, in West Africa, weave belts of ginger root to restore their mates' sexual potency.

Indications: Arthritis, rheumatism, indigestion, digestive disorders, motion sickness.

Other Uses: Ginger may be used for alcoholism, loss of appetite, arthritis, chills, respiratory infections, congestion, coughs, digestive disorders, infectious diseases, muscular aches/pains, nausea, rheumatism, sinusitis, sore throats, and sprains.

Application: Diffuse and apply topically. May be added to food or water as a dietary supplement or flavoring.

Fragrant Influence: Gentle, stimulating, endowing physical energy, and courage.

Safety Data: If pregnant or under a doctor's care, consult your physician. Repeated use can possibly result in contact sensitization. Avoid direct sunlight after use.

Companion Oils: All spice oils, all citrus oils, eucalyptus, frankincense, geranium, myrtle, rosemary, and spearmint.

Grapefruit (*Citrus paradisi*)

Botanical Family: Rutaceae (citrus)

Plant Origin: California.

Extraction Method: Cold press from rind.

Chemical Constituents: Monoterpenes: limonene (96-98%); Aldehydes; Coumarins and furocoumarins.

Action: Antiseptic, disinfecting, detoxifying, diuretic. Like many cold-pressed citrus oils, it has unique fat-dissolving characteristics. It is exceptionally cleansing for oily skin. Psychologically, it is antidepressant and emotionally uplifting.

Found In: Citrus Fresh

Historical Use: Grapefruit is actually a hybrid between *Citrus maxima* and *Citrus sinesis*.

Indications: Helps with acne, cellulite, digestion, and fluid retention.

Other Uses: Grapefruit oil may help with depression, drug withdrawal, eating disorders, fatigue, jet lag, liver disorders, migraine headaches, pre-menstrual tension, and stress. It may also have a cleansing effect on the kidneys, the lymphatic system, and the vascular system.

Application: Diffuse and apply topically. Add to food or water as a dietary supplement or flavoring. Grapefruit is not photosensitizing unlike other oils with furocoumarins.

Fragrant Influence: Refreshing and uplifting.

Safety Data: If pregnant or under a doctor's care, consult physician.

Companion Oils: Basil, bergamot, cedarwood, chamomile, cypress, frankincense, geranium, juniper, lavender, peppermint, rosemary, rosewood, and ylang ylang.

Helichrysum (*Helichrysum italicum*)

Botanical Family: Asteraceae or Compositae (daisy)

Plant Origin: Yugoslavia, Corsica

Extraction Method: Steam distilled from flower.

Chemical Constituents: Sesquiterpenes; Monoterpenols: nerol; Terpene esters; neryle acetate (75%); Ketones.

Action: Anticoagulant, anaesthetic, dissolves hematomas (blood clots), mucolytic, expectorant, antispasmodic, stimulates liver, reduces scar tissue and skin discoloration. It balances blood pressure, chelates chemicals and toxins.

Found In: Aroma Life, Brain Power, Forgiveness, JuvaFlex, M-Grain, PanAway, Passion, and Trauma Life.

Traditional Uses: Helichrysum has been studied by European researchers for regenerating tissue and nerves and improving circulation and skin conditions.

Indications: Hematoma (swelling or blood-filled tumor), bleeding, arteriosclerosis, atherosclerosis, hypertension, congestive heart failure, cardiac arrhythmias, thrombosis, embolisms, liver disorders, phlebitis, sciatica, sinus infection, skin conditions (eczema, dermatitis, psoriasis).

Other Uses: This oil may help blood circulation, hearing loss, pain (acute), respiratory conditions, scar tissue, varicose veins. It may regenerate tissue, detoxify and stimulate the liver cell function.

Application: Diffuse. Apply topically around outside of ear, temple, forehead, back of neck, or on location.

Fragrant Influence: It is uplifting to the subconscious.

Safety Data: If pregnant or under a doctor's care, consult physician.

Hyssop (*Hyssopus officinalis*)

Botanical Family: Lamiaceae or Labiatae (mint)

Plant Origin: France, Hungary

Extraction Method: Steam distilled from stems/leaves.

Chemical Constituents: Monoterpenes (25-30%); β–pinenes; Sesquiterpenes (12%); Sesquiterpenols (5-10%); Phenols methyl-ethers, methyl chavicol; Monoterpenones (45-58%); α and β– thujones, camphor, isopinocamphone (31-32%); pinocamphone (53%).

Action: Anticatarrhal, mucolytic, decongestant, expectorant, cleansing, purifying, and helps reduce fats and lipids in the tissue. Raises low blood pressure. regulates menstrual flow, and increases perspiration.

Found In: Exodus II, Harmony, ImmuPower, Relieve It, and White Angelica.

Traditional Uses: While there is some uncertainty that *Hyssopus officinalis* is the same species of plant as the hyssop referred to in the Old and New Testaments, there is no question that *H. officinalis* has been used medicinally for almost a millennia for its antiseptic, disinfecting, and anti-infectious properties. It has also been used for opening the respiratory system.

Indications: This oil may be beneficial for anxiety, arthritis, asthma, bruises, respiratory infections, coughs, cuts, dermatitis, indigestion, fatigue, nervous tension, parasites (expelling worms), rheumatism, sore throats, viral infections, and wounds.

Application: Diffuse and apply topically. May be added to food or water as a dietary supplement.

Fragrant Influence: Stimulates creativity and meditation.

Safety Data: If pregnant or under a doctor's care, consult your physician. Do not use if epileptic.

Companion Oils: All citrus oils, clary sage, sage, myrtle, geranium, and fennel.

Bible References:

Exodus 12:22— "And ye shall take a bunch of hyssop, and dip [it] in the blood that [is] in the bason, and strike the lintel and the two side posts with the blood that [is] in the bason; and none of you shall go out at the door of his house until the morning."

Leviticus 14:4— "Then shall the priest command to take for him that is to be cleansed two birds alive [and] clean, and cedar wood, and scarlet, and hyssop:"

Leviticus 14:6— "As for the living bird, he shall take it, and the cedar wood, and the scarlet, and the hyssop, and shall dip them and the living bird in the blood of the bird [that was] killed over the running water:"

Leviticus 14:49— "And he shall take to cleanse the house two birds, and cedar wood, and scarlet, and hyssop:"

Leviticus 14:51— "And he shall take the cedar wood, and the hyssop, and the scarlet, and the living bird, and dip them in the blood of the slain bird, and in the running water, and sprinkle the house seven times:"

Leviticus 14:52— "And he shall cleanse the house with the blood of the bird, and with the running water, and with the living bird, and with the cedar wood, and with the hyssop, and with the scarlet:"

Numbers 19:6— "And the priest shall take cedar wood, and hyssop, and scarlet, and cast [it] into the midst of the burning of the heifer."

Numbers 19:18— "And a clean person shall take hyssop, and dip [it] in the water, and sprinkle [it] upon the tent, and upon all the vessels, and upon the persons that were there, and upon him that touched a bone, or one slain, or one dead, or a grave:"

1 Kings 4:33— "And he spake of trees, from the cedar tree that [is] in Lebanon even unto the hyssop that springeth out of the wall: he spake also of beasts, and of fowl, and of creeping things, and of fishes."

Psalms 51:7— "Purge me with hyssop, and I shall be clean: wash me, and I shall be whiter than snow."

John 19:29— "Now there was set a vessel full of vinegar: and they filled a spunge with vinegar, and put [it] upon hyssop, and put [it] to his mouth."

Hebrews 9:19— "For when Moses had spoken every precept to all the people according to the law, he took the blood of calves and of goats, with water, and scarlet wool, and hyssop, and sprinkled both the book, and all the people."

Idaho Tansy (*Tanacetum vulgare*)

Botanical Family: Asteraceae or Compositae (daisy)

Plant Origin: Idaho, Washington

Extraction Method: Steam distilled from leaves.

Chemical Constituents: Thujone, Camphor, Sabinene, Camphene

Action: Insect repellent, analgesic, antitumoral, hemostat, immune stimulant.

Found In: ImmuPower and Into The Future

Traditional Uses: This antimicrobial oil has been used extensively as an insect repellent. According to E. Joseph Montagna's P.D.R. on herbal formulas, it may help numerous skin conditions and tone the entire system.

Indications: May help respiratory infections, stomach conditions, arthritis, irritable bowel syndrome, aneurysm, bruises, diarrhea, freckles, and gout.

Application: Diffuse or apply topically.

Safety Data: If pregnant or under a doctor's care, consult your physician.

Companion Oils: Clary sage, hyssop, myrtle, pine, valerian, elemi, birch, and vetiver

Jasmine (*Jasminum officinale*)

Botanical Family: Oleaceae (olive)

Plant Origin: India

Extraction Method: Absolute extraction from flower. Jasmine is actually an "essence" not an essential oil. The flowers must be picked at night to maximize fragrance.

Chemical Constituents: Benzyl Acetate, Benzyl Benzoate, Methyl Anthranilate, Linalol, Phytol, Methyl Palmitate.

Action: Beneficial for skin, uplifting, antidepressant, and stimulating.

Found In: Dragon Time, Inner Child, Into The Future, Passion, Sensation

Traditional Uses: Jasmine has been nicknamed as the "queen of the night" and "moonlight of the grove." For centuries, women have treasured jasmine for its beautiful, seductive fragrance.

Indications: Beneficial for dry, greasy, irritated, or sensitive skin. Helps anxiety, stress, depression.

Other Uses: This oil may help with eczema (when caused by emotions), frigidity, labor pains, laryngitis, lethargy (abnormal drowsiness), menstrual pain and problems, and stress. It is ideal for skin care (dry, greasy, irritated, and sensitive).

Application: Diffuse and apply topically. May be added to food or water as a dietary supplement.

Fragrant Influence: Uplifting and stimulating in times of hopelessness and nervous exhaustion. It helps to reduce anxiety, apathy, depression, dilemmas that deal with relationships, indifference, and listlessness. When worn as a cologne, it increases excitability.

Safety Data: If pregnant or under a doctor's care, consult physician.

Companion Oils: Bergamot, frankincense, geranium, helichrysum, lemongrass, mandarin, melissa, orange, palmarosa, rose, rosewood, sandalwood, and spearmint.

Note: One pound of jasmine oil requires about 1,000 pounds of jasmine or 3.6 million fresh unpacked blossoms. The blossoms must be collected before sunrise, or much of the fragrance will have evaporated. The quality of the blossoms may also be compromised if they are squashed. A single pound of pure jasmine oil may cost between $1,200 to $4,500. In contrast, synthetic jasmine oils can be obtained for $3.50 per pound, but it obviously does not possess the same therapeutic qualities as pure jasmine oil. The above-mentioned properties are based on pure jasmine oil, not synthetic oil.

Juniper Berry *(Juniperus communis)*

Botanical Family: Cupressaceae (cypress)

Plant Origin: Utah

Extraction Method: Steam distilled from berries and twigs.

Chemical Constituents: Monoterpenes: α pinene (34-46%), sabinene (9-28%), myrcene (6-8%); Sesquiterpenes; Terpene alcohols; Aldehydes; Ketones mono and sesquiterpenes: camphor, pinocamphone.

Action: Antiseptic, astringent, digestive stimulant, purifying, and detoxifying. It increases circulation through kidneys and promotes excretion of uric acid and toxins.

Found In: Di-Tone, Dream Catcher, En-R-Gee, Grounding, Hope, and Into the Future.

Traditional Uses: Bundles of juniper berries were hung over doorways to ward off witches during medieval times. It has been used for centuries as a diuretic. Until recently, French hospital wards burned sprigs of juniper and rosemary to protect from infection.

Indications: It may help acne, dermatitis, eczema, depression, fatigue, liver problems, sore muscles, rheumatism, ulcers, urinary infections, fluid retention, and wounds.

Other Uses: This oil may work as a detoxifier and a cleanser, as well as being beneficial for the skin. It may possibly assist with nerve regeneration.

Application: Diffuse and apply topically. May be added to food or water as a dietary supplement.

Fragrant Influence: Juniper evokes feelings of health, love, and peace and may help to elevate one's spiritual awareness.

Safety Data: If pregnant or under a doctor's care, consult physician.

Companion Oils: Bergamot, all citrus oils, cypress, geranium, lavender, melaleuca, Melrose, and rosemary.

Bible Reference:

Job 30:45— "Who cut up mallows by the bushes, and juniper roots [for] their meat."

Selected Research:

Takacsova M, et al. "Study of the antioxidative effects of thyme, sage, juniper and oregano." *Nahrung.* 1995;39(3):241-3.

Laurus nobilis

Botanical Family: Lauraceae

Plant Origin: France

Extraction Method: Steam distilled from leaves.

Chemical Constituents: Monoterpenes: α pinene, β–pinene, sabinene; Sesquiterpenes; Monoterpenols: linalol (8-16%); Terpene Esters; Phenols: eugenol (3%); Oxides: 1,8 cineol (35045%); Lactones sesquiterpenes.

Action: Antiseptic, antimicrobial, expectorant, mucolytic, anti-infectious, antibacterial (staph, strep, E. coli), candida, anticoagulant.

Traditional Uses: Both the leaves and the black berries were also used to alleviate indigestion, indigestion, and loss of appetite. During the Middle Ages, it was used for angina pectoris, asthma, gout, migraine, palpitations, and liver and spleen complaints.

Indications: Nerve regeneration, arthritis (rheumatoid), oral infections.

Other Uses: Laurel may help with loss of appetite, asthmatic conditions, chronic bronchitis, hair loss (after an infection), pediculosis, scabies, and viral infections.

Application: Diffuse or apply topically on the abdomen or on location. Add to food or water as a dietary supplement or flavoring.

Fragrant Influence: Laurel has been used as a fragrance component in cosmetics and perfumes.

Safety Data: If pregnant or under a doctor's care, consult your physician. Use in moderation.

Lavender *(Lavandula angustifolia)*

Botanical Family: Lamiaceae or Labiatae (mint)

Plant Origin: Utah, Idaho, France

Extraction Method: Steam distilled from flowering top.

Chemical Constituents: Monoterpene; α pinene, β–pinene, camphene; Sesquiterpenes; Non terpene alcohols (45%), geraniol, borneol, lavandulol; Esters: linalyl acetate (30-34%); lavanduyle, Oxides: 1,8 cineole; Ketones; Sesquiterpenones; Aldehydes; Lactones: Coumarins.

Action: Antiseptic, analgesic, antitumoral, anticonvulsant, sedative, anti-inflammatory. It is beneficial for cleansing cuts and wounds and is ideal for skin care, since it prevents the build up of excess sebum, a skin oil that bacteria feed on. Lavender has also been clinically evaluated for its relaxing effects.

Found In: Aroma Siez, Brain Power, Dragon Time, Envision, Forgiveness, Gathering, Gentle Baby, Harmony, Mister, Motivation, M-Grain, R.C., SARA, Surrender, and Trauma Life

Traditional Uses: The French scientist René Gatefossé was the first to discover lavender's ability to promote tissue regeneration and speed wound healing when he severely burned his arm in a laboratory accident. Today, lavender is one of the few to still be listed in the British Pharmacopoeia.

Indications: Burns (cell renewal), sunburns (including lips), dandruff, hair loss, allergies, convulsions, herpes, headaches, indigestion, insomnia, high blood pressure, menopausal conditions, nausea, phlebitis, tumors, premenstrual conditions, scarring (minimizes), skin conditions (acne, dermatitis, eczema, psoriasis, and rashes) and stretch marks. It may be used to cleanse cuts, bruises, and skin irritations.

Other Uses: Lavender is a universal oil with many different applications. It may help arthritis, asthma, bronchitis, convulsions, depression, earaches, heart palpitations, high blood pressure, hives (urticaria), insect bites, laryngitis, nervous tension, respiratory infections, rheumatism, and throat infections.

Application: Diffuse or apply topically. Has a wide range of uses. Apply where you would use a deodorant. Safe for use on small children. May also be added to food or water as a dietary supplement.

Fragrant Influence: Calming, relaxing, and balancing, both physically and emotionally.

Safety Data: If pregnant or under a doctor's care, consult physician.

Companion Oils: Most oils, especially citrus oils, chamomile, clary sage, and geranium.

Selected Research:

Larrondo JV, et al. "Antimicrobial activity of essences from labiates." *Microbios.* 1995; 82(332):171-2.

Guillemain J, et al. "Neurodepressive effects of the essential oil of Lavandula angustifolia Mill." *Ann Pharm Fr.* 1989;47(6):337-43.

Kim HM, et al. "Lavender oil inhibits immediate-type allergic reaction in mice and rats." *J Pharm Pharmacol.* 1999;51(2):221-6.

Vernet-Maury E, et al. "Basic emotions induced by odorants: a new approach based on autonomic pattern results." *J Auton Nerv Syst.* 1999;75(2-3):176-83.

Diego MA, et al. "Aromatherapy positively affects mood, EEG patterns of alertness and math computations." *Int J Neurosci.* 1998 Dec;96(3-4):217-24.

Hay IC, et al. "Randomized trial of aromatherapy. Successful treatment for alopecia areata." *Arch Dermatol.* 1998; 134(11):1349-52.

Bradshaw RH, et al. "Effects of lavender straw on stress and travel sickness in pigs." *J Altern Complement Med.* 1998;4(3):271-5.

Lantry LE, et al. "Chemopreventive effect of perillyl alcohol on 4-(methylnitrosamino)-1-(3-pyridyl)-1-butanone induced tumorigenesis in (C3H/HeJ X A/J)F1 mouse lung." *J Cell Biochem Suppl.* 1997;27:20-5.

Reddy BS, et al. "Chemoprevention of colon carcinogenesis by dietary perillyl alcohol." *Cancer Res.* 1997;57(3):420-5.

Cornwell S, et al. "Lavender oil and perineal repair." *Mod Midwife* 1995;5(3):31-3.

Dunn C, et al. "Sensing an improvement: an experimental study to evaluate the use of aromatherapy, massage and periods of rest in an intensive care unit." *J Adv Nurs.* 1995;21(1):34-40.

Yamada K, et al. "Anticonvulsive effects of inhaling lavender oil vapour." B*iol Pharm Bull.* 1994;17(2):359-60.

Buchbauer G, et al. "Aromatherapy: evidence for sedative effects of the essential oil of lavender after inhalation." *Z Naturforsch* [C]. 1991;46(11-12):1067-72.

Sysoev NP. "The effect of waxes from essential-oil plants on the dehydrogenase activity of the blood neutrophils in mucosal trauma of the mouth." *Stomatologiia* 1991;70(1):12-3.

Nikolaevskii VV, et al. "Effect of essential oils on the course of experimental atherosclerosis." *Patol Fiziol Eksp Ter.* 1990; (5):52-3.

Delaveau P, et al. "Neuro-depressive properties of essential oil of lavender." *C R Seances Soc Biol Fil.* 1989;183(4):342-8.

Lavandin (*Lavandula x hybrida*)

Botanical Family: Lamiaceae or Labiatae (mint)

Chemical Constituents: Lynalyl acetate (30-32%), linalol, cineol, camphene (8-12%), pinene, and others.

Action: Antibacterial, antifungal, and strong antiseptic. (See lavender for additional properties.)

Found In: Purification, Release

Traditional Uses: Also known as *Lavandula x intermedia*, lavandin is a hybrid plant developed by crossing true lavender with spike lavender or aspic (*Lavandula latifolia*). It has been used to sterilize the animal cages in veterinary clinics and hospitals throughout Europe.

Indications: There is not a long history of the therapeutic use of lavandin.

Other Uses: Lavendin is best used as an antiseptic. The greater penetrating qualities make it well suited to help with respiratory, circulatory, and muscular conditions.

Application: Diffuse or apply topically.

Fragrant Influence: It has the same calming effects as lavender.

Safety Data: If pregnant or under a doctor's care, consult your physician. **DO NOT USE FOR BURNS**.

Companion Oils: Bergamot, cinnamon, citronella, clove, cypress, clary sage, geranium, lime, patchouly, pine, rosemary, and thyme.

Lemon (*Citrus limon*)

Botanical Family: Rutaceae (citrus)

Plant Origin: California (organic), Italy

Extraction Method: Cold pressed from rind. It takes 3,000 lemons to produce a kilo of oil.

Chemical Constituents: Monoterpenes: limonene (54-72%); Sesquiterpenes; Aldehydes; Coumarins and furocoumarins, contains flavonoids, carotenoids, steroids.

Action: Anti-infectious, disinfectant, antibacterial (spores), antiseptic, antiviral, vitamin P-like action for improving microcirculation, promotes white blood cell formation, improves immune function.

Found In: Citrus Fresh, Joy, Raven, Surrender, and Thieves

Traditional Uses: Lemon has antiseptic-like properties and contains compounds that have been studied for their effects on immune function. According Jean Valnet, M.D., the vaporized essence of lemon can kill meningococcus bacteria in 15 minutes, typhoid bacilli in one hours, *Staphylococcus aureus* in two hours, and *Pneumococcus* bacteria within three hours. Even a .2 percent solution of lemon oil can kill diphtheria bacteria in 20 minutes and inactivate tuberculosis bacteria. Lemon oil has been widely used in skin care to cleanse skin and reduce wrinkles.

Indications: Anemia, asthma, herpes, warts, shingles, bleeding, malaria, parasites, rheumatism, throat infection, ureter infections, and varicose veins.

Other Uses: This oil may be beneficial for anxiety, blood pressure, digestive problems, respiratory infections, sore throats. It is helps promote leukocyte formation, improves memory, strengthens nails, cleans the skin, and promotes a sense of well-being. It may also help brighten a pale, dull complexion by removing the dead skin cells. It serves as an effective insect repellent and works well in removing gum, wood stain, oil, and grease spots.

Application: Diffuse or add a few drops to a spray bottle to deodorize and sterilize the air. Add 2 drops to water for purification or combine with peppermint (*Mentha piperita*) to provide a refreshing lift. Add to food or water as a dietary supplement or flavoring.

Fragrant Influence: It promotes clarity of thought and purpose, as well as health, healing, physical energy, and purification. Its fragrance is invigorating, enhancing, and warming.

Safety Data: If pregnant or under a doctor's care, consult your physician. Lemon oil is very slightly photosensitizing, so avoid applying it to skin that will be exposed to direct sunlight or UV light.

Companion Oils: Chamomile, eucalyptus, fennel, frankincense, geranium, juniper, peppermint, sandalwood, and ylang ylang.

Lemongrass (*Cymbopogon flexuosus*)

Botanical Family: Poaceae or Gramineae (grasses)

Plant Origin: India, Guatemala

Extraction Method: Steam distilled from leaves.

Chemical Constituents: Alcohol monoterpenes; α terpenol, borneol, geraniol; Alcohol sesquiterpenes: farnesol (12.8%); Monoterpene aldehydes (60-85%): citrals (75%), neral (27.7%), geranial (46.6%); Monoterpene aldehydes.

Action: Support digestion, tones and helps regenerate connective tissues and ligaments, dilates blood vessels, strengthens vascular walls, promotes lymph flow, and is anti-inflammatory and sedative.

Found In: Di-Tone, En-R-Gee, Inner Child, Purification

Traditional Uses: Lemongrass is used for purification and digestion. Research was published in *Phytotherapy Research* on topically applied lemongrass for its powerful antifungal properties.

Indications: Bladder infection, digestive disturbances, parasites, torn ligaments, edema, fluid retention, kidney disorders, and varicose veins.

Other Uses: This oil may help improve circulation, digestion, eyesight, as well as combat headaches, infections, respiratory problems, sore throats, and fluid retention. It aids in tissue regeneration.

Application: Diffuse or apply topically.

Fragrant Influence: Promotes psychic awareness and purification.

Safety Data: If pregnant or under a doctor's care, consult your physician. Skin test for sensitivity/ irritation.

Companion Oils: Basil, cedarwood, eucalyptus, geranium, lavender, melaleuca, and rosemary.

Selected Research:

Pattnaik S, et al. "Antibacterial and antifungal activity of ten essential oils in vitro." *Microbios.* 1996;86(349):237-46.

Lorenzetti BB, et al. "Myrcene mimics the peripheral analgesic activity of lemongrass tea." *J Ethnopharmacol.* 1991;34(1):43-8.

Elson CE, et al. "Impact of lemongrass oil, an essential oil, on serum cholesterol." Lipids. 1989;24(8):677-9.

Tiwari BK, et al. "Evaluation of insecticidal, fumigant and repellent properties of lemongrass oil." *Indian J Exp Biol.* 1966;4(2):128-9.

Mandarin *(Citrus reticulata)*

Botanical Family: Rutaceae (citrus)

Plant Origin: Madagascar, Italy, China

Extraction Method: Cold press from rind.

Chemical Constituents: Monoterpenes; limonene (65-94%); Esters; Aldehydes; Coumarins and furocoumarins. Contains flavonoids, carotenoids, and steroids.

Action: Light antispasmodic, digestive tonic (promoting good digestion), antiseptic, antifungal, stimulates gallbladder.

Found In: Citrus Fresh, Joy, and Awaken

Traditional Uses: This fruit was traditionally given to Imperial Chinese officials named the mandarins.

Other Uses: This oil may help acne, digestive problems, fluid retention, insomnia, intestinal problems, skin problems (congested and oily skin, scars, spots, tones the skin), stretch marks (when combined with either jasmine, lavender, sandalwood, and/or frankincense), nervous tension, restlessness. Recommended for children and pregnant women because it is very gentle.

Application: Diffuse or apply topically.

Fragrant Influence: It is appeasing, gentle, and promotes happiness.

Safety Data: If pregnant or under a doctor's care, consult your physician. Avoid direct sunlight after use.

Companion Oils: Lavender; neroli and other citrus oils; cinnamon, clove, nutmeg, and other spice oils.

Marjoram *(Origanum majorana)*

Botanical Family: Lamiaceae or Labiatae (mint)

Plant Origin: France

Extraction Method: Steam distilled from leaves.

Chemical Constituents: Monoterpenes (40%): α and β-pinenes, myrcene; Sesquiterpenes; Monoterpenols (50%): linalol; Terpene esters: terpenyle acetates, geranyle acetates.

Action: Anti-infectious, antibacterial, dilates blood vessels, regulates blood pressure, soothes muscles, promotes intestinal peristalsis, tones the parasympathetic nervous system, and supports respiratory system.

Found In: Aroma Life, Aroma Siez, Dragon Time, M-Grain, and R.C.

Traditional Uses: Known as the "herb of happiness" to the Romans and "joy of the mountains" to the Greeks. Believed to increase longevity.

Indications: Aches, arthritis, asthma, bronchitis, indigestion, constipation, cramps, insomnia, migraine headaches, neuralgia, rheumatism, sprains.

Other Uses: It may be relaxing and calming to the muscles that constrict and sometimes contribute to headaches. It may help anxiety, nervous tension, bruises, burns, sores, cuts, circulatory disorders, respiratory infections, fungal and viral infections, menstrual problems, ringworm, shingles, shock, sores, spasms, sunburns, and fluid retention.

Application: Diffuse or apply topically. Massage to calm stressed muscles. Add to food or water as a dietary supplement or flavoring.

Fragrant Influence: Assists in calming the nerves.

Safety Data: If pregnant or under a doctor's care, consult physician.

Companion Oils: Bergamot, cedarwood, chamomile, cypress, lavender, orange, nutmeg, rosemary, rosewood, ylang ylang.

Melaleuca alternifolia

Botanical Family: Myrtaceae (myrtle)

Plant Origin: Australia

Extraction Method: Steam distilled from leaves.

Chemical Constituents: Monoterpenes: α pinene, β–pinene, myrcene; Sesquiterpenes; Monoterpene alcohols (45-50%); Terpene oxides.

Action: Anti-infectious, antibacterial for large spectrum action of gram positive: staph and gram negative: e.coli., antifungal, antiviral, antiparasitic, antiseptic, anti-inflammatory, immunostimulant, antiaesthetic, cardio tonic, decongestant of the veins, reduces phlebitis, neuro tonic, analgesic, protects against radiation, analgesic (reduces pain).

Found In: Melrose, Purification

Traditional Uses: Highly regarded as an antimicrobial and antiseptic essential oil. It has high levels of terpinenol, which is the key active constituent.

Indications: Athlete's foot, fungal infections, bronchitis, respiratory infections, gum disease, rash, sore throat, sunburn, tonsillitis, vaginal thrush.

Other Uses: This oil may help acne, burns, candida, cold sores, inflammation, viral infections, ingrown nails, warts, and wounds (promotes healing).

Application: Diffuse or apply topically. Safe for use on children and pets.

Fragrant Influence: Promotes cleansing and purity.

Safety Data: If pregnant or under a doctor's care, consult your physician. Repeated use can possibly result in contact sensitization.

Companion Oils: All citrus oils, cypress, eucalyptus, lavender, rosemary, and thyme.

Selected Research:

Syed TA, et al. "Treatment of toenail onychomycosis with 2% butenafine and 5% Melaleuca alternifolia (tea tree) oil in cream." *Trop Med Int Health.* 1999;4(4):284-7.

Hammer KA, et al. "In vitro susceptibilities of lactobacilli and organisms associated with bacterial vaginosis to Melaleuca alternifolia (tea tree) oil." Antimicrob Agents Chemother. 1999;43(1):196.

Concha JM, et al. 1998 William J. Stickel Bronze Award. "Antifungal activity of Melaleuca alternifolia (tea-tree) oil against various pathogenic organisms." *J Am Podiatr Med Assoc.* 1998;88(10):489-92

Faoagali JL, et al. "Antimicrobial effects of melaleuca oil." *Burns.* 1998;24(4):383. No abstract available.

Nenoff P, et al. "Antifungal activity of the essential oil of Melaleuca alternifolia (tea tree oil) against pathogenic fungi in vitro." *Skin Pharmacol.* 1996;9(6):388-94.

Hammer KA, et al. "Susceptibility of transient and commensal skin flora to the essential oil of Melaleuca alternifolia (tea tree oil)." *Am J Infect Control.* 1996;24(3):186-9.

Carson CF, et al. "Antimicrobial activity of the major components of the essential oil of Melaleuca alternifolia." *J Appl Bacteriol.* 1995;78(3):264-9.

Bassett IB, et al. "A comparative study of tea-tree oil versus benzoylperoxide in the treatment of acne." *Med J Aust.* 1990;153(8):455-8.

Veal L. "The potential effectiveness of essential oils as a treatment for headlice, Pediculus humanus capitis." *Complement Ther Nurs Midwifery.* 1996;2(4):97-101.

Melaleuca ericifolia (Australian Rosalina)

Botanical Family: Myrtaceae (myrtle)

Plant Origin: Australia

Chemical Constituents: α-Pinene, 1,8 Cineol, Linalook, α-Terpineol, Limonene, para-Cymene.

Application: Diffuse or apply topically.

Safety Data: If pregnant or under a doctor's care, consult physician.

Note: This oil is still under study. It has been found beneficial for bronchitis, asthma, respiratory infection, cynitis, and sinus infection.

Melaleuca quinquenervia

Botanical Family: Myrtaceae (myrtle)

Plant Origin: Australia

Extraction Method: Steam distilled from leaves and limbs.

Chemical Constituents: Sesquiterpenes; Monoterpene alcohols: linalol; Sesquiterpene alcohols: (+)-trans- nerolidol (81-82%), farnesols; Terpene oxides: 1.9 cineol.

Action: Hormone-like (testicles), anti-inflammatory, anti-infectious, antibacterial, antiviral, antiparasitic (amoeba and parasites in the blood).

Found In: Melrose

Indications: Relieves mucous in the respiratory passages, urinary tract, and genital organs, digestive tonic, reduces hypertension (high blood pressure).

Other Uses: This oil may help with the respiratory tract and respiratory allergies, infections, and hemorrhoids.

Application: Diffuse or apply topically.

Fragrant Influence: Sweet and delicate.

Safety Data: If pregnant or under a doctor's care, consult your physician. Repeated use can possibly result in contact sensitization.

Melissa (Melissa officinalis)

Botanical Family: Lamiaceae or Labiatae (mint)

Plant Origin: Utah, Idaho, France

Extraction Method: Steam distilled from leaves and flowers.

Chemical Constituents: Monoterpenols: linalol, nerol, geraniol, citronnellol, α terpineol; Sesquiterpenols; Terpene esters: geranial acetates, Terpene oxides: 1,8 cineole; Monoterpenals: citrals, neral (15%) geranial (15%); Coumarins.

Action: Calming, sedative, hypotensive (low blood pressure), fights against cholera, anti-inflammatory.

Found In: Brain Power, Forgiveness, Hope, Humility, Passion, and White Angelica.

Traditional Uses: Melissa has powerful anti-microbial constituents. It is very gentle and delicate because of the nature of the plant and helps to bring out those characteristics within an individual.

Traditional Uses: Anciently, melissa was used for nervous disorders and many different ailments dealing with the heart or the emotions. It was also used to promote fertility. Melissa was the main ingredient in Carmelite water, distilled in France since 1611 by the Carmelite monks.

Indications: Dr. Dietrich Wabner, a professor at the Technical University of Munich, reported that a one-time application of true melissa oil led to complete remission of Herpes Simplex lesions.

Other Uses: Allergies, anxiety, asthma, bronchitis, chronic coughs, respiratory infections, cold-sore blisters (apply directly three times per day), indigestion, depression, dysentery, eczema, fevers, hypertension, indigestion, insect bites, insomnia, menstrual problems, migraine, nausea, nervous tension, palpitations, throat infections, and vertigo.

Application: Diffuse or apply topically.

Fragrant Influence: Melissa brings out gentle characteristics within people. It is calming and uplifting and may help to balance the emotions. It may also help to remove emotional blocks and instill a positive outlook on life.

Safety Data: If pregnant or under a doctor's care, consult physician.

Companion Oils: Geranium, lavender, and other floral and citrus oils.

Selected Research:

Yamasaki K, et al. "Anti-HIV-1 activity of herbs in Labiatae." *Biol Pharm Bull.* 1998;21(8):829-33.

Larrondo JV, et al. "Antimicrobial activity of essences from labiates." *Microbios.* 1995;82(332):171-2.

Kucera LS, et al. "Antiviral activities of extracts of the lemon balm plant." *Ann NY Acad Sci.* 1965 Jul 30;130(1):474-82.

Hausen BM, et al. "Comparative studies of the sensitizing capacity of drugs used in herpes simplex." *Derm Beruf Umwelt.* 1986;34(6):163-70.

Mountain Savory *(Satureja montana)*

Botanical Family: Lamiaceae or Labiatae

Plant Origin: France

Extraction Method: Steam distilled from flowering plant.

Chemical Constituents: Monoterpenes: α thujene, α and β–pinenes, camphene, sabinene, myrcene, limonene; Sesquiterpenes; Monoterpenes: linalol; Terpene alcohols, Terpene esters; Phenols: thymol, carvacrol (25-50%), eugenol; Phenols methyl-ethers: methyl carvacrol; Terpene oxides: 1,8 cineol; Ketones, camphor.

Action: Strong anti-infectious, antibacterial, antifungal, antiviral, antiparasitic, immunostimulant, general tonic and stimulant.

Found In: ImmuPower, Surrender

Traditional Uses: Mountain Savory has been used historically as a general tonic for the body.

Indications: Reduces acute pain, tonic for the nerves and circulatory systems.

Other Uses: Due to its high phenol content, Mountain Savory is a very strong antiseptic and has been used to hasten the formation of scar tissue, and to help with abscesses, burns, and cuts. It is also known to stimulate the adrenal gland. Recent research suggests that the extract may have anti-HIV activity.

Application: Diffuse or apply topically mixed with massage oil.

Fragrant Influence: It may produce strong psychological effects and may help revitalize and stimulate the nervous system. It is a powerful energizer and motivator.

Safety Data: If pregnant or under a doctor's care, consult your physician. Dilution is recommended when using topically. Always skin test for sensitivity.

Selected Research:

Yamasaki K, et al. "Anti-HIV-1 activity of herbs in Labiatae." *Biol Pharm Bull.* 1998; 21(8):829-33.

Panizzi L, et al. "Composition and antimicrobial properties of essential oils of four Mediterranean Lamiaceae." *J Ethnopharmacol.* 1993;39(3):167-70.

Myrrh *(Commiphora myrrha)*

Botanical Family: Burseraceae (Frankincense)

Plant Origin: Somalia

Extraction Method: Steam distilled from gum/resin.

Chemical Constituents: Hydrocarbons; Sesquiterpenes; Sesquiterpenes furanics; Sesquiterpenones furanics; Ketones; Aldehydes.

Action: Anti-infectious, antiviral, parasitic (worms), hormone-like, anti-inflammatory, soothes skin conditions, antihyperthyroid, supports immune system.

Found In: Abundance, Exodus II, Hope, Humility, 3 Wise Men, and White Angelica.

Traditional Uses: The Arabian people used it for many skin conditions, such as chapped and cracked skin and wrinkles. It has one of the highest levels of sesquiterpenes, a class of compounds that has direct effects on the hypothalamus, pituitary, and amygdala, the seat of our emotions. It is widely used today in oral hygiene products.

Indications: Bronchitis, diarrhea, dysentery, hyperthyroidism, stretch marks, thrush, ulcers, vaginal thrush, viral hepatitis.

Other Uses: This oil may help asthma, athlete's foot, candida, coughs, eczema, digestion, fungal infection, gingivitis, gum infections, hemorrhoids, mouth ulcers, ringworm, sore throats, skin conditions (chapped and cracked), wounds, and wrinkles.

Application: Apply topically on location or in a massage. May be added to food or water as a dietary supplement.

Fragrant Influence: It promotes spiritual awareness and is uplifting.

Safety Data: If pregnant or under a doctor's care, consult physician.

Companion Oils: Frankincense, lavender, patchouly, sandalwood, and all spice oils.

Bible References:

Genesis 37:25— "And they sat down to eat bread: and they lifted up their eyes and looked, and, behold, a company of Ishmeelites came from Gilead with their camels bearing spicery and balm and myrrh, going to carry [it] down to Egypt."

Genesis 43:11— "And their father Israel said unto them, If [it must be] so now, do this; take of the best fruits in the land in your vessels, and carry down the man a present, a little balm, and a little honey, spices, and myrrh, nuts, and almonds:"

Exodus 30:23— "Take thou also unto thee principal spices, of pure myrrh five hundred [shekels], and of sweet cinnamon half so much, [even] two hundred and fifty [shekels], and of sweet calamus two hundred and fifty [shekels],"

Esther 2:12— "Now when every maid's turn was come to go in to king Ahasuerus, after that she had been twelve months, according to the manner of the women, (for so were the days of their purifications accomplished, [to wit], six months with oil of myrrh, and six months with sweet odours, and with [other] things for the purifying of the women;)"

Psalms 45:8— "All thy garments [smell] of myrrh, and aloes, [and] cassia, out of the ivory palaces, whereby they have made thee glad."

Proverbs 7:17— "I have perfumed my bed with myrrh, aloes, and cinnamon."

Song Of Solomon 1:13— "A bundle of myrrh [is] my wellbeloved unto me; he shall lie all night betwixt my breasts."

Song Of Solomon 3:6— "Who [is] this that cometh out of the wilderness like pillars of smoke, perfumed with myrrh and frankincense, with all powders of the merchant?"

Song Of Solomon 4:6— "Until the day break, and the shadows flee away, I will get me to the mountain of myrrh, and to the hill of frankincense."

Song Of Solomon 4:14— "Spikenard and saffron; calamus and cinnamon, with all trees of frankincense; myrrh and aloes, with all the chief spices:"

Song Of Solomon 5:1— "I am come into my garden, my sister, [my] spouse: I have gathered my myrrh with my spice; I have eaten my honeycomb with my honey; I have drunk my wine with my milk: eat, O friends; drink, yea, drink abundantly, O beloved."

Song Of Solomon 5:5— "I rose up to open to my beloved; and my hands dropped [with] myrrh, and my fingers [with] sweet smelling myrrh, upon the handles of the lock."

Song Of Solomon 5:13— "His cheeks [are] as a bed of spices, [as] sweet flowers: his lips [like] lilies, dropping sweet smelling myrrh."

Matthew 2:11— "And when they were come into the house, they saw the young child with Mary his mother, and fell down, and worshiped him: and when they had opened their treasures, they presented unto him gifts; gold, and frankincense, and myrrh."

Mark 15:23— "And they gave him to drink wine mingled with myrrh: but he received [it] not."

John 19:39— "And there came also Nicodemus, which at the first came to Jesus by night, and brought a mixture of myrrh and aloes, about an hundred pound [weight]."

Selected Research:

Al-Awadi FM, et al. "Studies on the activity of individual plants of an antidiabetic plant mixture." *Acta Diabetol Lat.* 1987;24(1):37-41.

Dolara P, et al. "Analgesic effects of myrrh." *Nature.* 1996 Jan 4;379(6560):29.

Michie CA, et al. "Frankincense and myrrh as remedies in children." *J R Soc Med.* 1991;84(10):602-5.

Myrtle *(Myrtus communis)*

Botanical Family: Myrtaceae (myrtle)

Plant Origin: Tunisia, Morocco

Extraction Method: Steam distilled from leaves.

Chemical Constituents: Monoterpenes: α pinene (24-25%), β–pinene; Sesquiterpenes; Monoterpene alcohols: linalol, geraniol; Terpene esters: linalyle acetate, geranyle, bornyle; Terpene oxides: 1,8 cineole (45%); Aldehydes: Lactones.

Action: expectorant, anti-infectious, liver stimulant, prostate decongestant, light antispasmodic, hormone-like for the thyroid and ovary, tonic for the skin.

Found In: EndoFlex, Inspiration, Mister, Purification, and R.C.

Traditional Uses: Myrtle has been researched by Dr. Daniel Pénoël for normalizing hormonal imbalances of the thyroid and ovaries, as well as balancing the hypothyroid. It has also been researched for its soothing effects on the respiratory system.

Indications: Bronchitis, coughs, hypothyroidism, insomnia, ovaries (hormone-like effects), prostate decongestant, respiratory tract ailments, sinus infection, tuberculosis, ureter infections.

Other Uses: This oil may help anger, asthma, respiratory infections, cystitis, diarrhea, dysentery, dyspepsia (impaired digestion), flatulence (gas), hemorrhoids, hormonal imbalances, support immune system, infections, infectious diseases, pulmonary disorders, skin conditions (acne, blemishes, bruises, oily skin, psoriasis, etc.), and sinusitis. Useful on children for chest complaints and coughs.

Application: Apply topically, diffuse, or use in a humidifier. Suitable for use on children.

Fragrant Influence: Elevating and euphoric.

Safety Data: If pregnant or under a doctor's care, consult physician.

Companion Oils: Bergamot, lavender, lemon, lemongrass, rosewood, rosemary, spearmint, thyme, and melaleuca.

Bible Reference:

Nehemiah 8:15— "And that they should publish and proclaim in all their cities, and in Jerusalem, saying, Go forth unto the mount, and fetch olive branches, and pine branches, and myrtle branches, and palm branches, and branches of thick trees, to make booths, as [it is] written."

Isaiah 41:19— "I will plant in the wilderness the cedar, the shittah tree, and the myrtle, and the oil tree; I will set in the desert the fir tree, [and] the pine, and the box tree together:"

Isaiah 55:13— "Instead of the thorn shall come up the fir tree, and instead of the brier shall come up the myrtle tree: and it shall be to the Lord for a name, for an everlasting sign [that] shall not be cut off."

Zechariah 1:8— "I saw by night, and behold a man riding upon a red horse, and he stood among the myrtle trees that [were] in the bottom; and behind him [were there] red horses, speckled, and white."

Zechariah 1:10— "And the man that stood among the myrtle trees answered and said, These [are they] whom the Lord hath sent to walk to and fro through the earth."

Zechariah 1:11— "And they answered the angel of the Lord that stood among the myrtle trees, and said, We have walked to and fro through the earth, and, behold, all the earth sitteth still, and is at rest."

Neroli (*Citrus aurantium*)

Botanical Family: Rutaceae (citrus)

Plant Origin: Morocco, Tunisia

Extraction Method: Absolute extraction from flowers of the orange tree.

Chemical Constituents: Monoterpenes (35%); α pinene, β–pinenes (17.75%), limonene (11.45%); Alcols arom. (40%); linalol (30-32%); Esters; Aldehydes; Ketones: jasmone.

Action: Anti-infectious, antibacterial, antimycobacterial, antiparasitic, digestive tonic, anti-depressive, hypotensive (high blood pressure).

Found In: Acceptance, Humility, Inner Child, Awaken, Passion, and Present Time.

Traditional Uses: Regarded by the Egyptian people for its great attributes for healing the mind, body, and spirit.

Indications: It may support the digestive system and fight bacteria, infections, parasites, and viruses. It may also help with anxiety, depression, digestive spasms, fear, headaches, heart arrhythmia, hysteria, insomnia, nervous nervous tension, palpitations, PMS, poor circulation, scars, shock, stress-related conditions, stretch marks, tachycardia, thread veins, and wrinkles.

Other Uses: In support of the skin, it works at the cellular level to help shed the old skin cells and stimulate new cell growth. It is particularly beneficial for mature and sensitive skin.

Application: Diffuse or apply topically.

Fragrant Influence: As a natural tranquilizer, neroli has some powerful psychological effects. It has been used successfully to treat depression, anxiety, and shock. It is calming and relaxing to body and spirit. It may also help to strengthen and stabilize the emotions and bring relief to seemingly hopeless situations. It encourages confidence, courage, joy, peace, and sensuality. It brings everything into focus at the moment.

Safety Data: If pregnant or under a doctor's care, consult physician.

Companion Oils: Rose, lavender, sandalwood, jasmine, cedarwood, geranium, and lemon.

Nutmeg *(Myristica fragrans)*

Botanical Family: Myristicaceae

Plant Origin: Tunisia, Indonesia

Extraction Method: Steam distilled from fruits and seeds.

Chemical Constituents: Monoterpenes: α and β–pinenes 915-10%), myrcene (12%), sabinene (15%), limonene (4%); Monoterpenols: terpinene; Phenols.

Action: Antiseptic, antiparasitic, reduces pain, analgesic, promotes menstruation, improves circulation.

Found In: EndoFlex, En-R-Gee, and Magnify Your Purpose.

Traditional Uses: It has been used historically to benefit circulation, muscles, and joints, and relieve muscle pain. It also helps to support the nervous system, overcome fatigue, and support immune and nervous systems.

Indications: Appetite (loss of), chronic debility, digestion (helps with starchy foods and fats), gallstones, halitosis, and rheumatism.

Other Uses: This oil has adrenal cortex-like activity, which helps support the adrenal glands for increased energy. It may also help treat arthritis, bacterial infection, frigidity, gout, impotence, menstrual problems, nausea, neuralgia (severe pain along nerve), and nausea.

Application: Apply topically mixed with massage oil. Add to food or water as a dietary supplement or flavoring.

Safety Data: If pregnant or under a doctor's care, consult your physician. Do not use if epileptic. Dilute with massage oil or only apply a single undiluted drop at a time when applied topically.

Companion Oils: Cinnamon bark, clove, cypress, frankincense, lemon, orange, patchouly, rosemary, melaleuca, melissa.

Orange *(Citrus sinesis)*

Botanical Family: Rutaceae (citrus)

Plant Origin: USA, South Africa, Italy, China

Extraction Method: Cold pressed from rind.

Chemical Constituents: Monoterpenes (90-92%); limonene (90%); Esters; Aldehydes; Coumarins and furocoumarins; contains flavonoids, β–carotene, steroids, and acids.

Action: Calming, sedative, anti-inflammatory, antitumoral, anticoagulant, and improves circulation.

Found In: Abundance, Christmas Spirit, Citrus Fresh, Envision, Harmony, Inner Child, Into The Future, Peace & Calming, SARA.

Traditional Uses: Palpitation, scurvy, jaundice, bleeding, heartburn, relaxed throat, prolapse of the uterus and the anus, diarrhea, and blood in the feces.

Indications: Angina (false), cardiac spasm, insomnia, menopause, tumor growth.

Other Uses: This oil may help appetite, bones (rickety), bronchitis, respiratory infections, indigestion (dilute for infants; helps them sleep), complexion (dull and oily), dermatitis, digestive system, lowers high cholesterol, mouth ulcers, muscle soreness, sedation, tissue repair, fluid retention, and wrinkles.

Application: Diffuse, apply topically on location, or add to food or water as a dietary supplement flavoring.

Fragrant Influence: Uplifting, works as an antidepressant.

Safety Data: If pregnant or under a doctor's care, consult your physician. Citrus oils should NOT be applied to skin that will be exposed to direct sunlight or UV light within 72 hours.

Companion Oils: Cinnamon bark, clove, cypress, frankincense, geranium, juniper, lavender, nutmeg, rosewood.

Selected Research:

Reddy BS, et al. "Chemoprevention of colon carcinogenesis by dietary perillyl alcohol." *Cancer Res.* 1997;57(3):420-5.

Oregano *(Origanum compactum)*

Botanical Family: Lamiaceae or Labiatae (mint)

Plant Origin: Utah, Turkey, France

Extraction Method: Steam distilled from leaves and flowers.

Chemical Constituents: Monoterpenes (25%): α and β–pinenes, myrcene; Sesquiterpenes; Monoterpenols: linalol; Monoterpene phenols (60-72%): carvacrol, thymol: Phenols: methyl chavicol; Monoterpene ketones: camphor.

Action: Powerful anti-infectious agent (for respiratory, intestines, genital, nerves, blood, and lymphatics) with large-spectrum action against bacteria, mycovacteria, fungus, virus, and parasites. It is a general tonic and immune stimulant.

Found In: ImmuPower

Indications: Asthma, bronchitis (chronic), mental disease, pulmonary tuberculosis, rheumatism (chronic), whooping cough.

Other Uses: This oil may help respiratory infections, digestion problems, balance metabolism, viral and bacterial pneumonia, respiratory system problems, and strengthen the vital centers.

Application: Apply topically neat to bottom of feet. Mix with massage oil if applying elsewhere on the skin. May be used undiluted in Raindrop Therapy. Add to food or water as a dietary supplement or flavoring.

Fragrant Influence: Creates a feeling of security.

Safety Data: If pregnant or under a doctor's care, consult your physician. Skin test for sensitivity.

Companion Oils: Basil, fennel, geranium, lemongrass, myrtle, pine, thyme, rosemary.

Palmarosa *(Cymbopogon martinii)*

Botanical Family: Poaceae or Gramineae

Plant Origin: India, Conoros

Extraction Method: Steam distilled from leaves.

Chemical Constituents: Monoterpenes; limonene; Alcohols: geraniol (35-65%); Monoterpenones; carvone.

Action: Antimicrobial, antibacterial, antifungal, antiviral, uterine tonic, cardio tonic.

Found In: Gentle Baby

Traditional Uses: Helps with skin problems. A relative of lemongrass, it is antimicrobial and supportive to the nerves and circulation.

Indications: This oil may be beneficial for candida, cardiovascular system, circulation, digestion, infection, nervous system, and rashes. It is valuable for all types of skin problems because it stimulates new cell growth, regulates oil production, moisturizes, and speeds healing.

Application: Apply topically.

Fragrant Influence: Creates a feeling of security. It also helps to reduce stress and tension and promotes recovery from nervous exhaustion.

Safety Data: If pregnant or under a doctor's care, consult physician.

Companion Oils: Basil, fennel, geranium, lemongrass, myrtle, pine, thyme, rosemary.

Patchouly *(Pogostemon cablin)*

Botanical Family: Lamiaceae or Labiatae (mint)

Plant Origin: Indonesia, India

Extraction Method: Steam distilled from flowers.

Chemical Constituents: Monoterpenes; α and β–pinenes; Sesquiterpenes (40-45%); Sesquiterpenolnes: pathoulenone; Acids; Sesquiterpenes alkaloids.

Action: Tonic and stimulant, soothing to digestion, decongestant, anti-inflammatory, anti-infectious, antimicrobial, antiseptic, reduces soothes wrinkled or chapped skin.

Found In: Abundance, Di-Tone, Magnify Your Purpose, Passion, Peace & Calming.

Traditional Uses: It is very beneficial for the skin and may help prevent wrinkles or chapped skin. It is a general tonic and stimulant and helps the digestive system. It is also antimicrobial, antiseptic, and helps relieve itching.

Indications: Allergies, dermatitis, eczema, hemorrhoids, tissue regeneration.

Other Uses: This oil is a digester of toxic material in the body. It may also help acne, appetite (curbs), bites (insect and snake), cellulite, congestion, dandruff, depression, digestive system, relieve itching from hives, skin conditions (chapped and tightens loose skin), fluid retention, weeping wounds, weight reduction, and prevent wrinkles.

Application: Diffuse or apply topically.

Fragrant Influence: It is sedating, calming, and relaxing, allowing it to reduce anxiety. It may have some particular influence on sex, physical energy, and money.

Safety Data: If pregnant or under a doctor's care, consult physician.

Companion Oils: Bergamot, clary sage, frankincense, geranium, ginger, lavender, lemongrass, myrrh, pine, rosewood, sandalwood.

Pepper (Black) (*Piper nigrum*)

Botanical Family: Piperaceae

Plant Origin: Madagascar, Egypt, India

Extraction Method: Steam distilled from berries.

Chemical Constituents: Monoterpene: α and β–pinenes; Sesquiterpenes (85-90%); Terpene alcohols; Ketones; Acetophenones: Aldehydes.

Action: May help with toothache, expectorant, stimulates digestive secretions, reduces pain, dispels fever.

Found In: Dream Catcher, En-R-Gee, and Relieve It.

Traditional Uses: Pepper was used by the Egyptians in mummification as evidenced by the discovery of black pepper in the nostrils and abdomen of Ramses II. Indian monks ate several black pepper corns a day to maintain their incredible stamina and energy.

Other Uses: This oil may increase cellular oxygenation, support digestive glands, stimulate endocrine system, increase energy, and help rheumatoid arthritis. It may also help with loss of appetite, chills, cholera, respiratory infections, indigestion, constipation, coughs, diarrhea, dysentery, dysuria, flatulence (combine with fennel), heartburn, influenza, nausea, neuralgia, poor circulation, poor muscle tone, quinsy, sprains, toothache, vertigo, viruses, and vomiting.

Application: Apply topically to bottom of feet. Dilute with massage oil when applying topically elsewhere. Add to food or water as a dietary supplement or flavoring.

Fragrant Influence: Comforting and stimulating.

Safety Data: If pregnant or under a doctor's care, consult your physician. Skin test for irritation.

Companion Oils: Black cumin, fennel, frankincense, lavender, marjoram, rosemary, sandalwood, and other spice oils.

Selected Research:

Unnikrishnan MC, et al. "Tumour reducing and anticarcinogenic activity of selected spices." *Cancer Lett.* 1990;51(1):85-9.

Peppermint (*Mentha piperita*)

Botanical Family: Lamiaceae or Labiatae (mint)

Plant Origin: Utah

Extraction Method: Steam distilled from leaves, stems, and flower buds.

Chemical Constituents: Monoterpenes: α pinene, β–pinene, limonene: Monoterpenols: menthol (38-48%); Monoterpenones: menthone (20-30%); Terpene oxides: 1,8 cineol; Terpene esters: menthol acetate; Coumarins, Sulfurs: dimenthalsulfide.

Action: Anticarcinogenic, supports digestion, expels worms, decongestant, anti-infectious, antibacterial, antifungal, mucolytic, stimulant, hypertensive, cardiotonic, stimulates gallbladder, pain-relieving, expectorant, anti-inflammatory for the intestinal and urinary tract. It can heighten or restore the sense of taste by stimulating the trigeminal nerve (activated by menthol).

Found In: Aroma Siez, Clarity, Di-Tone, M-Grain, Mister, PanAway, R.C., Raven, and Relieve It.

Traditional Uses: Peppermint is one of the oldest and most highly regarded herbs for soothing digestion. Jean Valnet, M.D., studied peppermint's effect on the liver and respiratory systems. Other scientists have also researched peppermint's role in affecting impaired taste and smell when inhaled. Dr. Dember of the University of Cincinnati studied peppermint's ability to improve concentration and mental accuracy. Alan Hirsch, M.D., studied peppermint's ability to directly affect the brain's satiety center (the ventromedial nucleus of the hypothalamus) which triggers a sensation of fullness after meals.

Indications: Asthma, bronchitis, candida, diarrhea, digestive aid, fever (reduces), halitosis, heartburn, hemorrhoids, hot flashes, indigestion, menstrual irregularity, headaches, motion sickness, nausea, tumor growth, respiratory infections, shock, skin (itchy), throat infections, and varicose veins.

Other Uses: This oil may help arthritis, indigestion, depression, skin conditions (eczema, psoriasis, dermatitis), food poisoning, headaches, hives, hysteria, inflammation, morning sickness, nerve regeneration, rheumatism, elevate and open sensory system, toothaches, tuberculosis.

Application: Diffuse. Massage on the stomach or add to water or tea. Apply to bottom of feet or rub on the temples to treat headaches. To improve concentration, alertness, and memory, place several drops on the tongue. Add to food as a flavoring and preservative.

Fragrant Influence: It is purifying and stimulating to the conscious mind.

Safety Data: If pregnant or under a doctor's care, consult your physician. Avoid contact with eyes, mucus membranes, or sensitive skin areas. Do not apply neat to a fresh wound or burn.

Selected Research:

Gobel H, et al. "Effect of peppermint and eucalyptus oil preparations on neurophysiological and experimental algesimetric headache parameters." *Cephalalgia.* 1994; 14(3):228-34.

Juergens UR, et al. "The anti-inflammatory activity of L-menthol compared to mint oil in human monocytes in vitro: a novel perspective for its therapeutic use in inflammatory diseases." *Eur J Med Res.* 1998; 3(12):539-45.

Samman MA, et al. "Mint prevents shamma-induced carcinogenesis in hamster cheek pouch." *Carcinogenesis.* 1998;19(10):1795-801.

Lantry LE, et al. "Chemopreventive effect of perillyl alcohol on 4-(methylnitrosamino)-1-(3-pyridyl)-1-butanone induced tumorigenesis in (C3H/HeJ X A/J)F1 mouse lung." *J Cell Biochem Suppl.* 1997;27:20-5.

Veal L. "The potential effectiveness of essential oils as a treatment for headlice, Pediculus humanus capitis." *Complement Ther Nurs Midwifery.*1996;2(4):97-101.

Petitgrain (*Citrus aurantium*)

Botanical Family: Rutaceae (citrus)

Plant Origin: Italy

Extraction Method: Steam distilled from leaves and twigs.

Chemical Constituents: Monoterpenes (10%); myrcene; Terpene esters (50-70%), linalyle (45-55%).

Action: Antispasmodic, anti-inflammatory, anti-infectious, antibacterial (staph and pneumonia), re-establishes nerve equilibrium.

Traditional Uses: Petitgrain derives its name from the extraction of the oil, which at one time was from the green unripe oranges when they were still about the size of a cherry.

Other Uses: This oil may help re-establish nerve equilibrium. It may also help with acne, fatigue, greasy hair, insomnia, and excessive perspiration.

Application: Diffuse or apply topically.

Fragrant Influence: It is uplifting and refreshing and helps to refresh the senses, clear confusion, reduce mental fatigue, and reduce depression. It may also stimulate the mind, support memory, and gladden the heart.

Safety Data: If pregnant or under a doctor's care, consult physician.

Companion Oils: Bergamot, cistus, clary sage, clove, geranium, jasmine, lavender, neroli, orange, palmarosa, and rosemary.

Pine (*Pinus sylvestris*)

Botanical Family: Pinaceae (pine)

Plant Origin: Austria, Russia, Canada

Extraction Method: Steam distilled from needles.

Chemical Constituents: Monoterpenes: α and β–pinenes, limonene (25-30%); Sesquiterpenes; Monoterpenols: borneol; Sesquiterpenols; Terpene esters: bornyle acetate.

Action: Hormone-like, antidiabetic, cortisone-like, sexual stimulant, hypertensive (high blood pressure), anti-infectious, antifungal, antiseptic.

Found In: Grounding and R.C.

Traditional Uses: Pine was first investigated by Hippocrates, the father of Western medicine, for its benefits to the respiratory system. In 1990, Drs. Pénoël and Franchomme described pine oil's antiseptic properties in their medical textbook. Pine is used in massage for stressed muscles and joints. It shares many of the same properties as *Eucalyptus globulus*, enhancing the action of both oils when blended. American Indians stuffed mattresses with pine to repel lice and fleas. It was used to treat lung infections and even added to baths to revitalize those suffering from mental or emotional fatigue.

Indications: Asthma, pulmonary infections, bronchitis, diabetes, infections (severe), rheumatoid arthritis, sinusitis.

Other Uses: This oil may help dilate and open the respiratory system, particularly the bronchial tract. It may also help with respiratory infections, coughs, cuts, cysts, fatigue, gout, lice, nervous exhaustion, scabies, skin parasites, sores, stress, and urinary infection. Pine oil may also help increase blood pressure and stimulate the adrenal glands and the circulatory system. Pine is a good recommendation for any First Aid kit.

Application: Diffuse or apply topically. Dilute to avoid possible skin irritation. Put two drops in palms of hands, place over mouth and nose, and inhale. Add 2 to 4 drops to warm bathwater. Disperse with Bath Gel Base if desired.

Fragrant Influence: It helps soothe mental stress, relieve anxiety, freshen and deodorize a room, and revitalize the entire body.

Safety Data: If pregnant or under a doctor's care, consult your physician. Avoid oil adulterated with turpentine, a low-cost, but potentially hazardous filler.

Companion Oils: Cedarwood, eucalyptus, juniper, lavender, lemon, marjoram, melaleuca, and rosemary.

Bible Reference:

Nehemiah 8:15— "And that they should publish and proclaim in all their cities, and in Jerusalem, saying, Go forth unto the mount, and fetch olive branches, and pine branches, and myrtle branches, and palm branches, and branches of thick trees, to make booths, as [it is] written."

Isaiah 41:19— "I will plant in the wilderness the cedar, the shittah tree, and the myrtle, and the oil tree; I will set in the desert the fir tree, [and] the pine, and the box tree together:"

Isaiah 60:13— "The glory of Lebanon shall come unto thee, the fir tree, the pine tree, and the box together, to beautify the place of my sanctuary; and I will make the place of my feet glorious."

Ravensara *(Ravensara aromatica)*

Botanical Family: Lauraceae

Plant Origin: Madagascar

Extraction Method: Steam distilled from branches.

Chemical Constituents: Monoterpenes: α and β–pinene; Sesquiterpenes; Monoterpenols: Terpene esters: terpenyle acetate; Terpene oxides; 1,8 cineole.

Action: Anti-infectious, antiviral, antibacterial, expectorant, antimicrobial, supports nerves and respiratory system.

Found In: ImmuPower and Raven

Traditional Uses: Ravensara is referred to by the people of Madagascar as "the oil that heals." It is antimicrobial and supporting to the nerves and respiratory system.

Indications: Bronchitis, cholera, herpes, infectious mononucleosis, insomnia, muscle fatigue, rhinopharyngitis, shingles, sinusitis, viral hepatitis.

Other Uses: It may help asthma, cystitis, burns, cancer, respiratory infections, cuts, pneumonia, strengthen the respiratory system, scrapes, viral infections, and wounds.

Application: Diffuse or apply topically.

Safety Data: If pregnant or under a doctor's care, consult physician.

Rose *(Rosa damascena)*

Botanical Family: Rosaceae

Plant Origin: Bulgaria, Turkey

Extraction Method: Steam distilled from flower (a two-part process).

Chemical Constituents: Hydrocarbures; Monoterpenols: geraniol; Sesquiterpene alcohols: farnesol; Terpene esters; Phenols: eugenol, methyl eugenol; Oxides: rose oxides.

Action: Anti-inflammatory, prevents and reduces scarring, balances and elevates mind.

Found In: Envision, Forgiveness, Gathering, Gentle Baby, Humility, Harmony, Joy, SARA, Trauma Life, and White Angelica.

Traditional Uses: Rose has been used for the skin for thousands of years. The Arab physician, Avicenna, was responsible for first distilling rose oil, eventually authoring an entire book on the healing attributes of the rose water derived from the distillation of rose. Throughout much of ancient history, the oil was produced by enfleurage, a process of pressing the petals along with a vegetable oil to extract the essence. Today, however, almost all rose oils are solvent extracted.

NOTE: the Bulgarian *Rosa damascena* (high in citronellol) is very different from Morrocan *Rosa centifolia* (high in phenyl ethanol). They each have different colors, aromas, and therapeutic actions.

Other Uses: This oil may help asthma, chronic bronchitis, herpes simplex, impotence, scarring, sexual debilities, skin diseases, and wrinkles.

Application: Diffuse or apply topically.

Fragrant Influence: Its beautiful fragrance is intoxicating and aphrodisiac-like. It helps bring balance and harmony, allowing one to overcome insecurities. It is stimulating and elevating to the mind, creating a sense of well-being.

Safety Data: If pregnant or under a doctor's care, consult physician.

Selected Research:

Sysoev NP. "The effect of waxes from essential-oil plants on the dehydrogenase activity of the blood neutrophils in mucosal trauma of the mouth." *Stomatologiia* 1991;70(1):12-3.

Mahmood N, et al. "The anti-HIV activity and mechanisms of action of pure compounds isolated from Rosa damascena." *Biochem Biophys Res Commun.* 1996;229(1):73-9.

Rosemary *(Rosmarinus officinalis 1,8 Cineol CT)*

Botanical Family: Labiatae

Plant Origin: France, U.S.

Extraction Method: Steam distilled from leaves.

Chemical Constituents: Monoterpenes: α–pinene (12%), β–pinene, camphene (22%), myrcene (1.5%) α–and β–phellandrene, limonene (.5 to 2%) α–and γ–terpinenes, paracymene (2%); Sesquiterpenes: β–caryophyllene (3%); Monoterpenols: linalol (.5 to 1%), terpinen 1-ol-4, α–terpineol (1.5%), borneol (3.5%), isoborneol, cis and trans thujanol-4, p-cymene-8-ol; Terpene Esters: bornyl acetate (.2%) α–fenchyl acetate; Terpene Oxides: 1,8 cineole (30%) caryophyllene oxide, humulene epoxides I and II; Non-terpene Ketones: 3-hexanone, methyl heptanone; Monoterpenones: camphor (30%), verbenone, carvone (.4%).

Action: Antifungal, antibacterial, antiseptic, antiparasitic, general stimulant, enhances mental clarity, supports nerves and endocrine gland balance.

Found In: Clarity, En-R-Gee, JuvaFlex, Melrose, Purification, and Thieves.

Historical Use: Rosemary was part of the "Marseilles Vinegar" or "Four Thieves Vinegar" used by grave-robbing bandits to protect themselves during the 14th century plague. The name of the oil is derived from the latin words for dew of the sea (ros + marinus), According to folklore history, rosemary originally had white flowers; however they turned red after the Virgin Mary laid her cloak on the bush. Since the time of ancient Greece (about 1000 BC), rosemary was burnt as incense. Later cultures believed that it warded off devils, a practice that eventually became adopted by the sick who instead burned rosemary to protect against infection. Until recently, French hospitals continued to use rosemary this way in order to disinfect the air.

Indications: Rheumatism, arthritis, myalgia, hepatitis, liver conditions, menstrual disturbances, hypertension (weak doses), hypotension (strong doses), indigestion, bronchitis, respiratory and lung infections, hair loss (alopecia areata), asthma.

Other Uses: Improves concentration, stimulates the scalp.

Application: Diffuse, inhale, or apply topically on location. May also be added to food or water as a dietary supplement.

Fragrant Influence: Helps over come mental fatigue and improves mental clarity and focus.

Safety Data: Epileptics should use with caution. If pregnant or under a doctor's care, consult physician.

Companion Oils: Marjoram, lavender. eucalyptus, peppermint, basil, and pine.

Selected Research:

Larrondo JV, et al. "Antimicrobial activity of essences from labiates." *Microbios.* 1995; 82(332):171-2.

Panizzi L, et al. "Composition and antimicrobial properties of essential oils of four Mediterranean Lamiaceae." *J Ethnopharmacol.* 1993;39(3):167-70.

Diego MA, et al. "Aromatherapy positively affects mood, EEG patterns of alertness and math computations." *Int J Neurosci.* 1998; 96(3-4):217-24.

Hay IC, et al. "Randomized trial of aromatherapy. Successful treatment for alopecia areata." *Arch Dermatol.* 1998;134(11):1349-52.

Mangena T, et al. "Comparative evaluation of the antimicrobial activities of essential oils of Artemisia afra, Pteronia incana and Rosmarinus officinalis on selected bacteria and yeast strains." *Lett Appl Microbiol.* 1999;28(4):291-6.

Aqel MB. "Relaxant effect of the volatile oil of Rosmarinus officinalis on tracheal smooth muscle." *J Ethnopharmacol.* 1991;33(1-2):57-62.

Rosemary *(Rosmarinus officinalis Verbenon CT)*

Botanical Family: Labiatae

Plant Origin: France, U.S.

Extraction Method: Steam distilled from leaves.

Chemical Constituents: Monoterpenes: α–pinene (15-34%), β–pinene, camphene, myrcene, limonene α–terpinenes, terpinolene; Sesquiterpenes: β–caryophyllene; Monoterpenols: borneol (trace to 7%); Terpene Esters: bornyl acetate; Terpene Oxides: 1,8 cineole (trace to 20%); Monoterpenones: verbenon (15-37%), camphor (1-15%).

Action: Mucolytic, expectorant, antispasmodic, antibacterial, antiseptic, balance endocrine gland.

Found In: Clarity, En-R-Gee, JuvaFlex, Melrose, Purification, and Thieves.

Traditional Uses: The name of the oil is derived from the latin words for dew of the sea (ros + marinus), According to folklore history, rosemary originally had white flowers; however they turned red after the Virgin Mary laid her cloak on the bush. It has been used to lower cholesterol.

Indications: Respiratory infections, bronchitis, viral hepatitis, nervous tension, cardiac arrhythmia, cystitis, arthritis, and rheumatism.

Other Uses: Because of its lower camphor and higher verbenon content, this chemotype of rosemary is milder than the cineol chemotype and so is especially well-suited for chest, lung, and sinus infections. It is ideal for skin care, and can be used to combat hair loss.

Application: Diffuse, inhale, or apply topically on location. May also be added to food or water as a dietary supplement.

Fragrant Influence: Less stimulating than rosemary cineole, it can be clarifying for emotions and psychologically balancing.

Safety Data: Epileptics should use with caution. If pregnant or under a doctor's care, consult physician.

Companion Oils: Marjoram, lavender. eucalyptus, peppermint, basil, and pine.

Rosewood *(Aniba rosaeodora)*

Botanical Family: Lauraceae

Plant Origin: Brazil

Extraction Method: Steam distilled from wood.

Chemical Constituents: Monoterpenols: linalol (95%).

Action: Anti-infectious, antibacterial, antiviral, antiparasitic, antifungal, soothing to the skin.

Found In: Acceptance, Clarity, Gentle Baby, Humility, Inspiration, Magnify Your Purpose, Sensation, Valor, and White Angelica.

Traditional Uses: It has been researched at Weber State University for its inhibition rate against gram positive and gram negative bacterial growth.

Indications: Acne, candida, depression, eczema, oral infections, skin (dry), vaginitis.

Other Uses: This oil may create skin elasticity and is soothing to the skin. It is recognized for its ability to get rid of candida of the skin and slow the aging process. It may also be beneficial for cuts, nausea, tissue regeneration, and wounds. It helps to create a synergism with all other oils.

Application: Diffuse or apply topically.

Fragrant Influence: It is soothing and nourishing to the skin.

Safety Data: If pregnant or under a doctor's care, consult physician.

Sage *(Salvia officinalis)*

Botanical Family: Lamiaceae or Labiatae (mint)

Plant Origin: Spain, Croatia, France

Extraction Method: Steam distilled from leaves and flowers.

Chemical Constituents: Monoterpenes: α thujene, α pinene, β–pinene, camphene myrcene, limonene; Sesquiterpenes; Hydrocarbons; Esters; Phenols: thymol; Oxides (15%): 1,8 cineole; Monoterpenones (20-70%): α thujone (12-33%) β–Thujone (2-14%), camphor (1-26%); Aldehydes; Coumarins.

Action: Expectorant, mucolytic, anti-infectious, fights against cholera, estrogen-like, supports menstruation, prevents and reduces scarring, regulates circulation, soothes skin conditions and is a balancer and detoxifier of the body, It contains sclerol, balances estrogen levels, providing support during PMS and menopause.

Found In: EndoFlex, Envision, Magnify Your Purpose, and Mister.

Traditional Uses: Known as "herba sacra" or sacred herb by the ancient romans, sage's name is derived from the word for "salvation." Sage has been used in Europe for oral infections and skin conditions. It has been recognized for its benefits of strengthening the vital centers and supporting metabolism.

Indications: Asthma, bronchitis (chronic), digestion (sluggish), gingivitis, glandular disorders, menopause, and menstrual irregularity.

Other Uses: This oil may help improve estrogen, progesterone, and testosterone balance. It activates the nervous system and adrenal cortex and may help with illness that is related to digestion and liver problems. It may also be beneficial for acne, arthritis, bacterial infections, dandruff, depression, eczema, fibrosis, hair loss, low blood pressure, mental fatigue, metabolism, respiratory problems, rheumatism, skin conditions, sores, and sprains. It strengthens the vital centers of the body, balancing the pelvic chakra where negative emotions from denial and abuse are stored.

Application: Diffuse or apply topically mixed with massage oil. Add to food or water as a dietary supplement or flavoring.

Fragrant Influence: It is mentally stimulating and may help in coping with despair and mental fatigue.

Safety Data: If pregnant or under a doctor's care, consult your physician. Oral toxin due to thujone content. Do not use if epileptic. Use caution if suffering from high blood pressure.

Companion Oils: Bergamot, lemon, lavender, peppermint, rosemary, lemongrass, pine.

Sandalwood *(Santalum album)*

Botanical Family: Santalaceae (sandalwood)

Plant Origin: Indonesia, India

Extraction Method: Steam distilled from wood.

Chemical Constituents: Sesquiterpenes; Sesquiterpenols: α and β–santalols (67%); Sesquiterpenals; carbonic acid.

Action: Sandalwood is high in sesquiterpenes that have been researched in Europe for their ability to stimulate the pineal gland and the limbic region of the brain, the center of emotions. The pineal gland is responsible for releasing melatonin, a powerful antioxidant that enhances deep sleep. Sandalwood is similar to frankincense oil in its support of nerves and circulation.

Found In: Acceptance, Brain Power, Dream Catcher, Forgiveness, Gathering, Harmony, Inner Child, Inspiration, Magnify Your Purpose, Passion, Release, 3 Wise Men, Trauma Life, and White Angelica.

Traditional Uses: Sandalwood has been used for centuries in Ayurvedic medicine. It was used traditionally for skin revitalization, yoga, and meditation.

Indications: Bronchitis (chronic), herpes, cystitis, skin tumors.

Other Uses: Helps with cystitis and urinary tract infections. It may also be beneficial for acne, depression, meditation, pulmonary infections, menstrual problems, nervous tension, and skin infection. It help dry or dehydrated skin.

Application: Diffuse or apply topically. Add to food or water as a dietary supplement or flavoring.

Fragrant Influence: Enhances deep sleep, may help remove negative programming from the cells.

Safety Data: If pregnant or under a doctor's care, consult physician.

Companion Oils: Cypress, frankincense, lemon, myrrh, ylang ylang, patchouly, spruce.

Selected References:

Benencia F, et al. "Antiviral activity of sandalwood oil against herpes simplex viruses-1 and -2." *Phytomedicine.* 1999;6(2):119-23

Dwivedi C, et al. "Chemopreventive effects of sandalwood oil on skin papillomas in mice." *Eur J Cancer Prev.* 1997;6(4):399-401.

Spearmint *(Mentha spicata)*

Botanical Family: Lamiaceae or Labiatae (mint)

Plant Origin: Utah

Extraction Method: Steam distilled from leaves.

Chemical Constituents: Monoterpenes: α pinene, β-pinene, camphene, myrcene, limonene; Sesquiterpenes; Monoterpenols: menthol, linalol, borneol, Sesquiterpenols: farnesol: Terpene esters: Terpene oxides: 1,8 cineol: Monoterpenones: carvone (55-65%).

Action: Anti-inflammatory, calming, astringent, antiseptic, mucolytic, stimulates gallbladder, promotes menstruation.

Found In: Citrus Fresh and EndoFlex

Traditional Uses: Spearmint oil has been used to help support the respiratory and nervous systems.

Indications: Bronchitis, candida, cystitis, hypertension.

Other Uses: This oil may balance and increase metabolism. It may aid the glandular, nervous, and respiratory systems. It may also help with acne, appetite (stimulates), bad breath, balance, childbirth (promotes easier labor), depression, digestion, dry skin, eczema, headaches, intestines (soothes), menstruation (slow, heavy periods), nausea, sore gums, vaginitis, excess weight.

Application: Diffuse or apply topically. Add to food or water as a dietary supplement or flavoring.

Fragrant Influence: Its hormone-like activity may help open and release emotional blocks and bring about a feeling of balance and a lasting sense of well-being.

Safety Data: If pregnant or under a doctor's care, consult physician.

Companion Oils: Basil, lavender, peppermint, rosemary.

Spikenard *(Nardostachys jatamansi)*

Botanical Family: Valerianaceae

Plant Origin: India

Extraction Method: Steam distilled from roots.

Chemical Constituents: Sesquiterpenes (93%): Bomyl acetate, isobomyl valerianate, bomeol, terpinyl valerianate, terpineol, eugenol, pinene.

Action: Antibacterial, antifungal, antiinflammatory, deodorant, relaxing, and skin tonic.

Found In: Exodus II and Humility

Traditional Uses: Spikenard is highly regarded in India as a perfume, medicinal herb, and skin tonic. It was the one of the most precious oils in ancient times, used only by priests, kings, or high initiates. References in the New Testament described how Mary of Bethany used a salve of spikenard to anoint the feet of Jesus before the Last Supper.

Indications: The oil is known for helping in the treatment of allergic skin reactions.

Other Uses: It may also help with allergies, candida, flatulent indigestion, insomnia, menstrual difficulties, migraine, nausea, rashes, staph infections, stress, tachycardia, tension, and wounds that will heal. According to Dietrich Gumbel, Ph.D. it strengthens the heart and circulatory system.

Application: Apply to abdomen or on location for soothing and calming.

Fragrant Influence: Relaxing, soothing, and helps nourish and regenerate the skin.

Safety Data: If pregnant or under a doctor's care, consult physician.

Companion Oils: Cistus, lavender, patchouly, pine, and vetiver.

Bible References:

Song Of Solomon 1:12— "While the king [sitteth] at his table, my spikenard sendeth forth the smell thereof."

Song Of Solomon 4:13— "Thy plants [are] an orchard of pomegranates, with pleasant fruits; camphire, with spikenard,"

Song Of Solomon 4:14— "Spikenard and saffron; calamus and cinnamon, with all trees of frankincense; myrrh and aloes, with all the chief spices:"

Mark 14:3— "And being in Bethany in the house of Simon the leper, as he sat at meat, there came a woman having an alabaster box of ointment of spikenard very precious; and she brake the box, and poured [it] on his head."

John 12:3— "Then took Mary a pound of ointment of spikenard, very costly, and anointed the feet of Jesus, and wiped his feet with her hair: and the house was filled with the odour of the ointment."

Spruce (*Picea mariana*)

Botanical Family: Pinaceae (pine)

Plant Origin: Canada

Extraction Method: Steam distilled from leaves, needles, and twigs.

Chemical Constituents: Monoterpenes (50-55%): camphene (10-15%), tricyclene, α pinene (13-16%); Sesquiterpenes; Monoterpenols: borneol; Terpene esters (30-37%): bornyle acetate (30-37%); Sesquiterpenols.

Action: Antispasmodic, anti-infectious, antiparasitic, antiseptic, anti-inflammatory, hormone-like, cortisone-like; general tonic, stimulates thymus, releases emotional blocks.

Found In: Abundance, Christmas Spirit, Envision, Gathering, Grounding, Harmony, Hope, Inner Child, Inspiration, Motivation, Present Time, R.C., Relieve It, Sacred Mountain, Surrender, 3 Wise Men, Trauma Life, Valor, and White Angelica

Traditional Uses: The Lakota Indians used spruce to strengthen their ability to communicate with the Great Spirit.

Indications: Arthritis, candida, hyperthyroidism, immune-depression, prostatitis, rheumatism, solar plexus (balances).

Other Uses: It may be beneficial for bone pain, glandular imbalances, aching joints, and sciatica pain. It may help support the nervous system and respiratory system, and can be stimulating the pineal, thymus, and adrenal glands.

Application: Diffuse or apply topically. Add to food or water as a dietary supplement or flavoring.

Fragrant Influence: Helps to open and release emotional blocks, bringing about a feeling of balance. It also helps the respiratory and nervous systems.

Safety Data: If pregnant or under a doctor's care, consult physician.

Companion Oils: Birch, eucalyptus, frankincense, helichrysum, and ravensara

Tangerine *(Citrus nobilis)*

Botanical Family: Rutaceae (citrus)

Plant Origin: USA, South Africa

Extraction Method: Cold pressed from rind.

Chemical Constituents: Limonene, a-pinene, ß-pinene, mycene, linalol, nerol, p-cyrnene.

Action: Promotes happiness, helps with anxiety and nervousness.

Found In: Citrus Fresh, Dream Catcher, Inner Child, Peace & Calming.

Indications: Diffuse or apply topically. Add to food or water as a dietary supplement or flavoring.

Other Uses: It may help dissolve cellulite, improve circulation, and help digestive system disorders, dizziness, anxiety, insomnia, irritability, liver problems, parasites, stretch marks (smooths when blended with lavender), and fluid retention.

Application: Diffuse, take as dietary supplement, or apply topically.

Fragrant Influence: Calming, helps with anxiety and nervousness.

Safety Data: If pregnant or under a doctor's care, consult physician.

Companion Oils: Basil, bergamot, chamomile, clary sage, frankincense, geranium, grapefruit, lavender, lemon, orange.

Tansy (Blue) *(Tanacetum annuum)*

Botanical Family: Asteraceae or Compositae (daisy)

Plant Origin: Morocco, France

Extraction Method: Steam distilled from leaves and flowers.

Chemical Constituents: Monoterpenes: limonene; Sesquiterpenes polyinsatures: chamazulene.

Found In: Acceptance, Dream Catcher, JuvaFlex, Peace & Calming, Release, SARA, and Valor.

Action: Anti-inflammatory, reduces pain, relieves itching, sedating to the nerves, antihistamine, hypotensive (helps with low blood pressure), hormone-like.

Safety Data: If pregnant or under a doctor's care, consult physician.

Tarragon *(Artemisia dracunculus)*

Botanical Family: Asteraceae or Compositae (daisy)

Plant Origin: Slovenia, France

Extraction Method: Steam distilled from leaves.

Chemical Constituents: Methyl Chavicol (60-75%), Coumarins.

Action: Neuromuscular antispasmodic, anti-inflammatory, anti-infectious, antifermentation, and reduces allergies.

Found In: Di-Tone

Traditional Uses: Tarragon has been used in Europe for its antimicrobial and antiseptic functions.

Indications: Colitis, hiccups, intestinal spasms, parasites, rheumatic pain, sciatica.

Other Uses: It may be beneficial for abdominal discomfort and spasms, arthritis, digestive complaints, genital and urinary tract infection, nausea, pre-menstrual discomfort, and wounds. It may also balance the autonomic nervous system.

Application: Apply topically mixed with massage oil. Add to food or water as a dietary supplement or flavoring.

Safety Data: If pregnant or under a doctor's care, consult your physician. Do not use if epileptic.

Companion Oils: Chamomile, clary sage, fir, juniper, lavender, pine, rosewood, orange, and tangerine.

Thyme (*Thymus vulgaris*)

Botanical Family: Lamiaceae or Labiatae (mint)

Plant Origin: Utah, Idaho, France

Extraction Method: Steam distilled from leaves, stems, and flowers.

Chemical Constituents: Monoterpenols: geraniol; Terpene esters: geraniol acetate.

Action: Highly antimicrobial, antifungal, antiviral, uterine tonic, cardiotonic.

Traditional Uses: It has been used for respiratory problems, digestive complaints, the prevention and treatment of infection, gastritis, bronchitis, pertussis, asthma, laryngitis, and tonsillitis. The Egyptians used thyme for embalming.

Indications: Asthma, bronchitis, colitis, cystitis, dermatitis, anthrax, fatigue (general), pleurisy, psoriasis, sciatica, tuberculosis, vaginal candida.

Other Uses: This oil is a general tonic for the nerves and stomach. It may also help with bacterial infections, respiratory infections, circulation, depression, digestion, headaches, insomnia, rheumatism, urinary infections, and viruses along the spine.

Application: Apply topically mixed with massage oil.

Fragrant Influence: It t may be beneficial in helping to overcome fatigue and exhaustion after illness.

Safety Data: If pregnant or under a doctor's care, consult your physician.

Companion Oils: Bergamot, citrus oil, cedarwood, juniper, melaleuca, oregano, and rosemary.

Selected Research:

Panizzi L, et al. "Composition and antimicrobial properties of essential oils of four Mediterranean Lamiaceae." *J Ethnopharmacol.* 1993;39(3):167-70.

Youdim KA, et al. "Beneficial effects of thyme oil on age-related changes in the phospholipid C20 and C22 polyunsaturated fatty acid composition of various rat tissues." *Biochim Biophys Acta.* 1999;1438(1):140-6.

Inouye S, et al. "Antisporulating and respiration-inhibitory effects of essential oils on filamentous fungi." Mycoses. 1998;41(9-10):403-10.

Veal L. "The potential effectiveness of essential oils as a treatment for headlice, Pediculus humanus capitis." *Complement Ther Nurs Midwifery.* 1996;2(4):97-101.

Meeker HG, et al. "The antibacterial action of eugenol, thyme oil, and related essential oils used in dentistry." *Compendium.* 1988;9(1):32, 34-5, 38 passim.

Kulieva ZT. "Analgesic, hypotensive and cardiotonic action of the essential oil of the thyme growing in Azerbaijan." *Vestn Akad Med Nauk SSSR.* 1980;(9):61-3.

Valerian (*Valeriana officinalis*)

Botanical Family: Valerianaceae

Plant Origin: Belgium, Croatia, France

Extraction Method: Steam distilled from root.

Chemical Constituents: Monoterpenes: α-pinene, camphene; Sesquiterpenes; azulene; Monoterpenols: geraniol, α-terpineol, borneol, Terpene esters: acetate formiate, butyrate and bornyle isovalerate; Sesquiterpenals L valerenal; Sesquiterpenones: valeranon; Acids: isovaleric and acetoxyvaleric acid.

Action: Sedative and tranquilizing to the central nervous system. Its warming properties can help with hypothermia.

Found In: Trauma Life

Traditional Uses: During the last three decades, it has been clinically investigated for its tranquilizing properties. Researchers have pinpointed the sesquiterpenes, valerenic acid, and valerone as the active constituents that exerts a calming effect on the central nervous system. German health authorities (Commission E) have pronounced valerian to be an effective treatment for restlessness and for sleep disturbances resulting from nervous conditions.

Other Uses: Because of its effect on the nervous system, it may help with insomnia, nervous indigestion, migraine, restlessness, and tension.

Application: Diffuse or apply topically, especially in a soothing massage. May be added to food or water as a dietary supplement.

Fragrant Influence: Calming, relaxing, grounding, and emotionally balancing; sleep aid.

Safety Data: If pregnant or under a doctor's care, consult your physician. Repeated use can possibly result in contact sensitization.

Companion Oils: Cedarwood, lavender, mandarin, patchouly, petitgrain, pine, and rosemary.

Selected Research:

Wagner J, et al. "Beyond benzodiazepines: alternative pharmacologic agents for the treatment of insomnia." *Ann Pharmacother.* 1998;32(6):680-91.

Vetiver *(Vetiveria zizanioides)*

Botanical Family: Poaceae or Gramineae (grasses)

Plant Origin: Haiti, India

Extraction Method: Steam distilled from root.

Chemical Constituents: Ketones: Vitiverone; Terpenes: vitivene, cadinene; Terpene Alcohols: vetiverol.

Action: Antiseptic, antispasmodic, calming, grounding, rubefacient (locally warming), sedative (nervous system), stimulant (circulatory, production of red corpuscles).

Traditional Uses: Vetiver is distilled from roots of a scented grass native to India. It is well known for its anti-inflammatory properties and traditionally used for arthritic symptoms.

Other Uses: Vetiver may help acne, anxiety, arthritis, breasts (enlarge), cuts, depression (including postpartum), insomnia, rheumatism, stress, skin care (oily, aging, tired, irritated).

Application: Diffuse or apply topically, especially in a soothing massage. May be added to food or water as a dietary supplement.

Fragrant Influence: Vetiver has a heavy, earthy fragrance similar to patchouly with a touch of lemon. It is psychologically grounding, calming, and stabilizing. It helps us cope with stress and recover from emotional traumas and shocks.

Safety Data: If pregnant or under a doctor's care, consult physician.

Companion Oils: Clary sage, jasmine, lavender, patchouly, rose, sandalwood, and ylang ylang.

Vitex *(Vitex negundo)*

Botanical Family: Lamiaceae or Labiatae (mint)

Plant Origin: Turkey

Extraction Method: Steam distilled from the inner bark, small branches, and leaves of the Chaste tree.

Chemical Constituents: α-Terpinyl acetate, 1,8-Cineol, Caryophyllene Oxide, Limonene.

Traditional Uses: It has been extensively researched in Europe for its effects on Parkinson's and other neurological disorders.

Application: Diffuse or apply topically. Dilute with massage oil for massage. Put in palms and inhale. Add 2 to 4 drops to warm bath water.

Safety Data: If pregnant or under a doctor's care, consult physician.

Note: It is different from the extract of the chaste berry, which is used for PMS symptoms and hormone balance.

White Lotus *(Nymphaea lotus)*

Botanical Family: Nymphaeaceae

Plant Origin: Egypt

Extraction Method: Steam distilled from flower.

Action: Anticancerous

Traditional Uses: White lotus was traditionally used by the Egyptians for spiritual, emotional, and physical application. Research in

China found that white lotus contains anticancerous and strong immune supporting properties.

Other Uses: Inflamed eyes, jaundice, kidneys, liver spots, menstruation (promotes), palpitations, rheumatism, sciatica, sprains, sunburn, toothaches, tuberculosis, and vomiting.

Fragrant Influence: Stimulates a positive attitude and a general feeling of well-being.

Safety Data: If pregnant or under a doctor's care, consult your physician.

Companion Oils: Most oils

Note: This oil is only available periodically in very small amounts.

Yarrow *(Achillea millefolium)*

Botanical Family: Asteraceae or Compositae (daisy)

Plant Origin: Utah

Extraction Method: Steam distilled from flowering top.

Chemical Constituents: Monoterpenes: α and β–pinenes, campene, sabinene; Sesquiterpenes: chamazulene; Terpene oxides: 1,8 cineol (10%); Monoterpenones: isoartemisia ketone (9%), camphor (18%); Sesquiterpene lactones.

Action: Anti-inflammatory, reduces, indigestion, reduces or prevents scarring, promotes penetration, promotes healing of wounds.

Found In: Dragon Time, Mister

Traditional Uses: The Greek Achilles, hero of the Trojan Wars, was said to have used yarrow to help cure the injury to his Achilles tendon. Yarrow was considered sacred by the Chinese, who recognized the harmony of the Yin and Yang energies within it. It has been said that the fragrance of yarrow makes possible the meeting of heaven and earth. Yarrow was used by Germanic tribes for the treatment of battle wounds.

Indications: It is a powerful decongestant of the prostate and helps to balance hormones. It may also help with acne, amenorrhea, appetite (lack of), bladder or kidney weakness, cellulite, respiratory infections, digestion (poor), menstrual problems, eczema, gallbladder inflammation, gastritis, gout, hair (promotes hair growth), headaches, hemorrhoids, hypertension, liver, menopause problems, neuritis, neuralgia, pelvic and urinary infections, prostitis, rheumatism, sprains, sunburn, thrombosis, ulcers, vaginitis, varicose veins, and wounds.

Application: Diffuse or apply topically.

Fragrant Influence: Balancing highs and lows, both external and internal, yarrow may allow us to have our heads in the clouds while our feet remain firm on the ground. Its balancing properties may also make it useful during meditation. It is supportive to intuitive energies and helps reduce confusion and ambivalence.

Safety Data: If pregnant or under a doctor's care, consult physician.

Ylang Ylang *(Cananga odorata)*

Botanical Family: Annonaceae (custard-apple)

Plant Origin: Commores, Indonesia, Philippines

Extraction Method: Steam distilled from flowers. Flowers are picked early in the morning to maximize oil yield. The highest quality oil is drawn from the first distillation and is known as Ylang Ylang. The last distillation "known as the tail" is of inferior quality and is called "cananga."

Chemical Constituents: Sesquiterpenes: α farnesene; Alcools monoterpenes; linalol (55%); Esters; Phenols.

Action: Antispasmodic, balances blood pressure, regulates heartbeat. It is used in hair preparations to promote thick, shiny, lustrous hair (it is also reported to help control split ends).

Found In: Aroma Life, Dream Catcher, Gathering, Gentle Baby, Grounding, Harmony, Humility, Inner Child, Into The Future, Joy, Motivation, Peace & Calming, Present Time, Release, Sacred Mountain, SARA, Sensation, White Angelica.

Historical Use: Ylang Ylang is translated into Polynesian as "flower of flowers." Ylang ylang has been used to cover the beds of newlywed couples on their wedding night.

Indications: Helps treat skin conditions, insect bites, heart arrhythmias, cardiac problems, high blood pressure, anxiety, impotence, arterial hypertension, depression, fatigue (mental), frigidity, hair loss, hyperpnea (labored breathing), insomnia, palpitations, tachycardia.

Other Uses: Ylang ylang may help balance male-female energies so one can move closer towards being in spiritual attunement and allowing greater focus of thoughts, filtering out the ever-present negative frequencies. It may help lower blood pressure, rapid breathing, balance equilibrium, frustration, balance heart function, impotence, infection, intestinal problems, sex drive problems, shock, and skin problems.

Application: Diffuse or apply topically mixed with V-6 Mixing Oil or Massage Oil Base. Add to food or water as a dietary supplement or flavoring.

Fragrant Influence: It influences sexual energy and enhances relationships. It may help stimulate the adrenal glands. It is calming and relaxing and may also help with anger and possibly rage and low self-esteem. It brings back the feeling of self-love, confidence, joy and peace.

Safety Data: If pregnant or under a doctor's care, consult your physician. Repeated use can possibly result in contact sensitization.

Floral Waters

Floral Water is an exquisite by-product of the steam distillation of essential oils. It has the same properties as the essential oils, but in lower concentration. It is gentle, fragrant, and suitable for all ages. It provides rehydrating, nurturing, and refreshing benefits to the skin. It is also uniquely calming, soothing, and relaxing.

Use

1. Spray into the air to freshen the home of office.

2. Spray in an airplane or other enclosed environment to dispel stale air.

3. Spray on face to energize, and overcome fatigue and drowsiness.

4. Drink undiluted or diluted to taste with water or juice.

Basil Floral Water—stimulating, energizing, uplifting, and relaxing to the muscles.

Chamomile (German) Floral Water—soothing for sore muscles, tendons, ligaments, skin irritations, and swelling. It is also supportive of the liver.

Clary Sage Floral Water—supports the cells and hormones. It contains natural sclareol, which stimulates the body's production of estrogen.

Eucalyptus Floral Water—antiseptic and well suited for cleansing oily skin, soothing to respiration, and may be used as an insect repellent.

Juniper Floral Water—stimulating to the nervous system and excellent to detoxify and cleanse the skin.

Lavender Floral Water—soothing to the skin and calming. Spray on skin before bed as a lovely prelude to a peaceful night's rest.

Melissa Floral Water—exquisitely relaxing and uplifting. It soothes herpes-type sores. In lab tests, it has been shown to be antimicrobial against Streptococcus haemolytica, which can colonize in the throat and esophagus.

Peppermint Floral Water—uplifting, energizing, cooling, refreshing, and soothing to digestion.

Spearmint Floral Water—cooling and refreshing. It is cleansing for blemished and oily skin and soothing for digestion and headaches.

Tansy (Idaho) Floral Water—encourages an uplifting feeling, a positive attitude, and a general feeling of well-being. It is antimicrobial and supports the cleansing of the lymphatic system.

Thyme Floral Water—antiseptic, cleansing, energizing, and stimulating to the scalp.

Oil Blends

This section contains specific blends that were formulated as a result of years of research into both physical and emotional health. Each of these blends is formulated to maximize the synergistic effect between various oil chemistries and harmonic frequencies. When chemistry and frequency coincide harmonically, noticeable and measurable physical, spiritual, and emotional benefits can be attained.

NOTE: Please keep in mind there are many variables of frequency, based on the calibration and the type of instrument used.

Abundance

This blend was created to enhance the frequency of the energy field that surrounds us through the electrical stimulation of the somatides. Somatides transmit the frequency from the cells to the outside of the body when they are stimulated through fragrance and the thought process. This frequency, called the electrical field or the aura, creates what is called the "law of attraction," which we attract to ourselves. This might bring about an abundance of health, both physical and emotional. The oils in Abundance also contain tremendous antiviral and antifungal properties.

Contains:

Myrrh *(Commiphora myrrha)* is an antimicrobial oil referenced throughout the Old and New Testaments (A bundle of myrrh is my well-beloved unto me… Song of Solomon 1:13). It was also part of a formula the Lord gave Moses (Exodus 30:22-27). It was used traditionally in the royal palaces by the queens as an anti-infectious agent during pregnancy and birthing. It has one of the highest levels of sesquiterpenes, a class of compounds that has direct effects on the hypothalamus, pituitary, and amygdala, the emotional center of the brain. It has been used in eastern countries to enhance the feeling of spirituality or euphoria. Myrrh was a trade commodity which legends say possessed the frequency of wealth.

Cinnamon Bark *(Cinnamomum verum)* is the oil of wealth from the Orient and part of the formula the Lord gave Moses (Exodus 30:22-27). Cinnamon oil is anti-infectious, antibacterial, antiparasitic, antiviral, and antifungal. Researchers, including J. C. Lapraz, M.D., found that viruses could not live in the presence of cinnamon oil. Cinnamon oil was regarded by the emperors of China and India to have great value; their wealth was measured by the amount of oil they possessed. Traditionally, it was thought to have a frequency that attracted wealth and abundance. Physically, it has many attributes: (1) it is a powerful purifier (2) it is a powerful oxygenator, and (3) it enhances the action and the activity of other oils.

Frankincense *(Boswellia carteri)* was valued more than gold during ancient times, and only those with great wealth and abundance possessed it. It is considered the "holy anointing oil" in the Middle East and has been used in religious ceremonies for thousands of years. High in sesquiterpenes, it helps oxygenate the pineal and pituitary glands, which stimulate and elevate the mind, helping to overcome stress and despair. Frankincense is presently being studied for its help in improving its hGH (human growth hormone) receptivity. It relieves depression, builds immune function, and is antitumoral. In ancient times, it was known for its anointing and healing powers, and "was used to treat every conceivable ill known to man."

Patchouly *(Pogostemon cablin)* East Indian people use it to fragrance their clothing and their homes because of its natural insecticidal and anti-infectious properties. Legends indicate that it represented money and those who possessed it were considered to be wealthy. Patchouly is very beneficial for the skin, relieving itching and preventing wrinkles or chapped skin. It is a general tonic and stimulant and helps the digestive system. It is also antimicrobial, antiseptic.

Orange *(Citrus sinesis)* was believed to bring joy, peace, and happiness to those who possessed it. It contains limonene, an antiviral compound, and citral, an antibacterial compound. It prevents the growth of bacteria, stop free radicals, and enhance the absorption of vitamin C in the body. It is elevating to the mind and body and brings joy and peace. It has been recognized to help a dull, oily complexion.

Clove *(Syzygium aromaticum)* was another oil from the Orient associated with great abundance; those who possessed it were considered wealthy. This oil is one of the most antimicrobial and antiseptic of all essential oils. It is antifungal, antiviral, anti-infectious, and antibacterial.

Ginger *(Zingiber officinale)* is used to work against the effects of motion sickness and has been studied for its gentle, stimulating effects. It aids digestion and has been used for rheumatism, bronchitis, dyspepsia, constipation, impotence, and lowered libido.

Spruce *(Picea mariana)* helps the respiratory and nervous systems. It is anti-infectious, antiseptic, and anti-inflammatory. Its aromatic influences help to open and release emotional blocks, bringing about a feeling of balance and grounding. Traditionally, spruce oil was believed to possess the frequency of prosperity.

Safety Data: May be irritating to those with sensitive skin. Avoid eye contact. In case of accidental contact, put any vegetable oil or cream in the eye and call your doctor if necessary. Never use water. Avoid exposure to direct sunlight for 3 to 6 hours after use.

Application: Diffuse, wear on the wrists, behind ears, or as a perfume. Individuals with sensitive skin may want to dilute with V-6 Mixing Oil, AromaSilk and Body Lotion, Pharaoh or Rawhide Aftershave. Put a drop on your checkbook, car dash, computer, phone, or wallet, or put a drop on your bills when paying invoices or when expecting payment. Many people put a drop on a piece of felt attached to the back of their watch. Add a 15 ml. bottle of Abundance to 5 gallons of any color of paint to increase the attraction of abundance and success in the work area or at home.

Companion Oils: Release may be used first used first to help release the emotions that stop us from receiving abundance. Then follow with Acceptance, Motivation, Envision, Passion, Into the Future, Magnify and Joy.

Fragrant Influence: When focusing on issues of abundance and inhaling this oil, a memory link to the RNA template is created where the memory is blue printed and then passed to and stored in the DNA memory bank. Then every time you smell the oils the mental energy for abundance is created. The frequency of this blend has been believed to create a harmonic magnetic energy field around oneself.

Frequency: Approximately 78 MHz—approximately the same frequency as the brain.

Acceptance

This blend stimulates the mind, compelling it to open and accept new things in life, allowing one to reach a higher potential. It also helps to overcome procrastination and denial.

Contains:

Neroli *(Citrus aurantium)* has been highly regarded by ancient Egyptians for its ability to heal and calm the mind, body and spirit. It is stabilizing and strengthening to the emotions, promoting peace, confidence and awareness. It is antimicrobial and works both topically and by diffusing. It brings everything into focus at the moment.

Sandalwood *(Santalum album)* is high in sesquiterpenes, which have been researched for their ability to stimulate the pineal gland and the limbic region of the brain, the center of our emotions. The pineal gland is responsible for releasing melatonin, a hormone that enhances deep sleep. Used traditionally for skin revitalization, yoga, and meditation, sandalwood is similar to frankincense oil in its support of nerves and circulation.

Blue Tansy *(Tanacetum annuum)* may help cleanse the liver and calm the lymphatic system helping to overcome anger and negative emotions promoting a feeling of self-control. Its primary constituents are limonene and sesquiterpenes. European research shows that blue tansy works as an antihistamine, anti-inflammatory, and stimulant for the thymus gland reducing dermatitis, arthritis, sciatica, tuberculosis, and allergies.

Rosewood *(Aniba rosaeodora)* is soothing and nourishing to the skin. It has been researched at Weber State University for its inhibition rate against gram positive and gram negative bacterial growth. This oil is soothing, creates elasticity, and helps the skin rid itself of irritations and problems, such as candida. It is anti-infectious, antibacterial, antifungal, antiviral, and antiparasitic.

Geranium *(Pelargonium graveolens)* has been used for centuries for skin care. Its strength lies in the ability to revitalize tissue. It may help with hormonal balance and the discharge of toxins from the liver, the gland where fear and anger are stored.

Frankincense *(Boswellia carteri)* is considered the "holy anointing oil" in the Middle East and has been used in religious ceremonies for thousands of years. High in sesquiterpenes, it helps stimulate the limbic part of the brain, which elevates the mind, helping to overcome stress and despair.

Safety Data: May be irritating to those with sensitive skin. Avoid eye contact. In case of accidental contact, put any vegetable oil or cream in the eye and call your doctor if necessary. Never use water. Avoid exposure to direct sunlight for 3 to 6 hours after use.

Carrier Oil: Almond oil.

Application: Diffuse, apply over heart and thymus, on the wrists, behind the ears, on the neck, temples and on the face. May be worn as a perfume or cologne.

Fragrant Influence: May help calm a troubled mind and promote feelings of strength and confidence compelling one to accept new things in life striving toward a higher potential.

Frequency: Approximately 102 MHz.

AromaLife

This blend may support cardiovascular, lymphatic, and circulatory systems helping to lower high blood pressure, reduce stress, and alleviate hemorrhoids.

Contains:

Helichrysum *(Helichrysum italicum)* has been researched in Europe for regenerating tissue and nerves and improving circulation. It is anticoagulant, prevents phlebitis, helps regulate cholesterol, stimulates liver cell function, and may help to clean plaque and debris from the veins and arteries. It is mucolytic, expectorant, antispasmodic, and reduces scarring and discoloration. It may also stimulate nerve endings and improve conditions such as hearing loss. It may help release feelings of anger promoting forgiveness.

Ylang Ylang *(Cananga odorata)* has been used traditionally to balance heart function, having been used to treat tachycardia (rapid heart beat) and arterial hypertension (high blood pressure.)

Marjoram *(Origanum majorana)* is used for calming the respiratory system and soothing sore and aching muscles. Marjoram helps regenerate smooth muscle tissue, and assists in relieving spasms, sprains, bruises, migraine headaches and calming the nerves. It is antimicrobial, anti-infectious, antibacterial, antiseptic and may work as a diuretic.

Cypress *(Cupressus sempervirens)* is one of the oils most used for the circulatory and lymphatic systems. It may help with edema, cellulite, varicose veins and water retention. It is anti-infectious, antibacterial, antimicrobial, mucolytic, antiseptic, refreshing and relaxing. It may help improve the cardiovascular system and circulation as well as help relieve other lymphatic and capillary problems.

Safety Data: May be irritating to those with sensitive skin. Avoid eye contact. In case of accidental contact, put any vegetable oil or cream in the eye and call your doctor if necessary. Never use water. Avoid exposure to direct sunlight for 3 to 6 hours after use.

Carrier Oil: Sesame seed oil.

Application: Apply over the heart, on the feet, on the life line of the hand and under the ring finger, above the elbow, behind the ring toe on the left foot, and dilute with V-6 Mixing Oil for a full body massage. It may also help to apply this blend along the spine from the first to the fourth thoracic vertebrae, which correspond to the cardiopulmonary nerves.

Companion Oils: Helichrysum, Rosemary, Joy, Valor, Ylang Ylang.

Frequency: Approximately 84 MHz.

Aroma Siez

The special blend may help relax, calm and relieve tight, sore, tired, and aching muscles resulting from sports injuries, fatigue and stress. It may also help to relieve headaches.

Contains:

Basil *(Ocimum basilicum)* can be relaxing to smooth muscles as well as those involuntary muscles of the heart and digestive system. It may sooth insect bites such as bees, wasps and spiders and may also help with snakebites. It has been found to alleviate mental fatigue, spasms, rhinitis, and help when there is a loss of smell due to chronic nasal catarrh.

Cypress *(Cupressus sempervirens)* is one of the oils most used for the circulatory and lymphatic systems. It may help with edema, cellulite, varicose veins and water retention. It is anti-infectious, antibacterial, antimicrobial, mucolytic, antiseptic, refreshing and relaxing. It may help improve the cardiovascular system and circulation as well as help relieve other lymphatic and capillary problems.

Marjoram *(Origanum majorana)* is used for calming the respiratory system and soothing sore and aching muscles. Marjoram helps regenerate smooth muscle tissue, and assists in relieving spasms, sprains, bruises, migraine headaches and calming the nerves. It is antimicrobial, anti-infectious, antibacterial, antiseptic and may work as a diuretic.

Lavender *(Lavandula angustifolia)* is known as the universal oil because of its wide range of usage. It is beneficial for skin conditions, such as burns, rashes, and psoriasis. It is antispasmodic, hypotensive, anti-inflammatory, anti-infectious, and anticoagulant. It prevents scarring, stretch marks and relieves headaches and PMS symptoms.

Peppermint *(Mentha piperita)* is one of the oldest and most highly regarded herbs for soothing digestion. Jean Valnet, M.D. studied the effects of peppermint on the liver and respiratory systems. Other scientists have researched its effect on impaired taste and smell as well as improved concentration and mental accuracy. Alan Hirsch, M.D., studied its ability to directly affect the brain's satiety center, triggering a sensation of fullness after meals, which may help in weight loss by curbing the appetite. Daniel Penöél, M.D., reports that it may help to reduce fevers, candida, nausea, vomiting and strengthen the respiratory system. Adding peppermint to drinking water helps cool body temperature during hot weather.

Safety Data: May be irritating to those with sensitive skin. Avoid eye contact. In case of accidental contact, put any vegetable oil or cream in the eye and call your doctor if necessary. Never use water. Avoid exposure to direct sunlight for 3 to 6 hours after use.

Application: Apply on location for muscles, neck, feet, and to relax during stress headaches. Add to water or diluted with V-6 Mixing Oil for a full body massage. Peppermint oils is also a great addition to foods and desserts.

Companion Oils: Basil, Elemi, Spruce, Birch, Helichrysum, Tansy (wild Idaho), Marjoram, Ortho Ease Massage Oil and Ortho Sport Massage Oil.

Frequency: Approximately 64 MHz.

Awaken

This formulation is a combination of several other blends. It brings one to inner knowing in order to make changes and desirable transitions helping to reach one's highest potential.

Contains:

Joy is an exotic blend that produces a magnetic energy to enhance the frequency of self-love and bring joy to the heart. It inspires romance and may help overcome grief and depression.

Forgiveness is a blend that may help release negative memories through the electrical frequencies of the oils which may have powerful emotional effects helping people move past the barriers enabling them to achieve higher awareness compelling them to forgive and let go.

Present Time has an empowering fragrance, which gives a feeling of "being in the moment." One can only go forward and progress when in the present time.

Dream Catcher is an exotic formula that may help open the mind and enhance dreams and visualization, promoting greater potential for realizing your dreams and staying on your path. It also protects you from negative dreams that might cloud your vision.

Harmony is an exquisite blend of 12 oils for promoting physical and emotional healing by bringing about a harmonic balance to the energy centers of the body, allowing the energy to flow more efficiently. Harmony has been found to negate allergy symptoms. It is also beneficial in reducing stress and creating a general overall feeling of well-being.

Safety Data: May be irritating to those with sensitive skin. Avoid eye contact. In case of accidental contact, put any vegetable oil or cream in the eye and call your doctor if necessary. Never use water. Avoid exposure to direct sunlight for 3 to 6 hours after use.

Carrier Oil: Almond oil.

Application: Diffuse, add to bath water, diluted with V-6 Mixing Oil for a full body massage. Wear over the heart, the wrists, on the neck and use as an aftershave. For clearing allergies, rub over sternum.

Companion Oils: Passion, Into The Future, Dream Catcher, Envision, Motivation, Harmony, Joy, Valor, En-R-Gee.

Fragrant Influence: Stimulates the creativity of the right brain, enhancing the function of pineal and pituitary glands in balancing the energy centers of the body and bringing about a harmonious feeling that increases all body functions.

Frequency: Approximately 89 MHz.

Brain Power

The oils in this blend contain high sesquiterpene compounds that have been shown to increase oxygen around receptor sites around the pineal, pituitary and hypothalamus. They are responsible for the secretion of human growth hormone (hGH). Research indicates that they play a major role in dissolving petrochemicals known to plug the receptor sites and prevent receptivity. Brain Power may help clear the "brain fog" that people experience due to the ingestion of chemical foods, skin and hair care products with petrochemicals and breathing heavy chemical-laden air. Brain Power may increase mental potential, mental clarity, and long term use may retard the aging process. It may also support and strengthen immune function.

Contains:

Frankincense (*Boswellia carteri*) is considered the "holy anointing oil" in the Middle East and has been used in religious ceremonies for thousands of years. High in sesquiterpenes, it helps stimulate the limbic part of the brain, which elevates the mind, helping to overcome stress and despair.

Sandalwood (*Santalum album*) is high in sesquiterpenes, which have been researched for their ability to stimulate the pineal gland and the limbic region of the brain, the center of our emotions. The pineal gland is responsible for releasing melatonin, a hormone that enhances deep sleep. Used traditionally for skin revitalization, yoga, and meditation, sandalwood is similar to frankincense oil in its support of nerves and circulation.

Melissa *(Melissa officinalis)* is a powerful, antimicrobial oil, yet it is very gentle and delicate because of the nature of the plant, and helps to bring out those characteristics within the individual. It is calming and balancing to the emotions. Melissa is one of the highest in sesquiterpenes, much like cedarwood. It is very stimulating to the anterior pituitary and immune system.

Cedarwood *(Cedrus atlantica)* has calming and purifying properties. High in sesquiterpenes which can stimulate the limbic part of the brain (the center of our emotions), this conifer oil has been used by North American Indians to enhance spiritual awareness and communication. It also may help stimulate the pineal gland, which releases melatonin.

Blue Cypress, Australian *(Callitris intratropica)* improves circulation and increases the flow of oxygen to the brain, stimulating the amygdala, pineal gland, pituitary gland and hypothalamus.

Lavender *(Lavandula angustifolia)* has calming and relaxing properties that can improve concentration and mental acuity. High in sedating aldehydes and esters, its ability to help overcome insomnia, headaches, stress, and nervous tension can lead to a heightened ability to reason and remember.

Helichrysum *(Helichrysum italicum)* helps improve circulation and stimulate optimum nerve function, properties which can lead to enhanced awareness and cognition. On an emotional level, its ability to help release feelings of anger, can allow the mind to gain focus and concentration.

Safety Data: May be irritating to those with sensitive skin. Avoid eye contact. In case of accidental contact, put any vegetable oil or cream in the eye and call your doctor if necessary. Never use water. Avoid exposure to direct sunlight for 3 to 6 hours after use.

Application: Diffuse, wear as a perfume or cologne, apply on neck, throat, and under nose. Massage 1 or 2 drops with a finger on the insides of cheeks in the mouth. Doing this 1 or 2 times a day will immediately improve the smell sensory cortex.

Companion Oils: Clarity, Envision.

Fragrant Influence: Perfect for promoting deep concentration and channeling physical energy into mental energy.

Frequency: Approximately 78 MHz.

Christmas Spirit

This blend contains the oils of evergreens and spices, reminiscent of Christmas, bringing joy, happiness and security.

Contains:

Orange *(Citrus sinesis)* was believed to bring joy, peace, and happiness to those who possessed it. It contains limonene, an antiviral compound, and citral, an antibacterial compound. It prevents the growth of bacterial. It is elevating to the mind and body and bringing joy and peace. It has been recognized to help a dull, oily complexion.

Cinnamon Bark *(Cinnamomum cassia)* is the oil of wealth from the Orient and part of the formula the Lord gave Moses (Exodus 30:22-27). Emperors of China and India measured their wealth partly by the amount of cinnamon they possessed. Traditionally, it was thought to have a frequency that attracted wealth and abundance. It is highly antiviral, antifungal, and antibacterial.

Spruce *(Picea mariana)* helps the respiratory and nervous systems. It is anti-infectious, antiseptic, and anti-inflammatory. Its aromatic influences help to open and release emotional blocks, bringing about a feeling of balance and grounding. Traditionally, spruce oil was believed to possess the frequency of prosperity.

Safety Data: May be irritating to those with sensitive skin. Avoid eye contact. In case of accidental contact, put any vegetable oil or cream in the eye and call your doctor if necessary. Never use water. Avoid exposure to direct sunlight for 3 to 6 hours after use.

Application: Diffuse, sprinkle on logs in fireplace, on Christmas trees, on cedar chips for dresser drawers, or on potpourri. Use all year around

Fragrant Influence: This blend of oils has a delightful fragrance and is wonderful for creating the feeling of security that usually accompanies the holiday season. It is also nice for air purification.

Frequency: Approximately 104 MHz.

Citrus Fresh

This is a fragrance stimulates the right brain, bringing about more creativity, a sense of well-being, and joy. It has been found to be relaxing and calming, especially for children and works well as an air purifier.

Contains:

Orange *(Citrus aurantium)* was believed to bring joy, peace, and happiness to those who possessed it. It contains limonene, an antiviral compound, and citral, an antibacterial compound. It prevents the growth of bacterial. It is elevating to the mind and body and brings joy and peace. It has been recognized to help a dull, oily complexion.

Tangerine *(Citrus nobilis)* contains esters and aldehydes that are sedating and calming, helping with anxiety and nervousness. It is anti-inflammatory, anticoagulant, may help decongest the lymphatic system and works as a diuretic.

Lemon *(Citrus limon)* has antiseptic-like properties and contains compounds that have been studied for their effects on immune function. It has a vitamin P-like action, increasing microcirculation, which may improve vision. It may serve as an insect repellent and may be beneficial for the skin. It has been found to promote leukocyte formation, dissolve cellulite, increase lymphatic function, and promote a sense of well-being. Its fragrance is stimulating and invigorating.

Mandarin *(Citrus reticulata)* is appealing, gentle, and promotes happiness. Diffuse or apply topically, especially around meals and before sleep. Because of its sedative and slightly hypnotic properties, it may help with insomnia and is good for stress and irritability. It is antispasmodic, antiseptic, antifungal, supports hepatic duct function, and works as a digestive tonic.

Grapefruit *(Citrus paradisi)* works as a mild disinfectant. Like many cold-pressed citrus oils, it has unique fat-dissolving characteristics. It may be beneficial for digestive complaints, obesity, reducing water retention and cellulite.

Spearmint *(Mentha spicata)* oil helps support the respiratory and nervous systems. With its hormone-like activity, it may help open and release emotional blocks and bring about a feeling of balance. These oils may aid the respiratory, nervous, and glandular systems. It is antispasmodic, anti-infectious, antiparasitic, antiseptic, and anti-inflammatory. It has also been used to increase metabolism to burn fat.

Safety Data: May be irritating to those with sensitive skin. Avoid eye contact. In case of accidental contact, put any vegetable oil or cream in the eye and call your doctor if necessary. Never use water. Avoid exposure to direct sunlight for 3 to 6 hours after use.

Application: Diffuse, put in bath water, and dilute with V-6 Mixing Oil or Massage Base Oil for full body massage. It may be may be worn as a perfume or cologne and be applied over heart, on the wrists, and on the ears. It is excellent for children, although dilution with V-6 Mixing Oil is recommended.

Frgrant Influence: This blend creates an enjoyable aromatic fragrance at home or at work. Simple diffusion can be achieved by putting a few drops on a cotton ball and placing it on a desk or table.

Frequency: Approximately 90 MHz.

Note: A university in Japan experimented with diffusing different oils in the office. When they diffused lemon there were 54% fewer errors, with jasmine there were 33% fewer errors, and with lavender there were 20% fewer errors. When oils were diffused while studying and taking a test, test scores increased by as much as 50%. Different oils should be used for different tests, but the same oil should be used during the test as was used while studying for that particular test. The smell of the oil may help bring back the memory of what was studied.

115

Clarity

This blend has been used to promote a clear mind and mental alertness. Rosemary and peppermint, found in this blend, have been used for years to improve mental activity and vitality. Dr. Dember of the University of Cincinnati discovered in his research that inhaling peppermint oil increased the mental accuracy of the students tested by 28 percent. This blend may help keep one awake while driving and also keep one from going into shock during times of trauma.

Contains:

Cardamom *(Elettaria cardamomum)* is uplifting, refreshing and invigorating. It may be beneficial for clearing confusion.

Rosemary *(Rosmarinus officinalis)* is antiseptic and antimicrobial and may be beneficial for skin conditions and dandruff. It may help fight candida and is anti-infectious, antispasmodic, balances the endocrine system, and is an expectorant. It helps overcome mental fatigue stimulating memory and opening the conscious mind.

Peppermint *(Mentha piperita)* is one of the oldest and most highly regarded herbs for soothing digestion. Jean Valnet, M.D., studied the effects of peppermint on the liver and respiratory systems. Daniel Penöél, M.D., reports that it may help to reduce fevers, candida, nausea, vomiting and strengthen the respiratory system. adding peppermint to drinking water helps cool body temperature during hot weather.

Basil *(Ocimum basilicum)* can be relaxing to smooth muscles as well as those involuntary muscles of the heart and digestive system. It may sooth insect bites such as bees, wasps and spiders and may also help with snake bites. It has been found to alleviate mental fatigue, spasms, rhinitis and help when these is a loss of smell due to chronic nasal catarrh.

Rosewood *(Aniba rosaeodora)* is soothing and nourishing to the skin. It has been researched at Weber State University for its inhibition rate against gram positive and gram negative bacterial growth. This oil is soothing, creates elasticity, and helps the skin rid itself of irritations and problems, such as candida. It is anti-infectious, antibacterial, antifungal, antiviral, and antiparasitic.

Safety Data: May be irritating to those with sensitive skin. Avoid eye contact. In case of accidental contact, put any vegetable oil or cream in the eye and call your doctor if necessary. Never use water. Avoid exposure to direct sunlight for 3 to 6 hours after use.

Application: Diffuse, put in bath water, add a few 2 to 5 drops on a cotton ball and put in home and car air vents. Apply on temples, wrists, neck, and feet.

Companion Oils: En-R-Gee (when overly tired).

Frgrant Oils: The oils in this blend are known for their ability to help increase mental alertness.

Frequency: Approximately 101 MHz.

Comments: This blend contains cardamom and high levels of transphenol, which may cause headaches when inhaled or topically applied.

Di-Tone

These oils are blended to assist in relieving digestive irregularities and disturbances, such as an upset stomach, belching, heartburn, and bloating. Massage a drop or two on the outer ear to help alleviate morning sickness. It has been found to rid animals of parasites by applying it to their feet. It may also help dispel parasites by massaging and placing a compress across the stomach.

Contains:

Tarragon *(Artemisia dracunculus)* has been used in Europe for its antimicrobial and antiseptic functions. It helps to reduce dyspepsia, intestinal spasms, and genital urinary tract infection. It may reduce premenstrual discomfort and nerve pain. It is antispasmodic, anti-inflammatory, anti-infectious, antiviral, antibacterial, and prevents fermentation.

Ginger *(Zingiber officinale)* is used for relief from motion sickness, arthritis, rheumatism, sprains, muscle aches and pains, congestion, coughs, sinusitis, sore throats, diarrhea, colic, indigestion, loss of appetite, fever, flu, chills, and infectious disease.

Juniper berry *(Juniperus communis)* may work as a detoxifier, cleanser and promotes improved nerve and kidney function. It is also beneficial for the skin reducing dermatitis, eczema and acne.

Anisum *(Pimpinella anisum)* is antispasmodic, antiseptic, stimulates the increase of bile from the liver, expels worms, increases lactation, and helps calm gall bladder contractions. It may help with painful menstruation and irregularity, problems with menopause, dyspepsia, spastic colitis, flatulence, indigestion, lung congestion, asthmatic bronchitis, and intestinal pain.

Fennel *(Foeniculum vulgare)* is antiseptic and stimulating to the circulatory and respiratory systems. It is antispasmodic, antiseptic, and stimulating to the cardiovascular and respiratory systems. With its hormone-like activity, it may help facilitate childbirth and increase lactation after birthing.

Patchouly *(Pogostemon cablin)* was used in India in ancient times as a trade commodity because of its earthy, musty fragrance and its ability to mask many different odors. East Indian people use it to fragrance their clothing and their homes because of its natural insecticidal and anti-infectious properties. Legends indicate that it represented money, and those who possessed it were considered to be wealthy. Patchouly is very beneficial for the skin and may help prevent wrinkles or chapped skin. It is a general tonic and stimulant and helps the digestive system. It is also antimicrobial, antiseptic, and helps relieve itching.

Peppermint *(Mentha piperita)* is one of the oldest and most highly regarded herbs for soothing digestion. Jean Valnet, M.D., studied the effects of peppermint on the liver and respiratory systems. Daniel Penoël, M.D., reports that it may help to reduce fevers, candida, nausea, vomiting and strengthen the respiratory system. adding peppermint to drinking water helps cool body temperature during hot weather.

Lemongrass *(Cymbopogon flexuosus)* works well for purification. It is powerful in the regeneration of connective tissue. It is a vasodilator, anti-inflammatory, sedative and supportive to the digestive system. A study in *Phytotherapy Research* showed that this oil had strong antifungal properties when applied topically. It may also help increase the flow of oxygen and uplift the spirit.

Safety Data: May be irritating to those with sensitive skin. Avoid eye contact. For accidental contact put any vegetable oil or cream in the eye and call your doctor if necessary. Never use water. Avoid exposure to direct sunlight for 3 to 6 hours after use.

Application: May be applied to the Vita Flex points on the feet and ankles. Massage a drop or two on outer ear to help alleviate morning sickness. Massage 2 or 3 drops on the paws of your animals to expel parasites. Parasites may also be dispelled by massaging or placing a compress across the stomach. Add 1 or 2 drops to 8 ounces of water and sip slowly as a dietary supplement.

Fragrant Influence:

Companion Products: ComforTone(capsule), JuvaTone (tablet)

Frequency: Approximately 102 MHz.

Dragon Time

This blend helps soothe the discomfort associated with those uncomfortable times of the month including cramping and irregular periods.

Contains:

Clary Sage *(Salvia sclarea)* regulates the cells and balances the hormones. It contains natural sclareol, a phytoestrogen that mimics estrogen function. It may help with menstrual cramps, PMS, and pre-menopause symptoms and may help with circulatory problems.

Yarrow *(Achillea millefolium)* is a decongestant of the prostate and balances hormones. It is anti-inflammatory, and reduces scarring. It also helps with nerve inflammation.

Lavender *(Lavandula angustifolia)* is known as the universal oil because of its wide range of usage. It helps relieve headaches and PMS symptoms.

Jasmine *(Jasminum officinale)* is beneficial for dry, greasy, irritated, or sensitive skin. It is used for muscle spasms, sprains, coughs, laryngitis, frigidity, depression and nervous exhaustion.

Fennel *(Foeniculum vulgare)* is antiseptic and stimulating to the circulatory and respiratory systems. It is antispasmodic, antiseptic, and stimulating to the cardiovascular and respiratory systems. With its hormone-like activity, it may help facilitate childbirth and increase lactation after birthing.

Marjoram *(Origanum majorana)* is used for calming the respiratory system and soothing sore and aching muscles. Marjoram helps regenerate smooth muscle tissue, and also assists in relieving spasms and migraine headaches and calming the nerves. It is antimicrobial, anti-infectious, antibacterial, antiseptic and may work as a diuretic.

Safety Data: May be irritating to those with sensitive skin. Avoid eye contact. In case of accidental contact, put any vegetable oil or cream in the eye and call your doctor if necessary. Never use water. Avoid exposure to direct sunlight for 3 to 6 hours after use.

Application: Apply to the Vita Flex points on the feet and around the ankles, both inside and out. It may be diluted with V-6 Mixing Oil for application on the other Vita Flex points on the body. It may be applied as a hot compress over the lower abdomen, across the lower back, or anywhere it hurts.

Companion Oils: EndoFlex may help alleviate hot flashes (power surges) in women.

Fragrant Influence: This blend of oils may be beneficial in times of hormonal stress. It may be diffused in the home, the office, or put a few drops on a cotton ball and place in the car vent.

Frequency: Approximately 72 MHz.

Dream Catcher

This exotic formula may help open the mind and enhance dreams and visualization, promoting greater potential for realizing your dreams and staying on your path. It also protects you from negative dreams that might cloud your vision.

Contains:

Sandalwood *(Santalum album)* is high in sesquiterpenes, which have been researched for their ability to stimulate the pineal gland and the limbic region of the brain, the center of our emotions. The pineal gland is responsible for releasing melatonin, a hormone that enhances deep sleep. Used traditionally for skin revitalization, yoga, and meditation, sandalwood is similar to frankincense oil in its support of nerves and circulation.

Blue Tansy *(Tanacetum annuum)* may help cleanse the liver and calm the lymphatic system helping one to overcome anger and negative emotions promoting a feeling of self-control. Its primary constituents are limonene and sesquiterpenes. European research shows that it works as an antihistamine, anti-inflammatory, and stimulant for the thymus gland reducing dermatitis, arthritis, sciatica, tuberculosis, and allergies.

Juniper Berry *(Juniperus communis)* may work as a detoxifier, cleanser and promotes improved nerve and kidney function. It is also beneficial for the skin reducing dermatitis, eczema and acne. It elevates spiritual awareness creating feelings of love and peace.

Bergamot *(Citrus bergamia)* is one of the most uplifting fragrances, simultaneously energizing and calming, with a unique ability to relieve anxiety, stress and tension.

Anisum *(Pimpinella anisum)* is antispasmodic, antiseptic, stimulates the increase of bile from the liver, expels worms, increases lactation, and helps calm gall bladder contractions. It may help with painful menstruation and irregularity, problems with menopause, dyspepsia, spastic colitis, flatulence, indigestion, lung congestion, asthmatic bronchitis, and intestinal pain.

Tangerine *(Citrus nobilis)* contains esters and aldehydes that are sedating and calming, helping with anxiety and nervousness. It is anti-inflammatory, anticoagulant, may help decongest the lymphatic system and works as a diuretic.

Ylang Ylang *(Cananga odorata)* helps bring about a sense of relaxation and may help balance male and female energies. It balances equilibrium and restores confidence and self-love.

Pepper, Black *(Piper nigrum)* stimulates the endocrine system and increases energy while increasing cellular oxygenation. It is anti-inflammatory which may sooth deep tissue muscle aches. It is expectorant, supportive to the digestive glands, and has been traditionally used for rheumatoid arthritis.

Safety Data: May be irritating to those with sensitive skin. Avoid eye contact. In case of accidental contact, put any vegetable oil or cream in the eye and call your doctor if necessary. Never use water. Avoid exposure to direct sunlight for 3 to 6 hours after use.

Application: Diffuse, apply on forehead, ears, throat, under nose, eyebrow, and base of neck. Place a couple of drops on the pillow. This blend may be useful during meditation in sweat lodges, and in bath water.

Companion Oil: Envision, Passion, Motivation, Awaken, Gathering, Into the Future.

Fragrant Influence: This blend may be diffused during the day, but seems to be most effective during sleep.

Frequency: Approximately 98 MHz.

Note: Indian dream catchers have been used to help keep bad dreams away. If bad dreams occur, continue to use this oil, as something in the subconscious may need to be processed. Hold onto your dreams and visualize them into reality.

EndoFlex

This may help overall vitality. It contains oils associated with hormonal balance, improving and balancing metabolism and associated weight control.

Contains:

Spearmint *(Mentha spicata)* helps support the respiratory and nervous systems. With its hormone-like activity, it may help open and release emotional blocks and bring about a feeling of balance. This oil may aid the respiratory, nervous, and glandular systems. It is antispasmodic, anti-infectious, antiparasitic, antiseptic, and anti-inflammatory. It has also been used to increase metabolism to burn fat.

Myrtle *(Myrtus communis)* may help normalize hormonal imbalances of the thyroid and ovaries as well as balance the hypothyroid. It may help the respiratory system with chronic coughs and tuberculosis. It is suitable to use for coughs and chest complaints with children, and may support immune function in fighting cold, flu and infectious disease.

Nutmeg *(Myristica fragrans)* has adrenal cortex-like activity, which helps support the adrenal glands for increased energy. It may help with difficulties related to circulation, and aches and pains in muscles and joints related to stress, arthritis and gout. It may also help with digestive problems such as flatulence, indigestion, sluggish digestion, and nausea. It is antiseptic, antiparasitic, and a neurotonic.

German Chamomile *(Matricaria recutita)* has been a highly respected oil for over 3,000 years and has been used for helping skin conditions, such as dermatitis, boils, acne, rashes, and eczema. It is also used for hair care, burns, cuts, toothaches, teething pains, inflamed joints, menopausal problems, insomnia, migraine headaches and stress-related complaints. It has an electrical frequency that promotes peace and harmony, bringing about a feeling of security.

Geranium *(Pelargonium graveolens)* assists in balancing hormones. It is antispasmodic, relaxant, anti-inflammatory, anti-infectious, antibacterial, antifungal and stimulates the liver and pancreas.

Sage *(Salvia officinalis)* has been used in Europe for skin conditions such as eczema, acne, dandruff and hair loss. It has been recognized for its benefits of strengthening the vital centers. It may help in relieving depression and mental fatigue. Sage contains sclareol, which stimulates the body to produce its own estrogen, it may nutritionally support the body during PMS and menopause. The Lakota Indians used it for purification and healing and to dispel negative emotions from denial and sexual abuse, as well as a complete body tonic for healing and strength.

Carrier Oil: Sesame seed oil.

Safety Data: May be irritating to those with sensitive skin. Avoid eye contact. For accidental contact put any vegetable oil or cream in the eye and call your doctor if necessary. Never use water. Avoid exposure to direct sunlight for 3 to 6 hours after use.

Application: Apply over lower back, thyroid, kidneys, liver, feet, and glandular areas. It may also be applied to the Vita Flex points on the feet for these same areas of the body.

Frequency: Approximately 138 MHz.

En-R-Gee

Traditionally, the oils in this blend were used for increasing vitality, circulation and alertness in the body.

Contains:

Clove *(Syzygium aromaticum)* was another oil from the Orient haled as an oil of great abundance; those who possessed it were considered wealthy. This oil is one of the most antimicrobial and antiseptic of all essential oils. It is antifungal, antiviral, anti-infectious, and antibacterial. It works as a general stimulant and is used to treat sinusitis, bronchitis, cystitis, and cholera.

Juniper - berry and branches combined *(Juniperus communis)* may work as a detoxifier, cleanser and promotes improved nerve and kidney function. It is also beneficial for the skin reducing dermatitis, eczema and acne. It elevates spiritual awareness creating feelings of love and peace.

Fir *(Abies alba)* is antimicrobial. It has been researched for its ability to kill airborne germs and bacteria. It is antiseptic, antiarthritic, and stimulating. It supports the body and reduces the symptoms of arthritis, rheumatism, bronchitis, coughs, sinusitis, cold, flu and fevers. As a conifer oil, it creates a feeling of grounding, anchoring and empowerment.

Pepper, Black *(Piper nigrum)* stimulates the endocrine system and increases energy while increasing cellular oxygenation. It is anti-inflammatory which may soothe deep tissue muscle aches. It is expectorant, supportive to the digestive glands, and has been traditionally used for rheumatoid arthritis.

Nutmeg *(Myristica fragrans)* has adrenal cortex-like activity, which helps support the adrenal glands for increased energy. It may help with difficulties related to circulation, aches and pains is muscles and joints related to stress, arthritis and gout. It may also help with digestive problems such as flatulence, indigestion, sluggish digestion, and nausea. It is antiseptic, antiparasitic, analgesic, and a neurotonic.

Rosemary *(Rosmarinus officinalis* - Camphor, 1,8 Cineol) is antiseptic and antimicrobial and may be beneficial for skin conditions and dandruff. It may help fight candida and is anti-infectious, antispasmodic, balances the endocrine system, and is an expectorant. It helps overcome mental fatigue stimulating memory and opening the conscious mind.

Lemongrass *(Cymbopogon flexuosus)* works well for purification. It is powerful in the regeneration of connective tissue. It is a vaso-dilator, anti-inflammatory, sedative and supportive to the digestive system. A study in *Phytotherapy Research* showed that this oil had strong antifungal properties when applied topically. It may also help increase the flow of oxygen and uplift the spirit.

Safety Data: May be irritating to those with sensitive skin. Avoid eye contact. In case of accidental contact, put any vegetable oil or cream in the eye and call your doctor if necessary. Never use water. Avoid exposure to direct sunlight for 3 to 6 hours after use.

Application: Diffuse, apply 2 drops on the wrists or temples, back of neck, behind ears, or add to warm bath water with Bath Gel Base. Dilute with V-6 Mixing Oil or Massage Oil Base for an uplifting body massage. Massage on Vita Flex points of the feet. It may be worn as a perfume or cologne.

Companion Oils: One may feel like they have had eight hours of sleep by rubbing this blend on the feet and Awaken on the temples. This blend and Clarity together may help one stay awake while driving late at night.

Fragrant Influence: This blend of oils may help boost one's energy when diffused. It is also purifying when diffused. Simple diffusion can be achieved by applying a few drops on a cotton ball and placing in the air vent of a car or on the heat registers of the home or hotel room.

Frequency: Approximately 106 MHz.

Envision

This blend helps bring renewed faith in the future and maintain the emotional fortitude to achieve your goals and dreams. Many people suppress their own internal drive and creativity and can become a doormat or they may be shutting down out of fear of the unknown, fear of the responsibility that comes with getting out of the rut. Some people are in a relationship where the spouse may be very dominating. Envision helps in awakening and renewing your drive and independence, and overcoming the fear of experiencing new dimensions and letting the creativity flow, which will help you become a self-made person.

Contains:

Sage *(Salvia officinalis)* has been used in Europe for skin conditions such as eczema, acne, dandruff, and hair loss. It has been recognized for its benefits of strengthening the vital centers. It may help in relieving depression and mental fatigue. Sage contains sclareol, which stimulates the body to produce its own estrogen. It may nutritionally support the body during PMS and menopause. The Lakota Indians used it for purification and healing and to dispel negative emotions from denial and sexual abuse, as well as a complete body tonic for healing and strength.

Geranium *(Pelargonium graveolens)* helps release negative memories, thereby opening and elevating the mind.

Orange *(Citrus aurantium)* was believed to bring joy, peace, and happiness to those who possessed it. It contains limonene, an antiviral compound, and citral, an antibacterial compound. It prevents the growth of bacterial. It is elevating to the mind and body and bringing joy and peace. It has been recognized to help a dull, oily complexion.

Rose *(Rosa damascena)* possesses the highest frequency of the oils. It brings balance and harmony, and elevates the mind, creating a sense of well-being. It is antihemorrhaging, anti-infectious, and prevents scarring. It may help with chronic bronchitis, asthma, tuberculosis, sexual disabilities, frigidity, impotency, skin disease, ulcers, sprains, wrinkles, thrush, and gingivitis. It is also promotes healthy skin.

Lavender *(Lavandula angustifolia)* has sedative and calming properties that help overcome insomnia, headaches, stress, and nervous tension.

Spruce *(Picea mariana)* helps to open and release emotional blocks, bringing about a feeling of balance and grounding. Traditionally, spruce oil was believed to possess the frequency of prosperity.

Safety Data: May be irritating to those with sensitive skin. Avoid eye contact. In case of accidental contact, put any vegetable oil or cream in the eye and call your doctor if necessary. Never use water. Avoid exposure to direct sunlight for 3 to 6 hours after use.

Application: Diffuse, apply 2 drops on wrists or temples, or add to warm bath water with bath Gel Base. Dilute with V-6 Mixing Oil or Massage Oil Base for an uplifting massage.

Companion Oils: Motivation, Acceptance, Valor, Magnify Your Purpose, Into the Future, Clarity.

Fragrant Influence: Stimulate one's creative and intuitive abilities in a positive and progressive way—moving one to take action.

Frequency: Approximately 90 MHz.

Exodus II

These particular oils were used by Moses to protect the Israelites from the plague. Modern science shows that these oils contain either immune-stimulating or antiviral compounds or both, which explains why these various oils were chosen. Today viruses and bacteria are beginning to mutate in response to conventional drugs, becoming resistant. Because of the complex chemistry of essential oils, viruses and bacteria have a more difficult time becoming resistant. This blend was designed to work with the Exodus food supplement to help build the body's natural defenses.

Contains:

Cassia *(Cinnamomum cassia)* is anti-infectious, antibacterial, and anticoagulant. It was part of the formula the Lord gave Moses (Exodus 30:22-27) for protecting the Israelites.

Hyssop *(Hyssopus officinalis)* is anti-inflammatory and antiviral, supporting the respiratory system. It is antiparasitic, mucolytic, decongestant, antiasthmatic, anti-infectious, regulates lipid metabolism, and prevents scarring.

Frankincense *(Boswellia carteri)* is considered the "holy anointing oil" in the Middle East and has been used in religious ceremonies for thousands of years. High in sesquiterpenes, it helps stimulate the hypothalamus which can lead to heightened immune function. It is being researched and used therapeutically in European hospitals to build immunity and treat cancer. In ancient times, it was well-known for its healing powers, and "was used to treat every conceivable ill known to man."

Spikenard *(Nardostachys jatamansi)* was highly prized at the time of Christ and was used by Mary of Bethany to anoint the feet of Jesus. High in sesquiterpenes, spikenard is very supporting to the immune system. It strengthens and calms the cardiovascular system, stimulates under active ovaries, and helps with tachycardia, anemia, psoriasis and hemorrhoids.

Galbanum *(Ferula gummosa)* was used for both medicinal and spiritual purposes. It is antimicrobial and supporting to the body. When combined with frankincense and sandalwood, it's frequency increases dramatically. (And the Lord said unto Moses, Take unto thee sweet spices, stacte, and onycha, and galbanum; sweet spices with pure with frankincense: Exodus 30:34).

Myrrh *(Myrtus communis)* is an antimicrobial oil referenced throughout the Old and New Testaments (A bundle of myrrh is my well-beloved unto me... Song of Solomon 1:13). It was used traditionally in the royal palaces by the queens as an anti-infectious agent during pregnancy and birthing. It has one of the highest levels of sesquiterpenes, which is a class of compounds having direct effects on the hypothalamus and the pituitary, glands responsible for activating hormone and immune response. Today, myrrh is widely used in oral hygiene products.

Cinnamon Bark *(Cinnamomum verum)* is the oil of wealth from the Orient and part of the formula the Lord gave Moses (Exodus 30:22-27). Cinnamon oil is anti-infectious, antibacterial, antiparasitic, antiviral, and antifungal. Cinnamon oil was regarded by the emperors of China and India to have great value; their wealth was measured by the amount of oil they possessed. Traditionally, it was thought to have a frequency that attracted wealth and abundance. Physically, it has many attributes: (1) it is a powerful purifier (2) it is a powerful oxygenator, and (3) it enhances the action and the activity of other oils. Researchers, including J. C. Lapraz, M.D., found that viruses could not live in the presence of cinnamon oil.

Calamus *(Acorus calamus)* is part of the formula the Lord gave Moses (Exodus 30:22-27). It is antispasmodic, anti-inflammatory (gastrointestinal), and supportive for stomach disorders. Calamus also helps inflammation of the small intestine and colon, gastritis and spasms, asthmatic bronchitis, kidney congestion after intoxication, cystitis, gout, and arterial hypotension (low blood pressure). It is highly regarded as an aromatic stimulant and a tonic for the digestive system.

Carrier Oil: Olive oil.

Safety Data: May be irritating to those with sensitive skin. Avoid eye contact. For accidental contact put any vegetable oil or cream in the eye and call your doctor if necessary. Never use water. Avoid exposure to direct sunlight for 3 to 6 hours after use.

Application: Apply to Vita Flex points on feet and/or directly on area of concern. Put 2 drops on wrists, feet, or other non-sensitive areas of the body. Diffuse, apply to palms of hands, cup hands over nose and mouth, and inhale. It may also be applied along the spine raindrop style. However, dilution may be necessary because of the high sesquiterpenes and phenols, which may be caustic on the skin.

Companion Supplements: Exodus, Immune Tune.

Frequency: Approximately 180 MHz.

Forgiveness

This blend may help release negative memories through the electrical frequencies of the oils, which may have powerful emotional effects helping people move past the barriers, enabling them to achieve higher awareness compelling the to forgive and let go.

Contains:

Rose *(Rosa damascena)* possesses the highest frequency of the oils. It creates a sense of balance, harmony, and well-being and elevates the mind. It promotes healthy skin, reduces scarring, and may help with chronic bronchitis, asthma, tuberculosis, sexual disabilities, frigidity, impotency, skin disease, ulcers, sprains, wrinkles, thrush, and gingivitis. It is also promotes healthy skin.

Melissa *(Melissa officinalis)* is a powerful, antimicrobial oil, yet it is very gentle and delicate because of the nature of the plant, and helps to bring out those characteristics within the individual. It is calming and balancing to the emotions. Melissa is one of the highest in sesquiterpenes, much like cedarwood. It is very stimulating to the anterior pituitary and immune system.

Helichrysum *(Helichrysum italicum)* may help release feelings of anger promoting forgiveness.

Angelica *(Angelica archangelica)* helps to calm emotions and to bring memories back to the point of origin before trauma or anger was experienced, helping us to let go of negative feelings.

Frankincense *(Boswellia carteri)* is considered the "holy anointing oil" in the Middle East and has been used in religious ceremonies for thousands of years. High in sesquiterpenes, it helps oxygenate the pineal and pituitary glands, which stimulate and elevate the mind, helping to overcome stress and despair.

Sandalwood *(Santalum album)* is high in sesquiterpenes, which have been researched for their ability to stimulate the pineal gland and the limbic region of the brain, the center of our emotions. The pineal gland is responsible for releasing melatonin, a hormone that enhances deep sleep. Used traditionally for skin revitalization, yoga, and meditation, sandalwood is similar to frankincense oil in its support of nerves and circulation.

Lavender *(Lavandula angustifolia)* has sedative and calming properties that help overcome insomnia, headaches, stress, and nervous tension.

Safety Data: May be irritating to those with sensitive skin. Avoid eye contact. For accidental contact put any vegetable oil or cream in the eye and call your doctor if necessary. Never use water Avoid exposure to direct sunlight for 3 to 6 hours after use.

Carrier Oil: Sesame seed oil

Application: Massage over the navel and the heart. It may be worn as a perfume or cologne or added to Pharaoh or Rawhide Aftershave.

Companion Oils: Valor on feet, Gathering.

Fragrant Influence: Diffused or worn, this blend may stimulate the desire to forgive and let go of hurt feeling and negative emotions caused by others towards us.

Frequency: Approximately 192 MHz.

Gathering

This was created out of the need to help us overcome the bombardment of chaotic energy that alters our focus and take us off our path toward higher achievements. Galbanum, a favorite oil of Moses, has a strong effect when blended with frankincense and sandalwood in gathering our emotional and spiritual thoughts, helping us to focus to achieve our potential. These oils may help increase the oxygen around the pineal and pituitary gland, bringing greater harmonic frequency to receive the communication we desire. This blend may help bring people together on a physical, emotional and spiritual level for greater focus and clarity. It may help one stay focused, grounded, and clear in gathering ones potential for self-improvement.

Contains:

Galbanum *(Ferula gummosa)* was used for both medicinal and spiritual purposes. It is antimicrobial and supporting to the body. When combined with frankincense and sandalwood, its frequency increases dramatically. (And the Lord said unto Moses, Take unto thee sweet spices, stacte, and onycha, and galbanum; sweet spices with pure with frankincense: Exodus 30:34).

Frankincense *(Boswellia carteri)* is considered the "holy anointing oil" in the Middle East and has been used in religious ceremonies for thousands of years. It elevates the mind and helps overcome stress and despair. It is high in sesquiterpenes, which stimulate the limbic region of the brain, the center of emotions. In ancient times, it was known for its anointing and healing powers, and "was used to treat every conceivable ill known to man."

Sandalwood *(Santalum album)* is high in sesquiterpenes, which have been researched for their ability to stimulate the pineal gland and the limbic region of the brain, the center of our emotions. The pineal gland is responsible for releasing melatonin, a hormone that enhances deep sleep. Used traditionally for skin revitalization, yoga, and meditation, sandalwood is similar to frankincense oil in its support of nerves and circulation.

Rose *(Rosa damascena)* possesses the highest frequency of the oils. It creates a sense of balance, harmony, and well-being and elevates the mind. It promotes healthy skin, reduces scarring, and may help with chronic bronchitis, asthma, tuberculosis, sexual disabilities, frigidity, impotency, skin disease, ulcers, sprains, wrinkles, thrush, and gingivitis. It is also promotes healthy skin.

Lavender *(Lavandula angustifolia)* has sedative and calming properties that help overcome insomnia, headaches, stress, and nervous tension.

Cinnamon Bark *(Cinnamomum verum)* is the oil of wealth from the Orient and part of the formula the Lord gave Moses (Exodus 30:22-27). Cinnamon oil is anti-infectious, antibacterial, antiparasitic, antiviral, and antifungal. Cinnamon oil was regarded by the emperors of China and India to have great value; their wealth was measured by the amount of oil they possessed. Traditionally, it was thought to have a frequency that attracted wealth and abundance. Physically, it has many attributes: (1) it is a powerful purifier (2) it is a powerful oxygenator, and (3) it enhances the action and the activity of other oils. Researchers, including J. C. Lapraz, M.D., found that viruses could not live in the presence of cinnamon oil.

Spruce *(Picea mariana)* helps to open and release emotional blocks, bringing about a feeling of balance and grounding. Traditionally, spruce oil was believed to possess the frequency of prosperity.

Ylang Ylang *(Cananga odorata)* helps bring about a sense of relaxation and may help balance male and female energies. It balances equilibrium and restores confidence and self-love.

Geranium *(Pelargonium graveolens)* stimulates nerves and assists in balancing hormones. Its aromatic influence helps release negative memories, thereby opening and elevating the mind.

Safety Data: May be irritating to those with sensitive skin. Avoid eye contact. For accidental contact put any vegetable oil or cream in the eye and call your doctor if necessary. Never use water. Avoid exposure to direct sunlight for 3 to 6 hours after use.

Application: Diffuse, wear on temples, neck, wrists, or where needed. It may be worn as a perfume or cologne.

Companion Oils: Forgiveness on navel, Sacred Mountain on crown (to clear negative attitudes), Valor on crown or feet, Three Wise Men on the crown, Clarity on the temples, and Dream Catcher.

Fragrant Influence: A feeling of coming together for a higher purpose.

Frequency: Approximately 99 MHz.

Gentle Baby

This is a beautiful combination of therapeutic-grade essential oils for mothers and babies. It is comforting, soothing, relaxing, and may be beneficial during the birthing process and for reducing stress during pregnancy. It helps reduce stretch marks and scar tissue. Gentle Baby enhances a youthful appearance of the skin, improving skin elasticity and smoothing wrinkles. It is particularly soothing to dry, chapped skin, and even diaper rash (dilute 1-3 drops in 1/2 tsp. carrier oil).

Contains:

Palmarosa *(Cymbopogon martinii)* is helpful for all types of skin problems, such as candida, rashes, and scaly and flaky skin. It stimulates new cell growth, moisturizes and speeds the healing process. It is antimicrobial, antibacterial, antifungal, and antiviral. It is supportive to the nervous and cardiovascular system.

Geranium *(Pelargonium graveolens)* has been used for centuries for skin care, especially the skin of pregnant mothers. It revitalizes tissue and nerves and assists in balancing hormones. It is antispasmodic, relaxant, anti-inflammatory, anti-infectious, antibacterial, antifungal and supports the liver, pancreas, and kidneys. Its aromatic influence helps release negative memories thus opening and elevating the mind.

Roman Chamomile *(Chamaemelum nobile)* may calm and relieve restlessness, tension, insomnia, muscle tension, cuts, scrapes, bruises and is anti-infectious. It may relieve allergies and expel toxins from the liver. It is used extensively in Europe for the skin.

Rose *(Rosa damascena)* possesses the highest frequency of the oils. It creates a sense of balance, harmony, and well-being and elevates the mind. It promotes healthy skin, reduces scarring, and may help with chronic bronchitis, asthma, tuberculosis, sexual disabilities, frigidity, impotency, skin disease, ulcers, sprains, wrinkles, thrush, and gingivitis. It is also promotes healthy skin.

Lavender *(Lavandula angustifolia)* is known as the universal oil because of its wide range of usage. It is beneficial for skin conditions, such as burns, rashes, and psoriasis. Its sedative and calming properties help overcome insomnia, headaches, stress, and nervous tension. It is antispasmodic, hypotensive, anti-inflammatory, anti-infectious, and anticoagulant. It prevents scarring, stretch marks and relieves headaches and PMS symptoms.

Rosewood *(Aniba rosaeodora)* is soothing and nourishing to the skin. It has been researched at Weber State University for its inhibition rate against gram positive and gram negative bacterial growth. This oil is soothing, creates elasticity, and helps the skin rid itself of irritations and problems, such as candida. It is anti-infectious, antibacterial, antifungal, antiviral, and antiparasitic.

Ylang Ylang *(Cananga odorata)* helps bring about a sense of relaxation.

Safety Data: May be irritating to those with sensitive skin. Avoid eye contact. For accidental contact put any vegetable oil or cream in the eye and call your doctor if necessary. Never use water. Avoid exposure to direct sunlight for 3 to 6 hours after use.

Application: Diffuse, apply over mother's abdomen, on feet, lower back, face and neck areas. Dilute with V-6 Mixing Oil for Massage Oil Base for full body massage and for applying on baby's skin.

Baby: Dilute by 1/2 with V-6 Mixing Oil. Apply to the feet, abdomen, back, face and neck.

Pregnancy and Delivery: Use for massage throughout entire pregnancy for relieving stress and anxiety, and to prevent scarring and create a calm and peaceful feeling. Massage on the perineum to help it stretch for easier birthing.

Fragrant Influence: Relaxing, calming, creating memories of childhood.

Frequency: Approximately 152 MHz.

Grounding

This blend helps stabilize and ground us in order to deal logically with reality in a peaceful manner. When we're hurting emotionally we sometimes wish to leave this physical existence. When this happens, it is easy to make choices that lead to unfortunate circumstances, such as bad relationships and bad business decisions. We escape because we do not have anchoring or awareness to know how to deal with the emotions.

Contains:

Spruce *(Picea mariana)* helps to open and release emotional blocks, bringing about a feeling of balance and grounding. Traditionally, spruce oil was believed to possess the frequency of prosperity.

Fir *(Abies alba)* creates a feeling of grounding, anchoring and empowerment.

Ylang Ylang *(Cananga odorata)* helps bring about a sense of relaxation and it may help balance male and female energies. It balances equilibrium, restores confidence and self-love.

Pine *(Pinus sylvestris)* may help reduce stress, relieve anxiety, and energize the entire body.

Cedarwood *(Cedrus atlantica)* is high in sesquiterpenes which can stimulate the limbic part of the brain (the center of our emotions). This conifer oil has been used by North American Indians to enhance spiritual awareness and communication. It also may help stimulate the pineal gland, which releases melatonin.

Angelica *(Angelica archangelica)* helps to bring memories back to the point of origin before trauma or anger was experienced, helping us to release negative feelings.

Juniper berry *(Juniperus communis)* may work as a detoxifier and cleanser. It promotes improved nerve and kidney function. It is also beneficial for the skin reducing dermatitis, eczema and acne. It elevates spiritual awareness creating feelings of love and peace.

Safety Data: May be irritating to those with sensitive skin. Avoid eye contact. For accidental contact put any vegetable oil or cream in the eye and call your doctor if necessary. Never use water. Avoid exposure to direct sunlight for 3 to 6 hours after use.

Application: Diffuse, wear on back of neck and on temples.

Fragrant Influence: Creates a feeling of solidity and balance.

Frequency: Approximately 140 MHz.

Harmony

This is an exquisite blend of 12 oils promoting physical and emotional healing by bringing about a harmonic balance to the energy centers of the body, allowing the energy to flow more efficiently through the body. It is also beneficial in reducing stress and creating a general overall feeling of well-being. Harmony has also been found to stop allergy attacks and symptoms.

Contains:

Hyssop *(Hyssopus officinalis)* is very balancing for emotions.

Spruce *(Picea mariana)* helps to open and release emotional blocks, bringing about a feeling of balance and grounding. Traditionally, spruce oil was believed to possess the frequency of prosperity.

Lavender *(Lavandula angustifolia)* has sedative and calming properties that help overcome insomnia, headaches, stress, and nervous tension.

Geranium *(Pelargonium graveolens)* stimulates nerves and assists in balancing hormones. Its aromatic influence helps release negative memories, thereby opening and elevating the mind.

Frankincense *(Boswellia carteri)* is considered the "holy anointing oil" in the Middle East and has been used in religious ceremonies for thousands of years. High in sesquiterpenes, it helps stimulate the limbic part of the brain, which elevates the mind, helping to overcome stress and despair. It is used in European medicine to combat depression.

Ylang Ylang *(Cananga odorata)* helps bring about a sense of relaxation and may help balance male and female energies. It balances equilibrium and restores confidence and self-love.

Sandalwood *(Santalum album)* is high in sesquiterpenes, which have been researched for their ability to stimulate the pineal gland and the limbic region of the brain, the center of our emotions. The pineal gland is responsible for releasing melatonin, a hormone that enhances deep sleep. Used traditionally for skin revitalization, yoga, and meditation, sandalwood is similar to frankincense oil in its support of nerves and circulation.

Angelica *(Angelica archangelica)* helps to bring memories back to the point of origin before trauma or anger was experienced, helping us to release negative feelings.

Rose *(Rosa damascena)* possesses the highest frequency of the oils. It creates a sense of balance, harmony, and well-being and elevates the mind. It promotes healthy skin, reduces scarring, and may help with chronic bronchitis, asthma, tuberculosis, sexual disabilities, frigidity, impotency, skin disease, ulcers, sprains, wrinkles, thrush, and gingivitis. It is also promotes healthy skin.

Orange *(Citrus aurantium)* was believed to bring joy, peace, and happiness to those who possessed it. It contains limonene, an antiviral compound, and citral, an antibacterial compound. It prevents the growth of bacterial. It is elevating to the mind and body and bringing joy and peace. It has been recognized to help a dull, oily complexion.

Safety Data: May be irritating to those with sensitive skin. Avoid eye contact. For accidental contact put any vegetable oil or cream in the eye and call your doctor if necessary. Never use water. Avoid exposure to direct sunlight for 3 to 6 hours after use.

Application: Diffuse, wear on ears, feet, over the heart, on areas of poor circulation, and over or around the energy centers of the body. Wear it as a perfume or cologne or aftershave. If there is an irritation or allergic reaction to any oil or blend, the following may help: Rub a few drops of Harmony over the thymus with one hand and hold the other hand over the navel for about one minute. For allergies, rub three drops on sternum, breathing deeply.

Fragrant Influence: Uplifting and elevating to the mind creating a happy, positive attitude.

Frequency: Approximately 101 MHz.

Hope

Everyone needs hope in order to go forward in life. Hopelessness can cause a loss of vision of goals and dreams. This blend helps to reconnect with a feeling of strength and grounding, restoring hope for tomorrow and helping us to go forward. It may help overcome suicidal depression.

Contains:

Melissa *(Melissa officinalis)* is a powerful, antimicrobial oil, yet it is very gentle and delicate because of the nature of the plant, and helps to bring out those characteristics within the individual. It is calming and balancing to the emotions. Melissa is one of the highest in sesquiterpenes, much like cedarwood. It is very stimulating to the anterior pituitary and immune system.

Spruce *(Picea mariana)* helps to open and release emotional blocks, bringing about a feeling of balance and grounding. Traditionally, spruce oil was believed to possess the frequency of prosperity. Spruce is anti-infectious, antiseptic, and anti-inflammatory.

Juniper berry *(Juniperus communis)* may work as a detoxifier, cleanser and promotes improved nerve and kidney function. It is also beneficial for the skin reducing dermatitis, eczema and acne. It elevates spiritual awareness creating feelings of love and peace.

Myrrh *(Commiphora myrrha)* is referenced throughout the Old and New Testaments constituting a part of a holy anointing formula given Moses (Exodus 30:22-27). It has one of the highest levels of sesquiterpenes, a class of compounds that can stimulate the hypothalamus, pituitary, and amygdala, the control center for emotions and hormone in the brain. It has been used in eastern countries to enhance the feeling of spirituality or euphoria.

Carrier Oil: Almond oil.

Safety Data: May be irritating to those with sensitive skin. Avoid eye contact. For accidental contact put any vegetable oil or cream in the eye and call your doctor if necessary. Never use water. Avoid exposure to direct sunlight for 3 to 6 hours after use.

Application: Diffuse, massage 1 or 2 drops on outer edge of ears. Apply to wrists, neck, or wear as a perfume or cologne.

Fragrant Influence: A feeling of peace and security and the ability to live life.

Frequency: Approximately 98 MHz.

Note: A lady in Arkansas for whom a diagnosis could not be found was given the oil of melissa. She responded quickly and said that melissa "gave her hope." This blend was name after that experience because it contains the oil of melissa.

127

Humility

Having humility and forgiveness helps us to heal ourselves and our earth (Chronicles 7:14). Humility is an integral ingredient in having forgiveness and seeking a closer relationship with God. Through its frequency and fragrance, you may find that special place where your own healing may begin.

Contains:

Frankincense *(Boswellia carteri)* is considered the "holy anointing oil" in the Middle East and has been used in religious ceremonies for thousands of years. High in sesquiterpenes, it helps stimulate the pineal gland, which secretes melatonin. It also helps to overcome stress and despair, and is used in European medicine to combat depression.

Rose *(Rosa damascena)* possesses the highest frequency of the oils. It creates a sense of balance, harmony, and well-being and elevates the mind. It promotes healthy skin, reduces scarring, and may help with chronic bronchitis, asthma, tuberculosis, sexual disabilities, frigidity, impotency, skin disease, ulcers, sprains, wrinkles, thrush, and gingivitis. It is also promotes healthy skin.

Rosewood *(Aniba rosaeodora)* is soothing and nourishing to the skin. It has been researched at Weber State University for its inhibition rate against gram positive and gram negative bacterial growth. This oil is soothing, creates elasticity, and helps the skin rid itself of irritations and problems, such as candida. It is antiinfectious, antibacterial, antifungal, antiviral, and antiparasitic.

Ylang Ylang *(Cananga odorata)* helps bring about a sense of relaxation and may help balance male and female energies. It balances equilibrium and restores confidence and self-love.

Geranium *(Pelargonium graveolens)* stimulates nerves and assists in balancing hormones. Its aromatic influence helps release negative memories, thereby opening and elevating the mind.

Melissa *(Melissa officinalis)* is a powerful, antimicrobial oil, yet it is very gentle and delicate because of the nature of the plant, and helps to bring out those characteristics within the individual. It is calming and balancing to the emotions. Melissa is one of the highest in sesquiterpenes, much like cedarwood. It is very stimulating to the anterior pituitary and immune system.

Spikenard *(Nardostachys jatamansi)* was highly prized at the time of Christ and was used by Mary of Bethany to anoint the feet of Jesus. High in sesquiterpenes, it is very supporting to the immune system. It strengthens and calms the cardiovascular system, stimulates under active ovaries, and helps with tachycardia, anemia, psoriasis and hemorrhoids.

Myrrh *(Commiphora myrrha)* is referenced throughout the Old and New Testaments constituting a part of a holy anointing formula given Moses (Exodus 30:22-27). It has one of the highest levels of sesquiterpenes, a class of compounds that can stimulate the hypothalamus, pituitary, and amygdala, the control center for emotions and hormone release in the brain. It has been used in eastern countries to enhance the feeling of spirituality or euphoria.

Neroli *(Citrus aurantium)* has been highly regarded by the Egyptian people for its great attributes of healing and calming the mind, body and spirit. It is stabilizing and strengthening to the emotions, promoting peace, confidence and awareness, thereby bringing everything into focus at the moment.

Carrier Oil: Sesame seed oil.

Application: Diffuse, rub over the heart, on neck, temples, or as needed.

Companion Oils: Inspiration, Inner Child, Peace & Calming, Envision, Acceptance, Forgiveness.

Safety Data: May be irritating to those with sensitive skin. Avoid eye contact. For accidental contact put any vegetable oil or cream in the eye and call your doctor if necessary. Never use water. Avoid exposure to direct sunlight for 3 to 6 hours after use.

Fragrant Influence: Peaceful healing.

Frequency: Approximately 88 MHz.

ImmuPower

This is a powerful blend for building, strengthening and protecting the body and supporting its defense mechanism. Diffusing protects the home environment especially during the seasons of cold and flu. ImmuPower has been found to reverse symptoms of lupus and inner ear infections.

Contains:

Cistus or **Labdanum** (*Cistus ladaniferus*) also known as "rock rose," has been studied for its effects on cell regeneration. It is anti-infectious, antiviral, antibacterial, and prevents hemorrhaging and scarring. It is a tonic to the parasympathetic nervous system and may help with viral problems and auto-immune disorders, such as rheumatoid arthritis.

Frankincense (*Boswellia carteri*) is considered the "holy anointing oil" in the Middle East and has been used in religious ceremonies for thousands of years. High in sesquiterpenes, it helps stimulate the hypothalamus which can lead to heightened immune function. It is being researched and used therapeutically in European hospitals to build immunity and treat cancer. In ancient times, it was well-known for its healing powers, and "was used to treat every conceivable ill known to man."

Oregano (*Origanum compactum*) is one of the most powerful antimicrobial essential oils. Laboratory research as Weber State University showed it to have a 99% kill rate against in vitro colonies of *Streptococcus pneumoniae*, a microorganism responsible for many kinds of lung and throat infections. This oil is antiviral, antibacterial, antifungal and antiparasitic.

Idaho **Tansy** (*Tanacetum vulgare*) is antiviral, anti-infectious, antibacterial, and fights cold and flu and infections. According to E. Joseph Montagna's PDR on herbal formulas, tansy may improve weakness of the kidneys, heart, joints, digestive system, and may help tone the entire system.

Black Cumin (*Cuminum cyminum*), commonly found in Egypt, helps with digestion and supports the immune system. It is antiseptic, antispasmodic, and carminative.

Clove (*Syzygium aromaticum*) was another oil from the Orient haled as an oil of great abundance; those who possessed it were considered wealthy. This oil is one of the most antimicrobial and antiseptic of all essential oils. It is antifungal, antiviral, anti-infectious, and antibacterial. It works as a general stimulant and is used to treat sinusitis, bronchitis, cystitis, and cholera.

Hyssop (*Hyssopus officinalis*) has anti-inflammatory and antiviral properties and is antiparasitic, mucolytic, decongestant, antiasthmatic, and anti-infectious.

Ravensara (*Ravensara aromatica*) is referred to by the people of Madagascar as "the oil that heals." It is antiseptic, anti-infectious, antiviral, antibacterial, antifungal, expectorant and supporting to the nerves. Similar to clove and nutmeg, it may help aid the respiratory system and support the adrenal glands. It has shown to help with flu, sinusitis, bronchitis, viral hepatitis, cholera, herpes, infectious mononucleosis, insomnia, muscle fatigue and rhinopharyngitis.

Mountain Savory (*Satureja montana*) is antimicrobial and immune stimulating. It is antiviral, antibacterial, antifungal, antiparasitic, and a general tonic for the body.

Safety Data: May be irritating to those with sensitive skin. Avoid eye contact. For accidental contact, put any vegetable oil or cream in the eye and call your doctor if necessary. Never use water. Avoid exposure to direct sunlight for 3 to 6 hours after use.

Application: Diffuse daily for 15 to 30 minutes every 3 or 4 hours or as needed. Massage on bottom of feet and use in Raindrop application along the spine is needed. It may be necessary to dilute with V-6 Mixing Oil as this blend may be too warming to the skin. May also be rubbed on throat and chest. Apply 2 to 3 drops on thymus. Put 1 to 2 drops on a piece of cotton and place in the ear for earaches.

Companion Oils: Alternate with Thieves and Exodus II. Other single oils may be added for extra strength: Rosewood, Melissa, Oregano, Clove, Cistus, Frankincense, and Mountain Savory.

Companion Supplements: ImmuneTune (capsule), Exodus (capsule) Radex (tablet), Super C (tablet), ImmuGel (liquid taken through mouth to coat lining of throat), Megazyme (to help digest toxic waste), and ComforTone (to cleanse colon).

Frequency: Approximately 89 MHz.

Inner Child

This is created for those suffering from abuse. When children have been abused and misused, they become disconnected from their inner child, or identity, which causes confusion. This can contribute to multiple personalities. Sometimes these problems do not manifest themselves until early- to mid-adult years, often labeled as a mid-life crisis. This fragrance may stimulate memory response and help one reconnect with the inner-self or one's identity. This is one of the first steps to finding emotional balance.

Contains:

Orange *(Citrus sinesis)* was believed to bring joy, peace, and happiness to those who possessed it. It contains limonene, an antiviral compound, and citral, an antibacterial compound. It prevents the growth of bacterial. It is elevating to the mind and body and bringing joy and peace. It has been recognized to help a dull, oily complexion.

Tangerine *(Citrus nobilis)* contains esters and aldehydes that are sedating and calming, helping with anxiety and nervousness. It is anti-inflammatory, anticoagulant, may help decongest the lymphatic system and works as a diuretic.

Jasmine *(Jasminum officinale)* is beneficial for dry, greasy, irritated, or sensitive skin. It is used for muscle spasms, sprains, coughs, laryngitis, frigidity, depression and nervous exhaustion.

Ylang Ylang *(Cananga odorata)* helps bring about a sense of relaxation and may help balance male and female energies. It balances equilibrium and restores confidence and self-love.

Sandalwood *(Santalum album)* is high in sesquiterpenes, which have been researched for their ability to stimulate the pineal gland and the limbic region of the brain, the center of our emotions. The pineal gland is responsible for releasing melatonin, a hormone that enhances deep sleep. Used traditionally for skin revitalization, yoga, and meditation, sandalwood is similar to frankincense oil in its support of nerves and circulation.

Spruce *(Picea mariana)* helps to open and release emotional blocks, bringing about a feeling of balance and grounding. Traditionally, spruce oil was believed to possess the frequency of prosperity. Spruce is anti-infectious, antiseptic, and anti-inflammatory.

Lemongrass *(Cymbopogon flexuosus)* works well for purification. It is powerful in the regeneration of connective tissue. It is a vasodilator, anti-inflammatory, sedative and supportive to the digestive system. A study in *Phytotherapy Research* showed that this oil had strong antifungal properties when applied topically. It may also help increase the flow of oxygen and uplift the spirit.

Neroli *(Citrus aurantium)* has been highly regarded by the Egyptian people for its great attributes of healing and calming the mind, body and spirit. It is stabilizing and strengthening to the emotions, promoting peace, confidence and awareness. It brings everything into focus at the moment.

Safety Data: May be irritating to those with sensitive skin. Avoid eye contact. For accidental contact put any vegetable oil or cream in the eye and call your doctor if necessary. Never use water. Avoid exposure to direct sunlight for 3 to 6 hours after use.

Application: Apply around navel, chest, temples, and nose.

Companion Products: Citrus Fresh, Gentle Baby, Acceptance, Envision, Awaken, Surrender, Forgiveness.

Fragrant Influence: Calming to the nerves with a feeling of inner peace.

Frequency: Approximately 98 MHz.

Inspiration

This blend combines oils traditionally used by the Eastern and North American natives to increase spirituality, enhancing prayer and inner awareness. Inspiration brings us closer to our spiritual connection. It can also reverse bladder and kidney infections.

Contains:

Frankincense (*Boswellia carteri*) is considered the "holy anointing oil" in the Middle East and has been used in religious ceremonies for thousands of years. High in sesquiterpenes, it helps stimulate the limbic part of the brain, which elevates the mind, helping to overcome stress and despair. It is used in European medicine to combat depression.

Cedarwood (*Cedrus atlantica*) has calming and purifying properties. High in sesquiterpenes which can stimulate the limbic part of the brain (the center of our emotions), this conifer oil has been used by North American Indians to enhance spiritual awareness and communication. It also may help stimulate the pineal gland, which releases melatonin.

Spruce (*Picea mariana*) helps to open and release emotional blocks, bringing about a feeling of balance and grounding. Traditionally, spruce oil was believed to possess the frequency of prosperity. Spruce is anti-infectious, antiseptic, and anti-inflammatory.

Rosewood (*Aniba rosaeodora*) is soothing and nourishing to the skin. It has been researched at Weber State University for its inhibition rate against gram positive and gram negative bacterial growth. This oil is soothing, creates elasticity, and helps the skin rid itself of irritations and problems, such as candida. It is anti-infectious, antibacterial, antifungal, antiviral, and antiparasitic.

Sandalwood (*Santalum album*) is high in sesquiterpenes, which have been researched for their ability to stimulate the pineal gland and the limbic region of the brain, the center of our emotions. The pineal gland is responsible for releasing melatonin, a hormone that enhances deep sleep. Used traditionally for skin revitalization, yoga, and meditation, sandalwood is similar to frankincense oil in its support of nerves and circulation.

Myrtle (*Myrtus communis*) may help normalize hormonal imbalances of the thyroid and ovaries as well as balance an under-active thyroid. It may help the respiratory system with chronic coughs and tuberculosis. It is suitable to use for coughs and chest complaints with children, and may support immune function infighting cold, flu and infectious disease.

Mugwort (*Artemisia vulgaris*)

Safety Data: May be irritating to those with sensitive skin. Avoid eye contact. In case of accidental contact, put any vegetable oil or cream in the eye and call your doctor if necessary. Never use water. Avoid exposure to direct sunlight for 3 to 6 hours after use.

Application: Diffuse during times of meditation and prayer, put 2 or 3 drops on a cotton ball and put in car vent, wear on back of neck, sides of forehead, crown of head, bottom of feet, or along spine.

Companion Products: Humility, Surrender, Acceptance, Forgiveness, 3 Wise Men.

Fragrant Influence: A feeling of being wrapped in a cocoon of spiritual quietness.

Frequency: Approximately 141 MHz.

Into the Future

This helps one leave the past behind in order to go forward with vision and excitement. So many times we find ourselves settling for mediocrity and sacrificing our own potential and success because of the fear of the unknown and the future. This blend was formulated to allow determination and a pioneering spirit come through and to support the emotions in helping us create the feeling of moving forward. Living on the edge with tenacity and integrity brings the excitement of the challenge and the joy of success.

Contains:

Frankincense (*Boswellia carteri*) is considered the "holy anointing oil" in the Middle East and has been used in religious ceremonies for thousands of years. High in sesquiterpenes, it helps stimulate the limbic part of the brain, which elevates the mind, helping to overcome stress and despair. It is used in European medicine to combat depression.

Clary Sage *(Salvia sclarea)* regulates the cells and balances the hormones. It contains natural sclareol, a phytoestrogen that mimics estrogen function. It may help with menstrual cramps, PMS, and pre-menopause symptoms and may help with circulatory problems.

Jasmine *(Jasminum officinale)* is beneficial for dry, greasy, irritated, or sensitive skin. It is used for muscle spasms, sprains, coughs, laryngitis, frigidity, depression, and nervous exhaustion.

Juniper berry *(Juniperus communis)* may work as a detoxifier, cleanser and promotes improved nerve and kidney function. It is also beneficial for the skin, reducing dermatitis, eczema and acne. It elevates spiritual awareness creating feelings of love and peace.

Fir *(Abies alba)* is antimicrobial. It has been researched for its ability to kill airborne germs and bacteria. It is antiseptic, antiarthritic, and stimulating. It supports the body and reduces the symptoms of arthritis, rheumatism bronchitis, coughs, sinusitis, cold, flu, and fevers. As a conifer oil, it creates a feeling of grounding, anchoring, and empowerment.

Orange *(Citrus sinesis)* was believed to bring joy, peace, and happiness to those who possessed it. It contains limonene, an antiviral compound, and citral, an antibacterial compound. It prevents the growth of bacterial. It is elevating to the mind and body and brings joy and peace. It has been recognized to help a dull, oily complexion.

Cedarwood *(Cedrus atlantica)* has calming and purifying properties. High in sesquiterpenes which can stimulate the limbic part of the brain (the center of our emotions), this conifer oil has been used by North American Indians to enhance spiritual awareness and communication. It also may help stimulate the pineal gland, which releases melatonin.

Ylang Ylang *(Cananga odorata)* helps bring about a sense of relaxation and may help balance male and female energies. It balances equilibrium and restores confidence and self-love.

Idaho Tansy *(Tanacetum vulgare)* is antiviral, anti-infectious, antibacterial, and fights colds, flu and infections. According to E. Joseph Montagna's PDR on herbal formulas, tansy may help skin problems, strengthen the kidneys, heart, joints, digestive system.

Carrier Oil: Almond oil.

Safety Data: May be irritating to those with sensitive skin. Avoid eye contact. For accidental contact, put any vegetable oil or cream in the eye and call your doctor if necessary. Never use water. Avoid exposure to direct sunlight for 3 to 6 hours after use.

Application: Diffuse, put in bath water, over the heart, on wrists, neck, as a compress, and dilute with V-6 Mixing Oil for full body massage.

Companion Products: Envision, Awaken, Passion, Magnify Your Purpose, Clarity, Dream Catcher, Inspiration.

Fragrant Influence: A strong emotional feeling of being able to reach one's potential.

Frequency: Approximately 88 MHz.

Joy

Joy is an exotic blend that produces a magnetic energy to enhance the frequency of self-love and bring joy to the heart. It inspires romance and may help overcome grief and depression.

Contains:

Rose *(Rosa damascena)* possesses the highest frequency of the oils. It creates a sense of balance, harmony, and well-being and elevates the mind. It promotes healthy skin, reduces scarring, and may help with chronic bronchitis, asthma, tuberculosis, sexual disabilities, frigidity, impotency, skin disease, ulcers, sprains, wrinkles, thrush, and gingivitis. It is also promotes healthy skin.

Bergamot *(Citrus bergamia)* has been used in the Middle East for hundreds of years for acne, boils, cold sores, eczema, insect bites, psoriasis, scabies, spot varicose veins, ulcers, sore throat, thrush, oily complexion, infectious disease, and depression. It balances hormones calming the emotions relieving anxiety, stress, and tension.

Mandarin *(Citrus reticulata)* is appealing, gentle, and promotes happiness. Diffuse or apply topically, especially around meals and before sleep. Because of its sedative and slightly hypnotic properties, it may help with insomnia and is good for stress and irritability. It is antispasmodic, antiseptic, antifungal, supports hepatic duct function, and works as a digestive tonic.

Ylang Ylang *(Cananga odorata)* helps bring about a sense of relaxation and may help balance male and female energies. It balances equilibrium and restores confidence and self-love.

Lemon *(Citrus limon)* has antiseptic-like properties and contains compounds that have been studied for their effects on immune function. It has a vitamin P-like action, increasing microcirculation, which may improve vision. It may serve as an insect repellent and may be beneficial for the skin. It has been found to promote leukocyte formation, dissolve cellulite, increase lymphatic function, and promote a sense of well-being. Its fragrance is stimulating and invigorating.

Safety Data: May be irritating to those with sensitive skin. Avoid eye contact. For accidental contact, put any vegetable oil or cream in the eye and call your doctor if necessary. Never use water. Avoid exposure to direct sunlight for 3 to 6 hours after use.

Application: Diffuse, use as a perfume or cologne, apply over heart, thymus, temples, and wrists. Add to bath water or put a few drops in Pharaoh or Rawhide Aftershave. Dilute with V-6 Mixing Oil for a full body massage. Put two drops on a wet cloth and put in the dryer for fragrancing.

Companion Products: Hope, Valor, Motivation, Passion, Clarity, Magnify Your Purpose.

Fragrant Influence: Feelings of self-love and confidence.

Frequency: Approximately 188 MHz.

JuvaFlex

These oils have been known to support liver and lymphatic system detoxification as well as support digestion. Anger and hate are stored in the liver, creating toxicity leading to sickness and disease.

JuvaFlex supports breaking addictions such as coffee, alcohol, drugs, and tobacco.

Contains:

Geranium *(Pelargonium graveolens)* helps improve the flow of bile to and from the liver. It is antispasmodic, antibacterial, antifungal and supports the liver, pancreas, and kidneys.

Rosemary *(Rosmarinus officinalis)* is antiseptic and antimicrobial and may be beneficial for skin conditions and dandruff. It may help fight candida and is anti-infectious, antispasmodic, balances the endocrine system, and is an expectorant. It helps overcome mental fatigue stimulating memory and opening the conscious mind.

Roman Chamomile *(Chamaemelum nobile)* may calm and relieve restlessness, tension, insomnia, muscle tension, cuts, scrapes, bruises and is anti-infectious. It may relieve allergies and expel toxins from the liver. It is used extensively in Europe for the skin.

Fennel *(Foeniculum vulgare)* is antiseptic and stimulating to the circulatory and respiratory systems. It is antispasmodic, antiseptic, and stimulating to the cardiovascular and respiratory systems. With its hormone-like activity, it may help facilitate childbirth and increase lactation after birthing.

Helichrysum *(Helichrysum italicum)* has been researched in Europe for regenerating tissue and nerves and improving circulation. It is anticoagulant, prevents phlebitis, helps regulate cholesterol, stimulates liver cell function, and may help to clean plaque and debris from the veins and arteries. It is mucolytic, expectorant, antispasmodic, and reduces scarring and discoloration. It may also stimulate nerve endings and improve conditions such as hearing loss. It may help release feelings of anger promoting forgiveness.

Blue Tansy *(Tanacetum annuum)* may help cleanse the liver and calm the lymphatic system, helping one to overcome anger and negative emotions promoting a feeling of self-control. Its primary constituents are limonene and sesquiterpenes. European research shows that it works as an antihistamine, anti-inflammatory, and stimulant for the thymus gland reducing dermatitis, arthritis, sciatica, tuberculosis, and allergies.

Carrier Oil: Sesame seed oil.

Safety Data: May be irritating to those with sensitive skin. Avoid eye contact. In case of accidental contact, put any vegetable oil or cream in the eye and call your doctor if necessary. Never use water. Avoid exposure to direct sunlight for 3 to 6 hours after use.

Application: Apply over liver neat or use a hot compress. Massage the Vita Flex points on the feet or use Raindrop technique on the spine and dilute with V-6 Mixing Oil.

Companion Oils: Di-Tone

Companion Supplements: JuvaTone (tablet) and ComforTone (capsule) together for maximum results. However, these two supplements are best taken an hour apart from each other to avoid too much cleansing at the same time. Add Megazyme to digest toxic waste.

Frequency: Approximately 82 MHz.

Magnify Your Purpose

The oils in this blend were specifically chosen to stimulate the endocrine system, creating energy flow to the brain that activates the right hemisphere of creativity, desire, motivation, and focus. These areas are the ones required to bring about commitment to purpose, and magnify your desire and pure intentions until they become reality.

Contains:

Sandalwood (*Santalum album*) is high in sesquiterpenes, which have been researched for their ability to stimulate the pineal gland and the limbic region of the brain, the center of our emotions. The pineal gland is responsible for releasing melatonin, a hormone that enhances deep sleep. Used traditionally for skin revitalization, yoga, and meditation, sandalwood is similar to frankincense oil in its support of nerves and circulation.

Nutmeg (*Myristica fragrans*) has adrenal cortex-like activity, which helps support the adrenal glands for increased energy. It may help with difficulties related to circulation, aches and pains is muscles and joints related to stress, arthritis and gout. It may also help with digestive problems such as flatulence, indigestion, sluggish digestion, and nausea. It is antiseptic, antiparasitic, analgesic, and a neurotonic.

Patchouly (*Pogostemon cablin*) was used in India in ancient times as a trade commodity because of its earthy, musty fragrance and its ability to mask many different odors. East Indian people use it to fragrance their clothing and their homes because of its natural insecticidal and anti-infectious properties. Legends indicate that patchouly represented money and those who possessed it were considered to be wealthy. Patchouly is very beneficial for the skin and may help prevent wrinkles or chapped skin. It is a general tonic and stimulant and helps the digestive system. It is also antimicrobial, antiseptic, and helps relieve itching.

Rosewood (*Aniba rosaeodora*) is soothing and nourishing to the skin. It has been researched at Weber State University for its inhibition rate against gram positive and gram negative bacterial growth. This oil is soothing, creates elasticity, and helps the skin rid itself of irritations and problems, such as candida. It is anti-infectious, antibacterial, antifungal, antiviral, and antiparasitic.

Cinnamon Bark (*Cinnamomum verum*) is the oil of wealth from the Orient and part of the formula the Lord gave Moses (Exodus 30:22-27). Cinnamon oil is anti-infectious, antibacterial, antiparasitic, antiviral, and antifungal. Cinnamon oil was regarded by the emperors of China and India to have great value; their wealth was measured by the amount of oil they possessed. Traditionally, it was thought to have a frequency that attracted wealth and abundance. Physically, it has many attributes: (1) it is a powerful purifier (2) it is a powerful oxygenator, and (3) it enhances the action and the activity of other oils. Researchers, including J. C. Lapraz, M.D., found that viruses could not live in the presence of cinnamon oil.

Ginger (*Zingiber officinale*) is used for relief from motion sickness, arthritis, rheumatism, sprains, muscular aches and pains, congestion, coughs, sinusitis, sore throats, diarrhea, colic, indigestion, loss of appetite, fever, flu, chills, and infectious disease.

Sage *(Salvia officinalis)* has been used in Europe for skin conditions such as eczema, acne, dandruff and hair loss. It has been recognized for its benefits of strengthening the vital centers. It may help in relieving depression and mental fatigue. Sage contains sclareol, which stimulates the body to produce its own estrogen. It may nutritionally support the body during PMS and menopause. The Lakota Indians used it for purification and healing and to dispel negative emotions from denial and sexual abuse, as well as a complete body tonic for healing and strength.

Safety Data: May be irritating to those with sensitive skin. Avoid eye contact. In case of accidental contact, put any vegetable oil or cream in the eye and call your doctor if necessary. Never use water. Avoid exposure to direct sunlight for 3 to 6 hours after use.

Application: Diffuse, use as a perfume or cologne, apply over heart, thymus, temples, and wrists. Add to bath water or put a few drops in Pharaoh or Rawhide Aftershave. Dilute with V-6 Mixing Oil for a full body massage. Put two drops on a wet cloth and put in the dryer for fragrancing.

Companion Products: Into the Future, Gathering, Clarity, Passion, Sensation, Harmony.

Frequency: Approximately 99 MHz.

Melrose

This blend has antiseptic-like properties when used topically for cleansing cuts, scrapes, burns, rashes and bruised tissue. It may also help prevent growth of bacteria, fungus or infection. It is very strong in the regeneration of damaged tissue and helps fight infection and fungus. It is very beneficial for animals such as horses, dogs and cats in the same way it benefits humans.

Contains:

Melaleuca *(Melaleuca alternifolia* terpinene-4-ol) is antiseptic, anti-infectious, antibacterial, antifungal, antiviral, antiparasitic, antiseptic, anti-inflammatory, immune-stimulating, decongestant, neurotonic, and and protects against radiation.

Melaleuca *(Melaleuca quinquenervia)* has a hormone-like action for the testicles. It is anti-inflammatory to the respiratory system and urinary genital tract, tonic to digestive system, antihypertensive, anti-infectious, antiviral, antiparasitic, and antibacterial. It has been used by European doctors for liver and pancreas deficiencies in children, viral hepatitis, colitis, ulcers, rheumatoid arthritis, hypertension of the arteries, and eczema.

Rosemary *(Rosmarinus officinalis)* has been research for its antiseptic and antimicrobial properties. It may be beneficial for skin conditions and dandruff. It may help fight candida and is anti-infectious, antispasmodic, balances the endocrine system, and is an expectorant. It helps overcome mental fatigue stimulating memory and opening the conscious mind.

Clove *(Syzygium aromaticum)* was another oil from the Orient haled as an oil of great abundance; those who possessed it were considered wealthy. This oil is one of the most antimicrobial and antiseptic of all essential oils. It is antifungal, antiviral, anti-infectious, and antibacterial. It works as a general stimulant and is used to treat sinusitis, bronchitis, cystitis, and cholera.

Safety Data: May be irritating to those with sensitive skin. Avoid eye contact. In case of accidental contact, put any vegetable oil or cream in the eye and call your doctor if necessary. Never use water. Avoid exposure to direct sunlight for 3 to 6 hours after use.

Application: Diffuse to dispel odors, apply topically on areas where the skin is broken, including cuts, scrapes, burns, rashes and infection. Put 1 to 2 drops on a piece of cotton and place in the ear for earaches.

Companion Products: Rose Ointment (to keep wounds soft and promote healing),

Fragrant Influence: Dispels odors.

Frequency: Approximately 48 MHz.

Mister

This may help to decongest the prostate and promote greater hormonal balance. Some women have found it reduces hot flashes. It has been beneficial for both men and women. Generally, Mister is good for women age 30 and older and Dragon Time is for teenagers and young women.

Contains:

Yarrow *(Achillea millefolium)* is a decongestant of the prostate and balances hormones. It is anti-inflammatory, and reduces scarring. It also helps with nerve inflammation.

Sage *(Salvia officinalis)* has been used in Europe for skin conditions such as eczema, acne, dandruff and hair loss. It has been recognized for its benefits of strengthening the vital centers. It may help in relieving depression and mental fatigue. Sage contains sclareol, which stimulates the body to produce its own estrogen. It may nutritionally support the body during PMS and menopause. The Lakota Indians used it for purification and healing and to dispel negative emotions from denial and sexual abuse, as well as a complete body tonic for healing and strength.

Myrtle *(Myrtus communis)* may help normalize hormonal imbalances of the thyroid and ovaries. It may help the respiratory system with chronic coughs and tuberculosis. It is suitable to use for coughs and chest complaints with children, and may support immune function in fighting cold, flu and infectious disease.

Fennel *(Foeniculum vulgare)* is antiseptic and stimulating to the circulatory and respiratory systems. It is antispasmodic, antiseptic, and stimulating to the cardiovascular and respiratory systems. With its hormone-like activity, it may help facilitate childbirth and increase lactation after birthing.

Lavender *(Lavandula angustifolia)* is known as the universal oil because of its wide range of usage. It is antispasmodic, hypotensive, anti-inflammatory, anti-infectious, and anticoagulant. It relieves headaches and PMS symptoms.

Peppermint *(Mentha piperita)* is one of the oldest and most highly regarded herbs for soothing digestion. Jean Valnet, M.D., studied the effects of peppermint on the liver and respiratory systems. Daniel Penöel, M.D., reports that it may help to reduce fevers, candida, nausea, vomiting and strengthen the respiratory system. Adding peppermint oil to drinking water helps cool body temperature during hot weather.

Carrier Oil: Sesame seed oil.

Safety Data: May be irritating to those with sensitive skin. Avoid eye contact. For accidental contact, put any vegetable oil or cream in the eye and call your doctor if necessary. Never use water. Avoid exposure to direct sunlight for 3 to 6 hours after use.

Application: This blend is effective for both men and women. Apply to Vita Flex points on ankles. Massage over lower pelvis, apply as a hot compress. Use directly on areas of concern. May be used diluted on prostate.

Companion Oils: Dragon Time, Clary Sage, Sage.

Companion Supplements: EssPro 7 (cream), Femigen (capsule), Femalin (tincture), Estro tincture).

Frequency: Approximately 147 MHz.

Motivation

This has an electrical frequency, which may help enable one to overcome the feelings of fear and procrastination and help stimulate feelings of moving forward and accomplishing new things.

Contains:

Roman Chamomile *(Chamaemelum nobile)* may calm and relieve restlessness, tension, insomnia, muscle tension, cuts, scrapes, bruises and is anti-infectious. It may relieve allergies and expel toxins from the liver. It is used extensively in Europe for the skin.

Spruce *(Picea mariana)* helps to open and release emotional blocks, bringing about a feeling of balance and grounding. Traditionally, spruce oil was believed to possess the frequency of prosperity. Spruce is anti-infectious, antiseptic, and anti-inflammatory.

Ylang Ylang *(Cananga odorata)* helps bring about a sense of relaxation and may help balance male and female energies. It balances equilibrium and restores confidence and self-love.

Lavender *(Lavandula angustifolia)* is known as the universal oil because of its wide range of usage. It has sedative and calming properties that help overcome insomnia, tension, and stress.

Safety Data: May be irritating to those with sensitive skin. Avoid eye contact. For accidental contact, put any vegetable oil or cream in the eye and call your doctor if necessary. Never use water. Avoid exposure to direct sunlight for 3 to 6 hours after use.

Application: Diffuse, apply on ears, feet (big toe), on chest or the nap of the neck, behind ears, wrists, around navel, or as needed. May be worn as a perfume or cologne.

Fragrant Influence: Creates a feeling of action and accomplishment.

Frequency: Approximately 103 MHz.

M-Grain

This contains oils that were traditionally used to relieve headaches, nausea, depression and problems related to severe migraine headaches.

Contains:

Marjoram (*Origanum majorana*) is used for calming the respiratory system and soothing sore and aching muscles. Marjoram helps regenerate smooth muscle tissue, and also assists in relieving spasms and migraine headaches and calming the nerves. It is antimicrobial, anti-infectious, antibacterial, antiseptic and may work as a diuretic.

Lavender (*Lavandula angustifolia*) is relaxing and calming. helping to overcome insomnia, nervous tension, headaches, and stress. It is antispasmodic, hypotensive, anti-inflammatory, anti-infectious, and anticoagulant

Peppermint (*Mentha piperita*) is one of the oldest and most highly regarded herbs for soothing digestion. Jean Valnet, M.D., studied the effects of peppermint on the liver and respiratory systems. Other scientists have researched its effect on impaired taste and smell as well as improved concentration and mental accuracy. Alan Hirsch, M.D., studied its ability to directly affect the brain's satiety center, triggering a sensation of fullness after meals, which may help in weight loss by curbing the appetite. Daniel Penöél, M.D., reports that it may help to reduce fevers, candida, nausea, vomiting and strengthen the respiratory system. Adding peppermint oil to drinking water helps cool body temperature during hot weather.

Basil (*Ocimum basilicum*) can be relaxing to smooth muscles as well as those involuntary muscles of the heart and digestive system. It may sooth insect bites such as bees, wasps and spiders and may also help with snakebites. It has been found to alleviate mental fatigue, spasms, rhinitis and help when these is a loss of smell due to chronic nasal catarrh.

Roman Chamomile (*Chamaemelum nobile*) may calm and relieve restlessness, tension, insomnia, muscle tension, cuts, scrapes, bruises and is anti-infectious. It may relieve allergies and expel toxins from the liver. It is used extensively in Europe for the skin.

Helichrysum (*Helichrysum italicum*) has been researched in Europe for regenerating tissue and nerves and improving circulation. It is anticoagulant, prevents phlebitis, helps regulate cholesterol, stimulates liver cell function, and may help to clean plaque and debris from the veins and arteries. It is mucolytic, expectorant, antispasmodic, and reduces scarring and discoloration. It may also stimulate nerve endings and improve conditions such as hearing loss. It may help release feelings of anger promoting forgiveness.

Safety Data: May be irritating to those with sensitive skin. Avoid eye contact. In case of accidental contact, put any vegetable oil or cream in the eye and call your doctor if necessary. Never use water. Avoid exposure to direct sunlight for 3 to 6 hours after use.

Application: It is most effective when inhales. Place 2 drops in palm of hand and cup over nose and inhale. Massage along the brain stem. Apply on forehead, crown, shoulders, back of neck, temples and Vita Flex points on the feet.

Companion Oils: Aroma Siez, Clarity, PanAway.

Frequency: Approximately 72 MHz.

PanAway

This blend was created as a result of an injury whereby the ligaments in the leg were severely torn. It helps reduce inflammation, increasing circulation and healing thus reducing pain. Many people have had relief from arthritis symptoms, sports injuries, sprains, muscle spasms, bumps and bruises.

Contains:

Helichrysum *(Helichrysum italicum)* has been researched in Europe for regenerating tissue and nerves and improving circulation. It is anticoagulant, prevents phlebitis, helps regulate cholesterol, stimulates liver cell function, and may help to clean plaque and debris from the veins and arteries. It is mucolytic, expectorant, antispasmodic, and reduces scarring and discoloration. It may also stimulate nerve endings and improve conditions such as hearing loss. It may help release feelings of anger promoting forgiveness.

Birch *(Betula alleghaniensis)* contains 99% methyl salicylate that has a cortisone-like activity. It is beneficial for bone, muscle and joint discomfort. It has been helpful in decreasing pain from arthritis, tendonitis and rheumatism.

Clove *(Syzygium aromaticum)* was another oil from the Orient hailed as an oil of great abundance; those who possessed it were considered wealthy. This oil is one of the most antimicrobial and antiseptic of all essential oils. It is antifungal, antiviral, anti-infectious, and antibacterial. It works as a general stimulant and is used to treat sinusitis, bronchitis, cystitis, and cholera.

Peppermint *(Mentha piperita)* is one of the oldest and most highly regarded herbs for soothing digestion. Jean Valnet, M.D., studied the effects of peppermint on the liver and respiratory systems. Daniel Penöél, M.D., reports that it may help to reduce fevers, candida, nausea, vomiting and strengthen the respiratory system. Adding peppermint oil to drinking water helps cool body temperature during hot weather.

Safety Data: May be irritating to those with sensitive skin. Avoid eye contact. For accidental contact, put any vegetable oil or cream in the eye and call your doctor if necessary. Never use water. Avoid exposure to direct sunlight for 3 to 6 hours after use.

Application: Apply to bottom of the feet first working the Vita Flex points and then topically on location. Rub on temples, back of neck, forehead or use as a compress on back. Apply on location for sore muscles, cramps, bruises, or wherever it may hurts.

Companion Oils: Relieve It (deep tissue pain), Melrose, add helichrysum (to enhance), birch (bone pain), or use with Ortho Ease or Ortho Sport Massage Oil.

Frequency: Approximately 112 MHz.

Passion, Live With

One of the reasons people fail to be successful in business, work, or personal accomplishment, is due to a lack of passion. The oils in this blend stimulate a feeling of passion. It has often been said that the lack of passion is the creation of disease in the body. The feeling of passion overcomes depression, mood swings, and loss of drive. Live life with passion and make a difference in the world.

Contains:

Melissa *(Melissa officinalis)* is a powerful, antimicrobial oil, yet it is very gentle and delicate because of the nature of the plant, and helps to bring out those characteristics within the individual. It is calming and balancing to the emotions. Melissa is one of the highest in sesquiterpenes, much like cedarwood. It is very stimulating to the anterior pituitary and immune system.

Helichrysum *(Helichrysum italicum)* has been researched in Europe for regenerating tissue and nerves and improving circulation. It is anticoagulant, prevents phlebitis, helps regulate cholesterol, stimulates liver cell function, and may help to clean plaque and debris from the veins and arteries. It is mucolytic, expectorant, antispasmodic, and reduces scarring and discoloration. It may also stimulate nerve endings and improve conditions such as hearing loss. It may help release feelings of anger promoting forgiveness.

Clary Sage *(Salvia sclarea)* regulates the cells and balances the hormones. It contains natural sclareol, a phytoestrogen that mimics estrogen function. It may help with menstrual cramps, PMS, and pre-menopause symptoms and may help with circulatory problems.

Cedarwood *(Cedrus atlantica)* has calming and purifying properties. High in sesquiterpenes, which can stimulate the limbic part of the brain (the center of our emotions), this conifer oil has been used by North American Indians to enhance spiritual awareness and communication.

Angelica *(Angelica archangelica)* helps to bring memories back to the point of origin before trauma or anger was experienced, helping us to release negative feelings.

Ginger *(Zingiber officinale)* is used for relief from motion sickness, arthritis, rheumatism, sprains, muscular aches and pains, congestion, coughs, sinusitis, sore throats, diarrhea, colic, indigestion, loss of appetite, fever, flu, chills and infectious disease.

Neroli *(Citrus aurantium)* has been highly regarded by the Egyptian people for its great attributes of healing and calming the mind, body and spirit. It is stabilizing and strengthening to the emotions, promoting peace, confidence and awareness. It brings everything into focus at the moment.

Sandalwood *(Santalum album)* is high in sesquiterpenes, which have been researched for their ability to stimulate the pineal gland and the limbic region of the brain, the center of our emotions. Used traditionally for skin revitalization, yoga, and meditation, sandalwood is similar to frankincense oil in its support of nerves and circulation.

Patchouly *(Pogostemon cablin)* was used in India in ancient times as a trade commodity because of its earthy, musty fragrance and its ability to mask many different odors. Its fragrance reestablishes equilibrium while simultaneously quieting emotion and energizing the mind.

Jasmine *(Jasminum officinale)* exudes an exquisite fragrance that revitalizes spirits.

Safety Data: May be irritating to those with sensitive skin. Avoid eye contact. For accidental contact, put any vegetable oil or cream in the eye and call your doctor if necessary. Never use water. Avoid exposure to direct sunlight for 3 to 6 hours after use.

Application: Diffuse, use as a perfume or cologne, apply over heart, thymus, temples, and wrists. Add to bath water or put a few drops in Pharaoh or Rawhide Aftershave. Dilute with V-6 Mixing Oil for a full body massage. Put two drops on a wet cloth and put in the dryer for fragrancing.

Companion Oils: Acceptance, Motivation, Clarity, Gathering, Harmony, Inspiration, 3 Wise Men, Magnify Your Purpose.

Frequency: Approximately 89 MHz.

Peace & Calming

This gentle fragrance is specifically designed for diffusing. It promotes relaxation and a deep sense of peace, helping to dampen tensions and uplift spirits. When massaged on the bottom of the feet, it can be a wonderful prelude to a peaceful night's rest. It may calm overactive and hard-to-manage children. The oils in this blend have historically been used to help reduce depression, anxiety, stress, and insomnia. This blend along with Mineral Essence may be a healthy alternative to Ritalin.

Contains:

Blue Tansy *(Tanacetum annuum)* may help cleanse the liver and calm the lymphatic system, helping one to overcome anger and negative emotions promoting a feeling of self-control. It contains sesquiterpenes that can stimulate the pineal gland, which secretes the hormone melatinin.

Patchouly *(Pogostemon cablin)* was used in India in ancient times as a trade commodity because of its earthy, musty fragrance and its ability to mask many different odors. Its fragrance reestablishes equilibrium while simultaneously quieting emotion and energizing the mind.

Tangerine *(Citrus nobilis)* contains esters and aldehydes that are sedating and calming, helping with anxiety and nervousness.

Orange *(Citrus sinesis)* was believed to bring joy, peace, and happiness to those who possessed it. It is elevating to the mind and body.

Ylang Ylang (*Cananga odorata*) helps bring about a sense of relaxation and may help balance male and female energies. It balances equilibrium and inspires confidence and self-love.

Safety Data: May be irritating to those with sensitive skin. Avoid eye contact. In case of accidental contact, put any vegetable oil or cream in the eye and call your doctor if necessary. Never use water. Avoid exposure to direct sunlight for 3 to 6 hours after use.

Application: Diffuse, wear as a perfume, apply on bottom of the feet, on wrists, and outside of ears. Put in bath water. Dilute with V-6 Mixing Oil for a full body massage.

Companion Oils: Lavender (for insomnia), chamomile (for calming).

Fragrant Influence: A feeling of calming and emotional well-being.

Frequency: Approximately 105 MHz.

Present Time

This blend has an empowering fragrance, which gives a feeling of "being in the moment." Disease develops when we live in the past and with regret. One can only go forward and progress when in the present time.

Contains:

Neroli (*Citrus aurantium*) has been highly regarded for its ability to heal the mind, body, and spirit. It is stabilizing and strengthening to the emotions, promoting peace, confidence and awareness. It brings everything into focus at the moment.

Ylang Ylang (*Cananga odorata*) helps bring about a sense of relaxation and may help balance male and female energies. It balances equilibrium and restores confidence and self-love.

Spruce (*Picea mariana*) helps to open and release emotional blocks, bringing about a feeling of balance and grounding. Traditionally, spruce oil was believed to possess the frequency of prosperity.

Carrier Oil: Almond oil.

Safety Data: May be irritating to those with sensitive skin. Avoid eye contact. In case of accidental contact, put any vegetable oil or cream in the eye and call your doctor if necessary. Never use water. Avoid exposure to direct sunlight for 3 to 6 hours after use.

Application: Rub over the sternum and thymus area, neck and forehead. Add a few drops to Pharaoh and Rawhide as an aftershave.

Companion Oils: Harmony, Hope.

Frequency: Approximately 98 MHz.

Purification

This is an antiseptic blend formulated for diffusing to help purity the home and work environment. It cleanses the air and neutralizes mildew, cigarette smoke, and disagreeable odors. When applied directly to the skin, Purification may be used to cleanse cuts and scrapes and neutralize the poison of insect bites, such as spiders, bees, hornets, wasps, scorpions, and rattlesnakes.

Contains:

Citronella (*Cymbopogon nardus*) is antiseptic, antibacterial, antispasmodic, anti-inflammatory, insecticidal, antispasmodic, and soothing to the tissues.

Lemongrass (*Cymbopogon flexuosus*) has strong antifungal properties when applied topically.

Lavandin (*Lavandula* x *hybrida*) is an antifungal, an anti-bacterial, a strong antiseptic, and a tissue regenerator.

Rosemary (*Rosmarinus officinalis*) is antiseptic and antimicrobial and may be beneficial for skin conditions and dandruff. It may help fight candida and is anti-infectious and antispasmodic.

Melaleuca (*Melaleuca alternifolia* terpinene-4-ol) is antiseptic, anti-infectious, antibacterial, antifungal, antiviral, antiparasitic, antiseptic, anti-inflammatory, immune-stimulating, decongestant, neurotonic, and and protects against radiation.

Myrtle (*Myrtus communis*) is antibacterial and may support immune function infighting cold, flu and infectious disease.

Safety Data: May be irritating to those with sensitive skin. Avoid eye contact. In case of accidental contact, put any vegetable oil or cream in the eye and call your doctor if necessary. Never use water. Avoid exposure to direct sunlight for 3 to 6 hours after use.

Application: Diffuse 15 to 30 minutes every 3 to 4 hour. Apply topically to disinfect and cleanse. Put on cotton balls to place in air vents home, car, hotel room, office, enclosed areas, etc. Put on cotton balls in air vents for purifying and repelling insects at home or at work.

Companion Products: Melrose, Citrus Fresh, Thieves.

Frequency: Approximately 46 MHz.

Raven

This combination gives strength in fighting respiratory disease and infections; and may help alleviate symptoms of tuberculosis, asthma, and pneumonia.

Contains:

Ravensara *(Ravensara aromatica)* is referred to by the people of Madagascar as "the oil that heals." It is antiseptic, anti-infectious, antiviral, antibacterial, antifungal, expectorant and supporting to the nerves. Similar to clove and nutmeg, it may help aid the respiratory system. It has shown to help with flu, sinusitis, bronchitis, herpes, infectious mononucleosis, and rhinopharyngitis.

Eucalyptus *(Eucalyptus radiata)* may have a profound antiviral effect upon the respiratory system. It may also help reduce inflammation of the nasal mucous membrane.

Peppermint *(Mentha piperita)* is useful for many kinds of respiratory conditions, including bronchitis and pneumonia. High in menthol and menthone, it helps suppress coughs and clear lung and nasal congestion.

Birch *(Betula alleghaniensis)* contains 99% methyl salicylate that has a cortisone-like activity.

Lemon *(Citrus limon)* has antiseptic-like properties and contains compounds that have been studied for their effects on immune function. It has a vitamin P-like action, increasing microcirculation.

Safety Data: May be irritating to those with sensitive skin. Avoid eye contact. In case of accidental contact, put any vegetable oil or cream in the eye and call your doctor if necessary. Never use water. Avoid exposure to direct sunlight for 3 to 6 hours after use.

Application: Diffuse, massage on Vita Flex points on the feet. Apply topically over throat and lung area. Put on pillow at night. Use in a suppository with V-6 Mixing Oil and retain during the night. With this method, the benefits go directly to the lungs in seconds.

Companion Oils: R.C., Thieves, Melrose.

Frequency: Approximately 70 MHz.

R.C.

This blend was formulated to help give relief from colds, bronchitis, sore throats, sinusitis and respiratory congestion. Diffusing may help decongest and relieve allergy-type symptoms, such as coughs and sore throats. It has also been reported to help dissolve bone spurs.

Contains:

Eucalyptus *(Eucalyptus globulus)* has shown to be a powerful antimicrobial agent containing a high percentage of eucalyptol (a key ingredient in many antiseptic mouth rinses.) It is expectorant, mucolytic, antimicrobial, antibacterial, antifungal, antiviral, and antiseptic. It helps reduce infections with the throat and lungs, such as rhinopharyngitis, laryngitis, flu, sinusitis, bronchitis, bronchial asthma, bronchial pneumonia.

Eucalyptus *(Eucalyptus radiata)* is anti-infectious, antibacterial, antiviral, expectorant, and anti-inflammatory. It has strong action against bronchitis and sinusitis.

Eucalyptus *(Eucalyptus australiana)* is antiviral, antibacterial, and antifungal.

Eucalyptus *(Eucalyptus citriodora)* helps decongest and disinfect the sinuses and lungs. It is anti-inflammatory, anti-infectious, and mildly antispasmodic.

Myrtle *(Myrtus communis)* supports the respiratory system and help treat chronic coughs and tuberculosis. It is suitable to use for coughs and chest complaints with children.

Pine *(Pinus sylvestris)* opens and disinfects the respiratory system, particularly the bronchial tract. It has been used since the time of Hippocrates to support respiratory function and fight infection. According to Daniel Penoël, M.D., it is one of the best oils for bronchitis and pneumonia.

Spruce *(Picea mariana)* helps the respiratory and nervous systems. It is anti-infectious, antiseptic, and anti-inflammatory.

Marjoram *(Origanum majorana)* supports the respiratory system and reduces spasms. It is antimicrobial, anti-infectious, antibacterial, antiseptic and may work as a diuretic.

Lavender *(Lavandula angustifolia)* is antispasmodic, hypotensive, anti-inflammatory, and anti-infectious. It prevents scarring, stretch marks and relieves headaches and PMS symptoms.

Cypress *(Cupressus sempervirens)* promotes blood circulation and lymph flow. It is anti-infectious, antibacterial, antimicrobial, mucolytic, and antiseptic, refreshing and relaxing.

Peppermint *(Mentha piperita)* is one of the oldest and most highly regarded herbs for soothing digestion. Jean Valnet, M.D., studied the effects of peppermint on the liver and respiratory systems. Other scientists have researched its effect on impaired taste and smell as well as improved concentration and mental accuracy. Daniel Penoël, M.D., reports that it may help to reduce fevers, candida, nausea, vomiting and strengthen the respiratory system. Adding peppermint oil to drinking water helps cool body temperature during hot weather.

Safety Data: May be irritating to those with sensitive skin. Avoid eye contact. In case of accidental contact, put any vegetable oil or cream in the eye and call your doctor if necessary. Never use water. Avoid exposure to direct sunlight for 3 to 6 hours after use.

Application: Diffuse, apply on chest, neck, ears, bottom of feet, and may be used in a humidifier. Dilute with V-6 Mixing Oil and massage on chest and back and Vita Flex points on the body. Use as a hot compress. Put on sinuses or up nasal passages with a cotton swab. Rub around ears and on feet, neck and throat. May help with headache with just deep breathing. Run hot, steaming water in sink, put Raven, R.C., or birch in water, put towel over head, and inhale to open sinuses. May help relieve difficulties breathing related to flu, colds and pneumonia.

Companion Oils: Raven (alternating morning and night), Thieves.

Fragrant Influence: R.C. is very beneficial in the diffuser to decongest and relieve allergy-type symptoms such as coughs, sore throat, and lung congestion.

Frequency: Approximately 75 MHz

Release

This oil may stimulate a sense of harmony and balance within the mind and body, and help release anger and memory trauma from the cells of the liver bring about a sense of peace and emotional well-being. Letting go of negative emotions and releasing frustration enables one to progress in a positive way.

Contains:

Ylang Ylang *(Cananga odorata)* helps bring about a sense of relaxation and may help balance male and female energies. It balances equilibrium and restores confidence and self-love.

Lavandin *(Lavandula* x *hybrida)* is an anti-fungal, an anti-bacterial, a strong antiseptic, and a tissue regenerator.

Geranium *(Pelargonium graveolens)* stimulates nerves and assists in balancing hormones. Its aromatic influence helps release negative memories, thereby opening and elevating the mind.

Sandalwood *(Santalum album)* is high in sesquiterpenes, which have been researched for their ability to stimulate the pineal gland and the limbic region of the brain, the center of our emotions. The pineal gland is responsible for releasing melatonin, a hormone that enhances deep sleep. Used traditionally for skin revitalization, yoga, and meditation, sandalwood is similar to frankincense oil in its support of nerves and circulation.

Blue Tansy (*Tanacetum annuum*) may help cleanse the liver and calm the lymphatic system helping one to overcome anger and negative emotions promoting a feeling of self-control. Its primary constituents are limonene and sesquiterpenes. European research shows that it works as an antihistamine, anti-inflammatory, and stimulant for the thymus gland reducing dermatitis, arthritis, sciatica, tuberculosis, and allergies.

Carrier Oil: Olive oil.

Safety Data: May be irritating to those with sensitive skin. Avoid eye contact. In case of accidental contact, put any vegetable oil or cream in the eye and call your doctor if necessary. Never use water. Avoid exposure to direct sunlight for 3 to 6 hours after use.

Application: Apply over liver or as a compress. Massage on bottom of feet and put behind ears. May be worn as a perfume or cologne.

Companion Oils: Valor, Harmony, and JuvaFlex on the feet.

Fragrant Influence: A feeling of being free and unburdened.

Frequency: Approximately 102 MHz.

Relieve It

This blend contains high anti-inflammatory action for the benefit of relieving deep tissue pain. It is calming to the nerves and alleviates skin and muscle soreness.

Contains:

Spruce (*Picea mariana*) helps the respiratory and nervous systems. High in terpenes, it is anti-infectious, antiseptic, and anti-inflammatory.

Pepper, Black (*Piper nigrum*) stimulates the endocrine system and increases energy while increasing cellular oxygenation. It is anti-inflammatory which may soothe deep tissue muscle aches. It has been traditionally used to treat rheumatoid arthritis.

Peppermint (*Mentha piperita*) is one of the oldest and most highly regarded herbs for soothing digestion. Jean Valnet, M.D., studied the effects of peppermint on the liver and respiratory systems. Daniel Penöél, M.D., reports that it may help to reduce fevers, candida, nausea, vomiting and strengthen the respiratory system. Adding peppermint to drinking water helps cool body temperature during hot weather.

Hyssop (*Hyssopus officinalis*) is anti-inflammatory and anti-infectious.

Safety Data: May be irritating to those with sensitive skin. Avoid eye contact. In case of accidental contact, put any vegetable oil or cream in the eye and call your doctor if necessary. Never use water. Avoid exposure to direct sunlight for 3 to 6 hours after use.

Application: Apply on location, anywhere there is pain.

Companion Oils: PanAway, Melrose, Aroma Siez, cypress, helichrysum.

Frequency: Approximately 56 MHz.

Sacred Mountain

This is a blend of oils extracted from the conifer trees representing the sacred feeling of the mountains. They bring about a feeling of protection, strength, grounding empowerment and security. It is antibacterial and soothing to the respiratory system.

Contains:

Spruce (*Picea mariana*) helps to open and release emotional blocks, bringing about a feeling of balance and grounding. Traditionally, spruce oil was believed to possess the frequency of prosperity. Spruce is anti-infectious, antiseptic, and anti-inflammatory.

Fir (*Abies alba*) has been researched for its ability to kill airborne germs and bacteria. As a conifer oil, it creates a feeling of grounding, anchoring and empowerment.

Cedarwood (*Cedrus atlantica*) has calming and purifying properties. High in sesquiterpenes which can stimulate the limbic part of the brain (the center of our emotions), this conifer oil has been used by North American Indians to enhance spiritual awareness and communication. It also may help stimulate the pineal gland, which releases melatonin.

Ylang Ylang *(Cananga odorata)* helps bring about a sense of relaxation and may help balance male and female energies. It balances equilibrium and restores confidence and self-love.

Safety Data: May be irritating to those with sensitive skin. Avoid eye contact. In case of accidental contact, put any vegetable oil or cream in the eye and call your doctor if necessary. Never use water. Avoid exposure to direct sunlight for 3 to 6 hours after use.

Application: Diffuse, put on crown of head, back of neck, behind ears, on thymus and wrists. Wear as a perfume or cologne.

Fragrant Influence: A feeling of strength, empowerment, grounding and protection.

Frequency: Approximately 176 MHz.

SARA

The blend produces a beautiful fragrance that may enable one to relax into a mental state whereby one may be able to release the trauma of Sexual And/or Ritual Abuse. SARA also helps unlock other traumatic experiences such as physical and emotional abuse.

Contains:

Geranium *(Pelargonium graveolens)* helps release negative memories, thereby opening and elevating the mind.

Lavender *(Lavandula angustifolia)* has sedative and calming properties that help overcome headaches, stress, and nervous tension.

Rose *(Rosa damascena)* possesses the highest frequency of the oils. It creates a sense of balance, harmony, and well-being and elevates the mind.

Blue Tansy *(Tanacetum annuum)* may help cleanse the liver and calm the lymphatic system helping one to overcome anger and negative emotions promoting a feeling of self-control. Its primary constituents are limonene and sesquiterpenes.

Orange *(Citrus sinesis)* was believed to bring joy, peace, and happiness to those who possessed it. It is elevating to the mind and body and bringing joy and peace.

Cedarwood *(Cedrus atlantica)* has calming and purifying properties. This conifer oil was used by North American Indians to enhance their spiritual awareness and communication. It may help stimulate the pineal gland which is responsible for releasing melatonin, a hormone associated with deep sleep.

Ylang Ylang *(Cananga odorata)* helps bring about a sense of relaxation and may help balance male and female energies. It balances equilibrium and restores confidence and self-love.

Carrier Oil: Almond oil.

Safety Data: May be irritating to those with sensitive skin. Avoid eye contact. In case of accidental contact, put any vegetable oil or cream in the eye and call your doctor if necessary. Never use water. Avoid exposure to direct sunlight for 3 to 6 hours after use.

Application: Apply over energy centers and areas of abuse, on Vita Flex points, navel, lower abdomen, temples and nose.

Companion Oils: Hope, Forgiveness, Valor, Inner Child, Trauma Life, White Angelica, Joy, Inspiration, Magnify Your Purpose, 3 Wise Men.

Fragrant Influence: Peace to the soul and freedom to go forward in life with joy.

Frequency: Approximately 102 MHz.

Sensation

This has a beautiful and romantic fragrance that is extremely uplifting, refreshing, and arousing. Sensation is also very nourishing and hydrating for the skin and is beneficial for various skin problems.

Contains:

Ylang Ylang *(Cananga odorata)* helps bring about a sense of relaxation and may help balance male and female energies. It balances equilibrium and restores confidence and self-love.

Rosewood (*Aniba rosaeodora*) is soothing and nourishing to the skin. It has been researched at Weber State University for its inhibition rate against gram positive and gram negative bacterial growth. This oil is soothing, creates elasticity, and helps the skin rid itself of irritations and problems, such as candida. It is anti-infectious, antibacterial, antifungal, antiviral, and antiparasitic.

Jasmine (*Jasminum officinale*) is beneficial for dry, greasy, irritated, or sensitive skin. It is used for muscle spasms, sprains, coughs, laryngitis, frigidity, depression and nervous exhaustion.

Safety Data: May be irritating to those with sensitive skin. Avoid eye contact. In case of accidental contact, put any vegetable oil or cream in the eye and call your doctor if necessary. Never use water. Avoid exposure to direct sunlight for 3 to 6 hours after use.

Application: Apply on location, use for massage, and add to Sensation Bath and Shower Gel. May also be used with a compress over the abdomen, or worn as a perfume or cologne.

Companion Oils: Passion, Into the Future, Joy, Dream Catcher, Awaken.

Fragrant Influence: Excitement of experiencing new heights of self-expression and awareness.

Frequency: Approximately 88 MHz.

Surrender

This blend is a combination of oils that may create the feeling of surrendering one's aggression, emotion, and controlling attitude. Stress and tension are released very quickly when we surrender our own will.

Contains:

Lavender (*Lavandula angustifolia*) has sedative and calming properties help overcome insomnia, headaches, stress, and nervous tension.

Roman Chamomile (*Chamaemelum nobile*) may calm and relieve restlessness, tension, insomnia, muscle tension, cuts, scrapes, bruises and is anti-infectious. It may relieve allergies and expel toxins from the liver. It is used extensively in Europe for the skin.

German Chamomile (*Matricaria recutita*) has been a highly respected oil for over 3,000 years and has been used for helping skin conditions, such as dermatitis, boils, acne, rashes, and eczema. It is also used for hair care, burns, cuts, toothaches, teething pains, inflamed joints, menopausal problems, insomnia, migraine headaches, and stress-related complaints. It has an electrical frequency that promotes peace and harmony bringing about a feeling of security.

Angelica (*Angelica archangelica*) helps to calm emotions and bring memories back to the point of origin before trauma or anger was experienced, helping us to let go of negative feelings.

Mountain Savory (*Satureja montana*) is antimicrobial and immune stimulating. It is antiviral, antibacterial, antifungal, antiparasitic, and a general tonic for the body.

Lemon (*Citrus limon*) has antiseptic-like properties and contains compounds that have been studied for their effects on immune function. It has a vitamin P-like action, increasing microcirculation, which may improve vision. It may serve as an insect repellent and may be beneficial for the skin. It has been found to promote leukocyte formation, dissolve cellulite, increase lymphatic function, and promote a sense of well-being. Its fragrance is stimulating and invigorating.

Spruce (*Picea mariana*) helps to open and release emotional blocks, bringing about a feeling of balance and grounding. Traditionally, spruce oil was believed to possess the frequency of prosperity. Spruce is anti-infectious, antiseptic, and anti-inflammatory.

Safety Data: May be irritating to those with sensitive skin. Avoid eye contact. In case of accidental contact, put any vegetable oil or cream in the eye and call your doctor if necessary. Never use water. Avoid exposure to direct sunlight for 3 to 6 hours after use.

Application: Diffuse. Apply on forehead, solar plexus, along the ear rim, on the chest and nape of the neck. Add 2-4 drops to warm bath water with or without Bath Gel Base.

Companion Oils: Peace & Calming, Forgiveness, Grounding, Sacred Mountain, Clarity.

Fragrant Influence: Let go of the need to control. Allow the need to be alone.

Frequency: Approximately 98 MHz.

Thieves

This blend was created from research about a group of 14th century thieves who rubbed oils on themselves to avoid contracting the plague while they robbed the bodies of the dead and dying. When apprehended, these thieves disclosed the formula of herbs, spices, and oils they used to protect themselves in exchange for more lenient punishment.

This blend of therapeutic-grade essential oils was tested at Weber State University for it potent antimicrobial properties. Thieves was found to have a 99.96% kill rate against airborne bacteria. The oils are highly antiviral, antiseptic, antibacterial, anti-infectious and help to protect the body against such illnesses as flu, colds, sinusitis, bronchitis, pneumonia, sore throats, cuts, etc.

Contains:

Clove *(Syzygium aromaticum)* was another oil from the Orient hailed as an oil of great abundance; those who possessed it were considered wealthy. This oil is one of the most antimicrobial and antiseptic of all essential oils. It is antifungal, antiviral, anti-infectious, and antibacterial. It works as a general stimulant and is used to treat sinusitis, bronchitis, cystitis, and cholera.

Lemon *(Citrus limon)* has antiseptic-like properties and contains compounds that have been studied for their effects on immune function. It has a vitamin P-like action, increasing microcirculation, which may improve vision. It may serve as an insect repellent and may be beneficial for the skin. It has been found to promote leukocyte formation, dissolve cellulite, increase lymphatic function, and promote a sense of well-being. Its fragrance is stimulating and invigorating.

Cinnamon Bark *(Cinnamomum verum)* is the oil of wealth from the Orient and part of the formula the Lord gave Moses (Exodus 30:22-27). Cinnamon oil is anti-infectious, anti-bacterial, antiparasitic, antiviral, and antifungal. Cinnamon oil was regarded by the emperors of China and India to have great value; their wealth was measured by the amount of oil they possessed. Traditionally, it was thought to have a frequency that attracted wealth and abundance. Physically, it has many attributes: (1) it is a powerful purifier (2) it is a powerful oxygenator, and (3) it enhances the action and the activity of other oils. Researchers, including J. C. Lapraz, M.D., found that viruses could not live in the presence of cinnamon oil.

Eucalyptus *(Eucalyptus radiata)* is anti-infectious, antibacterial, antiviral, expectorant, and anti-inflammatory. It has strong action against conjunctivitis, vaginitis, endometriosis, acne, bronchitis, and sinusitis.

Rosemary *(Rosmarinus officinalis)* is antiseptic and antimicrobial and may be beneficial for skin conditions and dandruff. It may help fight candida and is anti-infectious, antispasmodic, balances the endocrine system, and is an expectorant. It helps overcome mental fatigue stimulating memory and opening the conscious mind.

Safety Data: May be irritating to those with sensitive skin. Avoid eye contact. For accidental contact, put any vegetable oil or cream in the eye and call your doctor if necessary. Never use water. Avoid exposure to direct sunlight for 3 to 6 hours after use.

Application: Diffuse for 15 to 30 minutes every 3 to 4 hours in work or home environment. Apply to bottom of feet, or rub over feet, throat, stomach, and abdomen. Dilute one drop of Thieves in 15 drops of V-6 Mixing Oil and massage over thymus. It is best applied to the bottom of the feet as it may be caustic to the skin. It is best to dilute with V-6 Mixing Oil. For headaches put one drop on tongue and push tongue against the roof of the mouth.

Companion Oils: Immupower, Exodus II (to be alternated).

Frequency: Approximately 150 MHz.

Note: Studies conducted by Weber State University (Ogden, UT) during 1997 showed the anti-bacterial effectiveness of the Thieves blend against airborne microorganisms. One study showed a 90% reduction in the number of gram positive Micrococcus luteus organisms after diffusing Thieves for 12 minutes. After diffusing Thieves for a total of 20 minutes, there was a 99.3% reduction. Another study against the gram negative Pseudomonas aeruginosa showed a kill rate of 99.96% after just 12 minutes of diffusion.

3 Wise Men

This blend was formulated to open the subconscious mind through pineal stimulation to help release deep-seated trauma. The oils bring a sense of grounding and uplifting through emotional releasing and elevated spiritual consciousness.

Contains:

Sandalwood *(Santalum album)* is high in sesquiterpenes, which have been researched for their ability to stimulate the pineal gland and the limbic region of the brain, the center of our emotions. The pineal gland is responsible for releasing melatonin, a hormone that enhances deep sleep. Used traditionally for skin revitalization, yoga, and meditation, sandalwood is similar to frankincense oil in its support of nerves and circulation.

Juniper berry *(Juniperus communis)* may work as a detoxifier, cleanser and promotes improved nerve and kidney function. It is also beneficial for the skin reducing dermatitis, eczema and acne. It elevates spiritual awareness creating feelings of love and peace.

Frankincense *(Boswellia carteri)* is considered the "holy anointing oil" in the Middle East and has been used in religious ceremonies for thousands of years. High in sesquiterpenes, it helps stimulate the limbic part of the brain, which elevates the mind, helping to overcome stress and despair. It is used in European medicine to combat depression.

Myrrh *(Commiphora myrrha)* is referenced throughout the Old and New Testaments, constituting a part of a holy anointing formula given Moses (Exodus 30:22-27). It has one of the highest levels of sesquiterpenes, a class of compounds that can stimulate the hypothalamus, pituitary, and amygdala, the control center for emotions and hormone release in the brain. It has been used in eastern countries to enhance the feeling of spirituality or euphoria.

Spruce *(Picea mariana)* helps to open and release emotional blocks, bringing about a feeling of balance and grounding. Traditionally, this conifer oil was believed to possess the frequency of prosperity. Spruce is anti-infectious, antiseptic, and anti-inflammatory.

Carrier Oil: Almond oil.

Safety Data: May be irritating to those with sensitive skin. Avoid eye contact. In case of accidental contact, put any vegetable oil or cream in the eye and call your doctor if necessary. Never use water. Avoid exposure to direct sunlight for 3 to 6 hours after use.

Application: Apply 2 drops on the crown of the head, behind the ears, over the eyebrows, on the chest, over the thymus, and at the back of the neck. It may also be diffused.

Companion Oils: Frankincense, Myrrh, Sandalwood, Juniper, and Spruce.

Fragrant Influence: A feeling of reverence and spiritual awareness.

Frequency: Approximately 72 MHz.

Trauma Life

This blend was created at the request of Steven Seagal, renowned actor, director, and producer, who needed a blend for his volunteer work in hospital trauma centers. Trauma Life may help release buried emotional trauma as well as upsets, such as accidents, the death of a loved one, assault, abuse, etc. This blend of calming, grounding essential oils can help purge stress and uproot traumas that cause fatigue, anger, restlessness, and a weakened immune response. Seven Seagal is extremely pleased with the results that he has seen with this blend, using it even to help bring victims out of a coma.

Contains:

Valerian *(Valeriana officinalis)* has been used for calming, relaxing, grounding, and emotionally balancing influences. It has been clinically researched for its tranquilizing properties. German health authorities have pronounced valerian to be an effective treatment for restlessness and for sleep disturbances resulting from nervous conditions. It may help minimize shock, anxiety, and stress that accompanies traumatic situations.

Lavender *(Lavandula angustifolia)* has sedative and calming properties that can help overcome insomnia, headaches, stress, and nervous tension.

Frankincense *(Boswellia carteri)* elevates the mind and helps overcome stress and despair. It is high in sesquiterpenes, which stimulate the limbic region of the brain, the center of emotions. In ancient times, it was known for its anointing and healing powers, and "was used to treat every conceivable ill known to man."

Sandalwood *(Santalum album)* is high in sesquiterpenes, which have been researched for their ability to stimulate the pineal gland and the limbic region of the brain, the center of our emotions. The pineal gland is responsible for releasing melatonin, a hormone that enhances deep sleep. Used traditionally for skin revitalization, yoga, and meditation, sandalwood is similar to frankincense oil in its support of nerves and circulation.

Rose *(Rosa damascena)* possesses the highest frequency of the oils. It creates a sense of balance, harmony, and well-being and elevates the mind. It creates a magnetic energy that attracts love and brings joy to the heart.

Helichrysum *(Helichrysum italicum)* has been researched in Europe for regenerating tissue and nerves and improving circulation. It is anti-coagulant, prevents phlebitis, helps regulate cholesterol, stimulates liver cell function, and may help to clean plaque and debris from the veins and arteries. It is mucolytic, expectorant, antispasmodic, and reduces scarring and discoloration. It may also stimulate nerve endings and improve conditions such as hearing loss. It may help release feelings of anger promoting forgiveness.

Spruce *(Picea mariana)* helps to open and release emotional blocks, bringing about a feeling of balance and grounding. Traditionally, spruce oil was believed to possess the frequency of prosperity. Spruce is anti-infectious, antiseptic, and anti-inflammatory.

Geranium *(Pelargonium graveolens)* stimulates nerves and assists in balancing hormones. Its aromatic influence helps release negative memories, thereby opening and elevating the mind.

Davana *(Artemsia pallens)* is high in sesquiterpenes which are supporting to the immune system. It is mucolytic, antispasmodic, works to reduce painful scarring, and helps overcome anxiety.

Citrus hystrix is anti-infectious, antiseptic, liver decongestant, and neurotonic. With its hormone-like properties, it supports under active sexual glands. The constituents of aldehydes, esters, and coumarins make it calming and sedating.

Safety Data: May be irritating to those with sensitive skin. Avoid eye contact. In case of accidental contact, put any vegetable oil or cream in the eye and call your doctor if necessary. Never use water. Avoid exposure to direct sunlight for 3 to 6 hours after use.

Application: Diffuse, apply a few drops to the bottom of the feet, on the chest, behind the ears, on the forehead, and at the back of the neck. May also be applied along the spine using Raindrop technique.

Companion Oils: Peace and Calming, Joy Hope, Into the Future

Fragrant Influence: Promotes a feeling of calmness and a sense of awareness.

Frequency: Approximately 92 MHz.

Valor

Valor helps balance electrical energies within the body, giving courage, confidence, and self-esteem. It has been found to help the body self-correct its balance and alignment giving relief of pain. The oils in this blend empower the physical and spiritual bodies to overcome fear and opposition when facing adversity. It helps build courage, confidence, and self-esteem. Valor has been touted as a chiropractor in a bottle. It has improved scoliosis in as little as 30 minutes, where other individuals require several applications. Valor has also been shown to change anaerobic mutated cells back to their aerobic natural state.

Contains:

Rosewood *(Aniba rosaeodora)* is soothing and nourishing to the skin. It has been researched at Weber State University for its inhibition rate against gram positive and gram negative bacterial growth. This oil is soothing, creates elasticity, and helps the skin rid itself of irritations and problems, such as candida. It is anti-infectious, antibacterial, antifungal, antiviral, and antiparasitic.

Blue Tansy *(Tanacetum annuum)* may help cleanse the liver and calm the lymphatic system helping one to overcome anger and negative emotions promoting a feeling of self-control. Its primary constituents are limonene and sesquiterpenes. European research shows that it works as an antihistamine, anti-inflammatory, and stimulant for the thymus gland reducing dermatitis, arthritis, sciatica, tuberculosis, and allergies.

Frankincense *(Boswellia carteri)* is considered the "holy anointing oil" in the Middle East and has been used in religious ceremonies for thousands of years. High in sesquiterpenes, it helps stimulate the limbic part of the brain, which elevates the mind, helping to overcome stress and despair. It is used in European medicine to combat depression.

Spruce *(Picea mariana)* helps to open and release emotional blocks, bringing about a feeling of balance and grounding. Traditionally, spruce oil was believed to possess the frequency of prosperity. Spruce is anti-infectious, antiseptic, and anti-inflammatory.

Carrier Oil: Almond oil.

Safety Data: May be irritating to those with sensitive skin. Avoid eye contact. In case of accidental contact, put any vegetable oil or cream in the eye and call your doctor if necessary. Never use water. Avoid exposure to direct sunlight for 3 to 6 hours after use.

Application: Apply 4 to 6 drops on bottom of feet. Put on wrists, chest, and at the back of the neck, or along the spine in a Raindrop application. When using a series of oils, as in the Raindrop therapy application, apply Valor first and let it work for 5 to 10 minutes before applying other oils. This blend may be worn as a perfume or cologne. (For more detailed instruction, see Raindrop Therapy.)

Companion Oils:

Fragrant Influence: Gives a feeling of strength, courage and protection.

Frequency: Low to work with the physical body. Approximately 47 MHz.

White Angelica

This blend is a combination of 10 oils, some of which were used during ancient times to increase the aura around the body. It brings a delicate sense of strength and protection, creating a feeling of wholeness in the realm of one's own spirituality. Its frequency neutralizes negative energy. It is calming and soothing and brings a feeling of protection and security.

Contains:

Ylang Ylang *(Cananga odorata)* helps bring about a sense of relaxation and may help balance male and female energies. It balances equilibrium and restores confidence and self-love.

Rose *(Rosa damascena)* possesses the highest frequency of the oils. It creates a sense of balance, harmony, and well-being and elevates the mind. It promotes healthy skin, reduces scarring, and may help with sexual disabilities, frigidity, impotency, skin diseases, and wrinkles. It creates a magnetic energy that attracts love and brings joy to the heart.

149

Melissa *(Melissa officinalis)* is a powerful, antimicrobial oil, yet it is very gentle and delicate because of the nature of the plant, and helps to bring out those characteristics within the individual. It is calming and balancing to the emotions. Melissa is one of the highest in sesquiterpenes, much like cedarwood. It is very stimulating to the anterior pituitary and immune system.

Sandalwood *(Santalum album)* is high in sesquiterpenes, which have been researched for their ability to stimulate the pineal gland and the limbic region of the brain, the center of our emotions. The pineal gland is responsible for releasing melatonin, a hormone that enhances deep sleep. Used traditionally for skin revitalization, yoga, and meditation, sandalwood is similar to frankincense oil in its support of nerves and circulation.

Geranium *(Pelargonium graveolens)* stimulates nerves and assists in balancing hormones. Its aromatic influence helps release negative memories, thereby opening and elevating the mind.

Spruce *(Picea mariana)* helps to open and release emotional blocks, bringing about a feeling of balance and grounding. Traditionally, spruce oil was believed to possess the frequency of prosperity. Spruce is anti-infectious, antiseptic, and anti-inflammatory.

Myrrh *(Commiphora myrrha)* is referenced throughout the Old and New Testaments, constituting a part of a holy anointing formula given Moses (Exodus 30:22-27). It has one of the highest levels of sesquiterpenes, a class of compounds that can stimulate the hypothalamus, pituitary, and amygdala, the control center for emotions and hormone in the brain. It has been used in eastern countries to enhance the feeling of spirituality or euphoria.

Hyssop *(Hyssopus officinalis)* is strongly balancing for emotions.

Bergamot *(Citrus bergamia)* is one of the most uplifting fragrances, simultaneously energizing and calming, with a unique ability to relieve anxiety, stress and tension.

Rosewood *(Aniba rosaeodora)* is soothing and nourishing to the skin. It has been researched at Weber State University for its inhibition rate against gram positive and gram negative bacterial growth. This oil is soothing, creates elasticity, and helps the skin rid itself of irritations and problems, such as candida. It is anti-infectious, antibacterial, antifungal, antiviral, and antiparasitic.

Carrier Oil: Almond oil.

Safety Data: May be irritating to those with sensitive skin. Avoid eye contact. In case of accidental contact, put any vegetable oil or cream in the eye and call your doctor if necessary. Never use water. Avoid exposure to direct sunlight for 3 to 6 hours after use.

Application: Diffuse, apply on shoulders, along spine, on crown of head, on wrists, behind ears, back of neck, and may be added to bath water. Wear as perfume or cologne. .

Companion Oils: Valor, Inspiration, Awaken, Sacred Mountain, Joy, Aroma Life.

Fragrant Influence: A feeling of protection and security.

Frequency: Approximately 89 MHz.

Blood Types Relating to Food Supplements

People with blood type A and AB are natural vegetarians and have the easiest time converting to a vegetarian diet. However, these people also have a tendency for thyroid problems and tend to be overweight. For them, exercise that increases heartrate is necessary to have weight reduction.

People with type B blood are probably the most balanced in nutritional needs and can go either way

People with type 0 blood need additional protein, possibly through meat consumption. They have a more difficult time converting to vegetarianism. These people can get all the protein they need if they consume the correct portions of seeds, nuts and grains. VitaGreen should be a mainstay for this group. These people often have digestive deficiencies. They eat more but assimilate less, have excess gas, get full quickly but are hungry sooner, and tend to weigh less.

People who have type 0 blood tend to have poor circulation and as a result tend to be cold when fasting. Cayenne pepper improves this situation. One can also put some cayenne in one's shoes and socks when they are worn. Cayenne becomes damp from foot perspiration creating warmth to the feet.

During the fast, 0 blood types may require the more protein. During the first two weeks these people should take the Body Balance twice a day and should also take VitaGreen three times per day. These supplements will provide the necessary proteins. After 2 weeks, the supplements should be ceased, because protein intake must be zero in order to effect DNA memory change. The body will convert its minimal protein requirements as needed. Individuals can go 65 days on a water-only fast before there is tissue breakdown.

(See Building the Body and Cleansing.)

Health Issues

Sugars and Sweeteners

Nothing stresses the human body as much as refined sugar. Called a "skeletonized food" and "castrated carbohydrate" by Edward Howell, Ph.D., and a "metabolic freeloader" by Ralph Golan, M.D., sugar actually drains the body of vitamins, minerals, and nutrients in the process of being burned for energy. Sugar also stresses the pancreas, forcing it to pump out a surge of unneeded digestive enzymes.

Sugars also undermine and downregulate immune response. One study measured the effects of 100 grams of sugar (sucrose) on neutrophils, a form of white blood cell that comprises a central part of immunity. Within one hour of ingestion, neutrophil activity dropped 50 percent and remained below normal for another four hours (Castleman, 1997).

Population studies have also linked sugar consumption with diabetes and heart disease. According to researcher John Yudkin, the reason sugar elevates the risk of heart disease is due to an automatic built-in safety switch inside the body. To protect itself from being immediately poisoned from excess sugar, the body converts it into fats, like trigylcerides. So instead of killing you quickly, the body defends itself by clogging its arteries, thereby killing you on the installment plan.

The worst dangers, though, are not found in natural sugars but in the use of artificial sweeteners. Seventy-five percent of the adverse reactions reported to the U. S. Food and Drug Administration come from a single substance: the artificial sweetener Aspartame.

Aspartame is marketed today as NutraSweet, Equal, Spoonful and Equal-Measure. With so many Americans on one diet or another, the market for Aspartame is simply huge. And it matters not that aspartame users are suffering from symptoms ranging from headaches, numbness and seizures to joint pain, chronic fatigue syndrome, multiple sclerosis and epilepsy.

This toxic artificial sweetener is made up of three chemicals: aspartic acid, phenylalanine and methanol. What these chemicals do in our bodies is anything but "sweet."

Aspartame

A recent book by Dr. Russell L. Blaylock, professor of neurosurgery at the Medical University of Mississippi, *Excitotoxins: The Taste That Kills*, explains that aspartame is a neurotransmitter facilitating the transmission of information from one neuron to another. Aspartame allows too much calcium into brain cells, killing certain neurons, earning aspartate the name of "excitotoxin." With aspartame now in over 5,000 products such as instant breakfasts, breath mints, cereals, frozen desserts, "lite" gelatin desserts and even multivitamins, it is no surprise that there is a virtual epidemic of memory loss, Alzheimer's disease, and multiple sclerosis. In a move much like a telephone company selling your phone number to telephone solicitors and then charging you to block their calls, G. D. Searle (the Monsanto company that manufactures aspartame) is searching for a drug to combat memory loss caused by excitatory amino acid damage most often caused by aspartame.

Phenylalanine

The chemical phenylalanine is an amino acid normally found in the brain. You may have heard of testing infants for PKU, a condition where phenylalanine cannot be metabolized, which can lead to death. It has been shown that excessive amounts of phenylalanine in the brain can cause seratonin levels to decrease. Have you ever concluded that half the people you know are on Prozac? Perhaps the flooding of American foods and soft drinks with Aspartame is contributing to this need for drugs like Prozac and Zoloft.

But depression is not the most worrisome result of excessive phenylalanine levels in the brain. Dr. Blaylock writes that schizophrenia and susceptibility to seizures can occur as a result of these high levels. The Massachusetts Institute of Technology surveyed 80 people who suffered seizures following the ingestion of aspartame. The Community Nutrition Institute concluded that these cases met the FDA's own definition of an imminent hazard to the public health, but the FDA made no move to remove this dangerous product from the market.

It is hard not to become cynical when you find out that the commissioner of the FDA overruled the FDA's own scientific board of inquiry into the safety of aspartame and then took a position with the public relations firm that represents aspartame's manufacturer.

Do you fly the friendly skies? You may be interested to know that both the Air Force's magazine, *Flying Safety,* and *Navy Physiology,* the Navy's publication, detailed warnings about pilots being more susceptible to seizures after consuming aspartame. The Aspartame Consumer Safety Network notes that 600 pilots have reported acute reactions to aspartame including grand mal seizures in the cockpit. Many other publications have warned about aspartame, ingestion while flying, including a paper presented at the 57th Annual Meeting of the Aerospace Medical Association.

Methanol

If methanol were a criminal in a police lineup, it would wear a sign saying, "aka" wood alcohol. For those desperate enough to drink it, wood alcohol can lead to blindness and even death. It is not terribly reassuring to know that one quart of aspartame-sweetened beverage contains about 56 mg. of methanol. The EPA states that methanol is "considered a cumulative poison due to the low rate of excretion once it is absorbed."

Methanol is truly criminal after it enters your body. It breaks down into formic acid and formaldehyde. Methanol absorption is sped up when free methanol is ingested. Free methanol results when aspartame is heated higher than 86 degrees F. If you cook a sugar-free pudding that contains aspartame, you are creating free methanol.

Formaldehyde is a known carcinogen and can cause birth defects by interfering with DNA replication. Our Desert Storm troops were treated to free diet drinks that sat in the hot sun of Saudi Arabia. Many of the unusual symptoms found in Desert Storm veterans are similar to those of people chemically poisoned by formaldehyde.

The artificial sweetener aspartame would certainly not sell if people knew what kind of a toxic chemical stew they were ingesting.

Grade C Maple Syrup

Grade C maple syrup is the best sweetener and the most balanced sugar, since it contains a balance of positive and negative ions. It is processed in open kettles without formaldehyde. Other grades are processed in pressurized containers with formaldehyde added. It is also a low-glycemic index food, resulting in a slow, gradual rise in blood sugar levels.

Fructose

Fructose is a natural sweetener that has one of the lowest glycemic indexes of any food. A glycemic index measures the impact that a food has on blood sugar levels two to three hours after ingestion. The lower the glycemic level, the lower the rise in blood sugar levels.

With a glycemic index of only 20, fructose has one of the lowest of any food and many times lower than standard breads and processed grains. Fructose has a glycemic index that is only a third of glucose, a fourth of white bread, and a fifth of boiled potatoes.

Stevia

Known as *Stevia rebaudiana* by botanists and yerba dulce (honey leaf) by the Guarani Indians, stevia has been incorporated into many native medicines, beverages, and foods for centuries. The Guarani used stevia separately or combined with herbs like yerba mate and lapacho.

Fifteen times sweeter than sugar, stevia was introduced to the West in 1899, when M. S. Bertoni discovered natives using it as a sweetener and medicinal herb. With Japan's ban on the import of synthetic sweeteners in the 1960's, stevia began to be seriously researched by the Japanese National Institute of Health as a natural sugar substitute. In 1994, the U.S. Food and Drug Administration permitted the importation and use of stevia as a dietary supplement. However, its adoption by

American consumers as a noncaloric sweetener has been very slow because the FDA does not currently permit stevia to be marketed as a food additive. This means that stevia cannot be sold as a sweetener (all sweeteners are classified as food additives by the FDA). Moreover, stevia faces fierce opposition by both the artificial sweetener (aspartame) and sugar industry in the U.S.

Stevia, however, is more than just a non-caloric sweetener. Several modern clinical studies have documented the ability of stevia to lower and balance blood sugar levels, support the pancreas and digestive system, protect the liver, and combat infectious microorganisms. (Oviedo et al., 1971; Suzuki et al., 1977; Ishit et al., 1986; Boeckh, 1986; Alvarez, 1986.)

Water

There is nothing more refreshing when you are hot and thirsty than clear, cold spring water. Water is not only refreshing but absolutely essential to life. The only nutrient that is more important to the body than water is oxygen.

Water is the crucial ingredient in our body's self-cleansing system. We are very aware of the body's normal elimination processes, but may not realize that unwanted substances are also eliminated through exhaled breath and through perspiration, which also require water. Certainly our kidneys will not be able to cleanse efficiently if there is not enough water in our system to carry away waste.

Finding pure drinking water is becoming a challenge. Our increasingly polluted world has made it necessary for the Environmental Protection Agency to set water standards. The EPA screens for the presence of suspended solids, oil and grease, fecal coliform bacteria, chemicals and heavy metals. Unfortunately, the major source of pollution (65 percent in 1990) comes not from industrial sites which can be regulated, but from storm water run-off. Rainfall coming in contact with pollutants from agricultural and industrial operations absorbs these chemicals and transports them into lakes and rivers. Only 9 percent of water pollution came from actual industrial sites in 1990.

Municipal water should be avoided if possible. Most municipal waters have a high ppm (parts per million) concentration of aluminum due to the use of aluminum hydroxide as an accepted method of water treatment. Moreover, the addition of chlorine results in the creation of cancer-causing chemicals when dissolved organic solids are chemically altered by chlorination. While there is a trend toward replacing chlorination with peroxide treatment of water, it will be decades before peroxide is adopted as a standard.

We may turn to expensive bottled waters, but regulation in this industry is vague. Regardless of cost, the bottled water you buy may simply be tap water put through a filtration process. You may wish to invest in a water purifier for your home or drink distilled water to be sure you are getting pure water.

Distilled water washes out and flushes the system. With the help of essential oils, the body can excrete petroleum residues, metals, inorganic minerals, and other toxins.

Essential oils, like lemon, also make outstanding water purifiers. One drop per glass is generally enough. Put the oil in a glass or container first, then run the water in. Since oils do not mix with water, this will distribute them through the water. Or put several drops in the out end of the carbon filter of a water purification system. This can drop nitrate levels by up to 3,000 ppm.

Since chlorine shuts down thyroid function, drink water that has the chlorine removed. You can either distill the water or let it stand unsealed (which allows the chlorine to evaporate over time). You can also add a drop of lemon or other oil. To obtain chlorine-free water for showering and bathing, get a showerhead filter or aromatherapy showerhead like the RainSpa. Avoid public swimming pools. While carbon filters are good for removing chlorine from water, the best water distillers have pre-flash or pre-boiling chambers, to flash off volatile gases, such as chlorine, petroleum products, etc. Then the steam should rise at least 15 inches to balance the pH. and fall 15 inches to oxygenate again.

One very popular water purification system is the ion exchange used in areas of the country with "hard" water or water with dissolved minerals. Water is passed through a filter exchanging charged particles (ions) in the water for charged particles in the filter. Most units use salt, with sodium and chloride ions exchanging for the contaminated ions in the water. Since the minerals are replaced with salt, at least one cold water tap needs to be left out of the system so that drinking water is not loaded with sodium.

The ideal amount of water to consume is half your body weight in ounces per day. That means if you weight 160 pounds, you should drink 80 ounces of water (or about ten 8 ounce glasses per day. Avoid drinking any chlorinated water.

Microwaves

Microwaves can be found in almost every home and restaurant because they are extremely convenient for thawing and heating food. Yet we are paying a great price for this convenience. In a study by Dr. Radwan Farag of Cairo University, it was discovered that just two seconds of microwave energy destroys all the enzymes in a food, thus increasing our enzyme deficiency and altering the frequency of the food. Heating proteins in the microwave for 10 minutes or more may create a new, harmful species of protein. You may decide that this is a high price to pay for convenience.

Also, microwave radiation has been known to leak and could disrupt the delicate balances in cellular growth. Our bodies are regulated by electrical frequencies and electromagnetic fields. It would be wise to avoid disrupting these frequencies.

And there is this to think about: the University of Minnesota warned that microwaving a baby's bottle can cause slight changes in the milk. In the case of a hip-surgery patient in Oklahoma, microwaving blood for a transfusion killed the patient. Warming blood for a transfusion is routine; unfortunately, using a microwave caused enough changes in the blood to be deadly.

For those who cannot give up convenience, please remember that plastic molecules could end up in your food if you microwave in plastic dishes or use plastic wrap to cover open dishes.

A research project with 20 volunteers was conducted in 1980 with microwave cooking. Ten volunteers in group A and 10 in group B fasted on liquids for 10 days. Then both groups were fed the same foods for another 10 days with only one exception: Group A foods were steamed, while group B foods were microwaved. After 10 days, stool samples were taken and analyzed. Group A stools appeared to be normally digested, while group B stools were of a plastic texture. Ultrasound scans showed adhesive food particles stuck to the stomach wall. In the stool sample, altered enzymes were found, as well as protein with altered molecular structure which could not be absorbed.

pH Balance

The Importance of Alkalinity to Health

The unfriendly bacteria and fungi that populate our intestinal tracts thrive in an acid environment and are responsible for secreting mycotoxins, which are the root cause of many debilitating human conditions. In fact, many researchers believe that most diseases can be linked to blood and intestinal acidity, which contributes to an acid-based yeast and fungus dominance.

The symptoms of excess internal acidity include:
• Fatigue / Low energy
• Unexplained aches and pains
• Overweight conditions
• Low resistance to illness
• Allergies

• Unbalanced blood sugar
• Headaches
• Irritability / Mood swings
• Indigestion
• Colitis / Ulcers
• Diarrhea / Constipation
• Urinary tract infections
• Rectal itch / vaginal itch

The ideal pH for the human body ranges between 7.4 and 7.6. Preserving this alkalinity (pH balance) is the bedrock on which sound health and strong bodies are built. When the blood loses its alkalinity and starts to become more acidic, the foundation of health is undermined. This creates an environment where we become vulnerable to disease and runaway yeast and fungus overgrowth.

The naturally occurring yeast and fungi in the body thrive in an acid terrain. These same yeast and fungi are responsible for secreting a large number of poisons called mycotoxins, which are believed to be one of the root causes of many diseases and debilitating conditions.

When yeast and fungus decline in the body, so does their production of mycotoxins, the poisonous waste products and byproducts of their life cycles. There are numerous varieties of these mycotoxins, many of which are harmful to the body and must be neutralized by our immune systems. When our bodies are overwhelmed by large quantities of these toxins, our health becomes impaired, and we become susceptible to disease and illness.

Many cancers have been linked to mycotoxins. For example, the fungus *Aspergillus flavus*, which infests stored peanuts, not only generates cancer in laboratory animals but has been documented as the prime culprit in many liver cancers in humans.

By balancing the body's pH and creating a more alkaline environment, you rein in the microbial overgrowth and choke off the production of disease-producing mycotoxins. With pH balance restored, the body can regain newfound vigor and health.

How to Restore Alkalinity

1. **Carefully monitor your diet.** Avoiding yeast- and fungus-promoting foods is a crucial factor in combating excess acidity and fungus overgrowth. Meats, sugars, dairy products, mushrooms, and pickled and malted products can be especially acidic. On the other hand, garlic is excellent for controlling fungi and yeast. Other high-alkaline, fungus-inhibiting foods include green and yellow vegetables, beans, and whole uncracked nuts. The natural ratio between acid and alkaline foods in the diet should be 4:1—four parts alkaline foods to one part acid. In his book, THE YEAST SYNDROME, Dr. Morton Walker outlines some antifungal diets.

   The pH of a raw food does not always determine its acidity or alkalinity in the digestive system. Some foods, like lemons, might be acidic in their natural state but when consumed and digested are converted into highly alkaline residues. Thus, the true determinant of a food's pH is whether it is an alkaline-ash or acid-ash food. In this case, lemons are an alkaline-ash food.

2. **Avoid the use of antibiotics.** The overuse of antibiotics for incidental, minor, or cosmetic conditions not only increases the resistance of pathogenic microorganisms, but it kills the beneficial bacteria in your body, leaving the mycotoxin-generating yeast and fungi intact. This is why many women suffer outbreaks of yeast infections after antibiotic use.

3. **Use essential oils.** Many essential oils possess important antimicrobial, antibacterial and antifungal properties. French medical researchers in study after study have documented the healing properties of plant extracts and their ability to stimulate the immune system and inhibit bacterial growth.

   Essential oils work best when the body's blood and tissues are alkaline. When our systems become more acidic—due to improper diet or excessive levels of stress—the essential oils lose some of their effects. So the best way to enhance the action of essential oils is to alkalize your body, and AlkaLime is a first-rate tool to accomplish this.

4. **Using alkaline salts.** AlkaLime is an outstanding source of alkaline salts that can help reduce internal acidity. An alkaline environment is hostile to fungi, which require acidity to survive and thrive. Lowered yeast and fungus populations translate into lower levels of body-damaging, disease-inducing mycotoxins.

5. **Lower stress.** Emotional and psychological tension can be especially damaging to bodily systems and act as a prime promoter of acid formation in the body. To properly appreciate how acidic stress can be, just think back to the last time you were seriously stressed-out and had to reach for an antacid tablet to soothe your heartburn or stomach discomfort.

Some of the most common varieties of negative bacteria, yeast, and fungi that live in the intestines are inactive. However, when the body is weakened by illness, stress, and excess acidity caused by stress, these bacteria become active, damaging and assuming an invasive mycelic form.

Blends of essential oils high in sesquiterpenes, such as frankincense, myrrh, and sandalwood, can produce profound balancing and calming effects on emotions. They work by affecting the limbic system of our brain, the seat of our emotions.

6. **Boost friendly flora.** From three to four pounds of beneficial bacteria permanently reside in the intestines of the average adult. Not only are they the first line of defense against foreign invaders, but they are absolutely essential for health, energy, and optimum digestive efficiency. These intestinal houseguests not only control mucus and debris, but they produce B vitamins, vitamin K, and maintain the all-important pH balance of the body.

These friendly flora are also important in counteracting and opposing yeast and fungus overgrowth. When our natural cultures are compromised or disrupted by taking antibiotics or by poor dietary practices, yeast and fungus start growing unopposed and begin colonizing and invading larger swaths of our internal terrain, secreting ever-increasing volumes of poisonous mycotoxins.

Using an acidophilus or bifidus supplement, like Royaldophilus, may be especially valuable in boosting levels of naturally occurring beneficial bacteria in the body and preventing fungal and yeast overgrowth. They also help the body maintain proper pH balance for nutrient digestion and absorption. Ideally, the lactobacillus acidiphilus and bifidobacterium bifidus cultures must be combined with plantain to promote implantation on the intestinal wall.

Research indicates a significant proportion of bacteria from many acidophilus supplements do not reach the lower intestine alive, or they arrive in such a weakened state that they are not of much benefit. This is why combining the acidophilus and bifidus cultures with plantain is so important because plantain helps these cultures stick to the intestinal walls.

An even more effective means of fortifying the friendly flora in our intestines is by consumption of fructooligosaccharides (also known as FOS). FOS is one of the most powerful natural agents for feeding our friendly flora. FOS is made up of medium-chain sugars that cannot be used by pathogenic yeast and fungi. The end result is that FOS starves fungi while feeding the acidophilus and bifidus cultures that are our first-line defense against disease.

But FOS is far more than just an outstanding means of rebuilding and protecting the beneficial bacteria inside the body. Over a dozen clinical studies have documented the ability of fructooligosaccharides to prevent constipation, lower blood sugar and cholesterol levels, and even prevent cancer. (Hidaka et al., 1991; Briet et al., 1995); Bouhnik et al., 1996; Kawaguchi et al., 1993; Luo et al., 1996); Rochat et al., 1994; Tokunaga et al., 1993).

Stevia Select is a supersweet supplement that combines stevia with FOS.

Testing Your pH

You can easily test your pH at home by purchasing small litmus-paper strips at your drug store or pharmacy. To get the most accurate reading, expose the strip to a sample of your saliva immediately after awakening in the morning and before eating breakfast. Color changes on the litmus paper will determine pH; check the instructions of your kit for specific details on how to read the litmus paper.

Health Programs with
Essential Oils and Supplements

Cleansing and Digestion

The Risks of Internal Pollution

As we grow older, we risk suffering a greater and greater buildup of chemical contamination in our bodies. As toxins accumulate, we are more likely to suffer the energy-robbing effects of poor health and degenerative changes. We feel sluggish, tired, and prone to illnesses.

This is why cleansing our bodies is so important. When we purge our systems of heavy metal contamination, undigested foods, and internal pollution, we relieve our organs and tissues of enormous stress.

Cleansing becomes especially important whenever we consume animal products, such as meats and dairy products. These foods are loaded with naturally-occurring, disease-related microbes. According to Robert O. Young, Ph.D., D.Sc., meats contain an average of 300,000 to 3,000,000 microorganisms per gram, or roughly 336,000,000 per serving. Cheese contains from 300,000 to 1,000,000 microorganisms per gram; milk, 20,000. These animal products can be a major source of internal pollution. Clean plant food, on the other hand, contains only 10 microbes per gram.

Man was built to be primarily a plant-eater, not a meat-eater. Our long intestinal tracts are uncannily similar to many plant-eating species and are specifically designed by nature to digest a high-fiber, high-roughage, plant-based diet. Its long length gives our enzymes a chance to unlock the nutrient value of our food. This contrasts markedly with the short intestines of flesh-eating animals, which are designed to quickly digest and pass through meats, without having them putrefying, feeding fungi, and creating illness.

What happens when we consume meats and dairy products? Lacking fiber, such proteins move through our lengthy intestines very slowly and easily become trapped in its many "nooks and crannies." Acting like toxic time bombs, putrefying pockets of undigested food gradually release their payload of heavy metals, chemicals, hormones and toxins directly into the blood and tissues. Even worse, this undigested debris is fermented by our body's naturally occurring yeast and fungi, polluting us with toxic by-products called mycotoxins. These mycotoxins have been linked to many diseases.

Who Needs Cleansing?

All of us are stressed, to a lesser or greater degree, by an ever-mounting buildup of toxins, chemicals, bacteria, and parasites. A distinguished medical researcher, Kenneth Bock, M.D., states that humans are "walking toxic dumps." Why? Because of the industrial wastes, herbicides, pesticides, additives, and heavy metals we unknowingly absorb from our food, cosmetics, air, and water—even the mercury fillings in our teeth. Moreover, our place at the top of the food chain means that we are subjected to concentrated doses of potentially harmful chemicals from the meats and dairy products we consume.

According to a large 1990 survey by the Environmental Protection Agency, every single person tested showed some evidence of petro-chemical pollution in their tissues and fats. Some of the chemicals found included styrene (used in plastics), xylene (a solvent in paint and gasoline), benzene (a chemical found in gasoline), and toluene (another carcinogenic solvent).

Understanding a Complete Cleansing

The ideal cleansing program should combine high water consumption with high-potency herbs, digestive enzymes, and therapeutic-grade essential oils. Essential oils have a special lipid-soluble makeup, which gives them a remarkable ability to penetrate cell walls, breakup undigested food, and oppose toxins. Essential oils also deliver oxygen, which has an unparalleled ability to inhibit the growth of many types of microbes. In fact, many essential oils have been studied for their unique antimicrobial, antifungal, and antiparasitic properties. Some oils, like rosemary, have demonstrated significant antiseptic activity, with documented research appearing in many scientific journals.

A cleansing program should target many different parts of the body (colon, intestine, stomach, liver, pancreas) and cover many different types of internal pollution, including waste buildup, heavy metals, parasites, fungi, and yeast.

When Should You Cleanse?

Cleansing your system should not be just a once- or twice-a-year event. It should be continuous.

Cleansing is especially important for anyone over 40. With age comes a greater buildup of debris in our bodies caused by a decreased production of the stomach acids and enzymes. Without proper enzyme production, we lack the ability to properly break down undigested proteins and other fermenting debris that obstruct our digestive system and impede the assimilation of nutrients.

To get the most out of any cleansing regimen, **drink plenty of water** throughout the day. A good rule of thumb is to drink half your body weight in ounces. So, if you weigh 150 lbs., drink 75 ozs. of water. The water must be distilled or purified. One should never drink chlorinated tap water.

The Stanley Burroughs Master Cleanse

The Master Cleanse is not a fast, but a cleansing program. A true fast consists only of water, while the Master Cleanse incorporates a lemon juice, maple syrup, and cayenne pepper mixture that is consumed throughout the day and is a source of calories, vitamins, and minerals.

The Master Cleanse is ideal for anyone who is not a diabetic and can safely cleanse for at least three to seven days. The ideal duration of a cleanse can extend from one to three weeks. As with any program of caloric restriction, however, it is strongly recommended that you consult with your health care professional before undertaking any extended fast or cleanse.

To Start

- Take juice of 1/2 fresh lemon (preferably organic)
- Mix juice into 8 oz. of distilled water
- Add 1-2 tablespoons of grade C maple syrup
- Add 1/8 to 1/4 tsp. cayenne pepper (red)

Drink as many 8-10 oz. glasses as required according to your body weight per day. If you weigh 100 pounds then you would drink half your weight in ounces which would be 50 ounces or 5 glasses.

Grade C maple syrup is one of the most balanced of all sugars, containing a balance of positive and negative ions. Unlike other grades, Grade C is processed in open kettles without formaldehyde. Grade C does not enter the bloodstream as rapidly as honey or sugar which is better for people who react adversely to sugars, (becoming restless, sleepless, and energetic after consuming sugar), or may be borderline or pre-diabetic. Diabetics should substitute blackstrap molasses for the maple syrup, using up to 1/4 tablespoon.

Contrary to popular belief, lemon is not acidic in the body. It turns alkaline in the mouth. If an acid-like reaction is observed when using lemon with water, it is because of the minerals in the water. Distilled water will not react in this manner.

Cayenne pepper is a blood vessel dilator, thermal warmer, and provides vitamin A. People who have type O blood tend to have poor circulation. As a result, their body temperature may drop during a cleanse. Because cayenne is an herb known for its ability to warm and restore circulation, it may be taken internally and used topically (especially on the feet).

For the deepest cleanse, it is recommended that you cleanse for at least two to three weeks. Exercise enhances the cleansing action of the program.

During the middle and later phases of the cleanse, the body chemistry changes, and energy levels may begin to increase. One may experience minor discomforts, such as headaches, upset stomach, or low energy, as toxins and parasites are released from the body. These symptoms will be short-lived.

It is important to have a positive attitude during cleansing or fasting. If you are unaccustomed to the process, you can prepare yourself by fasting one day a week. Sunday, or your Sabbath day, is a wonderful day for this purpose. The biggest obstacle to successful cleansing is fear of failure and not knowing what to expect.

To fast for 24 hours, it is easier if you begin at the 12:00 noon of one day and finish at the 12:00 noon of the next day or from one dinner to the next.

Again, drink plenty of water.

As you begin to fast, you may experience some unpleasant side effects of cleansing, such as a headache, nausea, bloating, or irritability. These symptoms are part of the cleansing response and are often a result of toxins and waste matter being purged from the body which usually takes place within 12 to 36 hours. In any case, you may want to consult your health care professional.

You may have an unexpected emotional clearing. There are various essential oil blends designed to help control your emotions; modulate and facilitate the emotional release. Herbs, like St. John's wort, kava kava, and hops extract, are excellent for managing stress and negative emotions. Ideally, these herbs should be taken using oral infusion therapy (sprayed into the inside of the mouth where they can be most efficiently delivered into the blood).

Tips

To aid the transition to vegetarianism and help re-program the system, take Body Balance three or four times per week. Also, for two weeks, take VitaGreen, then follow the master cleanse for another 30 days.

The first 2 to 4 days of the fast are often the most difficult, since you will be overcoming the powerful psychological need to eat. As your body is cleansed from parasites and putrefying toxins, you will experience a sudden surge in energy and well being. Tapeworms, pinworms, and roundworms often start to appear in your stools (after 4 to 6 days), physical hunger will fade away. As the cleansing progresses, your mind will become sharper, your memory will improve, and your spirit will become more buoyant.

Remember: It is crucial to drink plenty of distilled water throughout the day, at least 8 to 10 eight ounce glasses. Water is crucial for not only flushing out toxins, but maintaining the metabolic machinery of your cells and tissues in proper working condition.

Fasting

It has been called nature's single greatest healing therapy. Fasting is the avoidance of solid food with liquid intake varying from no liquids to just water to fresh juices. A fast can last 24 hours or several weeks. Fasting has long been a tradition in Judaism, Christianity and the Eastern religions. Religious fasting can involve purification, penitence or preparation for approaching God. An increasing number of doctors are recognizing that fasting can be physically healing while allowing us to focus our energy inward, bringing clarity and change.

Gabriel Cousens, M. D. writes that "fasting in a larger context, means to abstain from that which is toxic to mind, body and soul. A way to understand this is that fasting is the elimination of physical, emotional and mental toxins from our organs, rather than simply cutting down on or stopping food intake. Fasting for spiritual purposes usually involves some degree of removal of oneself from worldly responsibilities. It can mean complete silence and isolation during the fast which can be a great revival to those of us who have been putting our energy outward."

Fasting is generally safe but those with medical conditions should check with their health care professional.

Elson M. Haas, M. D. notes that fasting is a catalyst for change and an integral part of transformational medicine. He writes, "Fasting clearly improves motivation and creative energy; it also enhances health and vitality and lets many of the body systems rest."

An extremely important benefit of fasting is the elimination of toxins. By minimizing the work our digestive system must do, we allow it to repair itself and clean up stored toxins. In the beginning of a fast, the liver will convert stored glycogen to energy. As the fast continues, some proteins will be broken down unless juices provide calories.

Information on cleansing juice fasts is included in the chapter on Digestion and Cleansing.

The best way to convert to vegetarianism is by fasting. To be healthy, have energy, be free of sickness and disease, you must learn to discipline yourself and listen to the needs of your body.

Our bodies do not need meat to maintain good health, even though many of us have programmed ourselves through years of meat consumption to have the desire to eat meat. Our bodies can get all the protein required from a diet containing a wide variety of non-meat foods: beans, lentils, vegetables, whole grains, seeds, some cheeses, dairy products (preferably unpasteurized and natural colored), and occasionally eggs. However, you must be sure to eat enough protein to maintain a balanced, healthy body.

NOTE: Anyone can fast, whether young, old, or even lactating mothers. Wastes are eliminated through urine and stools. Mammary glands are filters, so the baby gets pure nutrients from a lactating mother.

The Hunza Diet - Limited Caloric Intake

A people living in the remote Hunza Valley in Northern Pakistan are renowned for their longevity. The Hunzakuts (as they call themselves) routinely live past ages 100, 110 and even 120. They also share another remarkable trait: the near absence of degenerative disease.

It is known that the diet of the Hunza people is high in potassium and low in sodium. Apricots, barley, millet, and buckwheat are the main staples of their diet along with mineral-rich water with a pH of 8.5. But there is yet another unusual factor that may protect the health of the Hunza people and increase their longevity: their limited food intake.

Because the land provides just enough food to cover their basic caloric expenditures, the Hunzakuts rarely indulge in overeating. In fact, prior to the construction of the Korakoram Highway, they annually endured near-fasting conditions for several weeks each spring, a time when the previous year's food was depleted and the current year's harvests had not yet begun.

Restricted caloric intake can have powerful effects on longevity because it increases blood levels of growth hormone which is one of the most significant anti-aging hormones to be identified during the last two decades. Secreted by the pituitary gland, growth hormone production steadily declines with age. By age 70, the human body produces less than one-tenth of the growth hormone it did at age 20.

Clinical studies have repeatedly shown that growth hormone production is stimulated by low glucose levels. Because fasting depresses glucose levels, it leads to a surge in natural growth hormone production (Khansari et al., 1991)

Other studies have shown that the practice of caloric restriction (providing all necessary nutrients but limiting calorie intake) results in increased longevity and postponement of disease. Clive McCay at Cornell University showed that rats fed a diet low in calories but high in vitamins, minerals, and nutrients lived up to *twice as long* as rats fed on a regular diet (McCay et al., 1939). Ray Walford of the University of California in Los Angeles found that in studies on mice, the greater the reduction in calories, the longer the animal lived—as long as the vitamin and mineral content remained constant and the calories consumed did not drop below 40 percent of the normal (Walford et al., 1987).

The Complete Cleanse

It is difficult to control internal pollution with a simple one-time fix or a single magic-bullet type solution. Complete cleansing requires a battery of different solutions all targeted at specific systems of the body. Cleansing the liver needs different herbs, oils and minerals than cleansing the colon which requires a different cleansing solution than the intestines.

Complete cleansing also requires a broad array of products that are effective against a wide variety of contaminants and microorganisms—not just one or two. Contaminants like heavy metals need a different set of tools to deactivate and purge them from the body than parasites do.

An important part of a complete cleansing program is essential oils. Highly antibacterial, antifungal, and antiviral, essential oils help dissolve and chelate toxic chemicals in the body. They also promote digestive function and enhance the intestinal contractions that are the cornerstone of waste elimination.

The Herbal Colon Cleanse: ComforTone

Some of the best natural laxative herbs include diatomaceous earth, buckthorn bark, licorice root, apple pectin, bentonite, and black current extract. These herbs are particularly effective in cleansing the colon (large intestine) and can help counteract bloating and constipation. Purging the colon of toxins and impurities is just as important as cleaning the small intestine. Waste products and gases that are held in the colon have a far higher concentration of toxic by-products. When these leach into the organs and tissues, they can wreak havoc in our bodies.

The essential oils of rosemary and tarragon are antimicrobial and combat fungal buildup in the colon. Peppermint oil promotes peristalsis, the wavelike motion of the intestines, that is pivotal in moving waste matter out of the body.

Program:

Begin: 2 capsules every morning and 2 every night for 2 days.

Bowel movements should increase to 3-4 daily.

If elimination does not improve, then increase capsules to 3 each night and morning.

Keep increasing amount each day by one more capsule until you have achieved results.

If you feel cramping without results, you may have a dehydrated colon, spastic colon, loss of peristalsis, or a collapsed colon.

Drink 8 oz. of aloe vera and/or prune juice daily, which will work as a lubricant.

You should drink half your body weight of water in fluid ounces daily. When cleansing, you need 20% more water. However, water is not a lubricant. It works to soften and flush. Clay-like stools indicate dehydration caused by not drinking enough.

When proper bowel function is established, start reducing the amount of ComforTone each day. You may completely reduce the amount to zero or you may find that you need 1-2 capsules daily for a few weeks until you feel that you do not need it any more.

If you experience diarrhea, you may be taking too much ComforTone or not have enough I.C.P. fiber.

ComforTone and JuvaTone should not be taken together as they might cause a release of too many toxins at the same time creating nausea, vomiting, dizziness or simple discomfort. They are best taken an hour apart to allow them to work separately within the body.

The Fiber Cleanse: I.C.P.

Coarsely ground grains rich in soluble and semi-soluble fiber are some of the best intestinal cleansers known. Psyllium powder and husks, rice bran, oat bran, and flax seed all help loosen and expel undigested and fermenting materials from the intestines that may block nutrient absorption and poison our internal environment.

Fibers act as a biochemical sponge for the body, absorbing impurities, gases, and toxins. They also speed up the flow of waste matter through the intestines, helping to minimize the exposure to harmful substances. The slower the "transit time," or movement of waste matter through the gastro-intestinal tract the higher the incidence of disease.

Fibers satisfy appetite by giving people a feeling of fullness without adding excessive calories. Fiber may also help balance blood sugar levels. They also help maintain regularity as we grow older, preventing and overcoming constipation, diarrhea, and gas. Essential oils, such as fennel, tarragon, ginger, lemongrass, and rosemary, not only help dissolve and chelate toxins, but they also combat pathological microorganisms that reside in the intestines.

Program:

Begin: 1 teaspoon morning and night for two or three days

Increase to 2 tablespoons morning and night while you cleanse and drink plenty of water.

Maintenance: 2 tablespoons 3-4 time per week.

The Enzyme Cleanse: Megazyme

Enzymes help break down foods and proteins that might otherwise ferment and putrefy in the gastrointestinal tract. Undigested foods tax our bodies, sap our energy, and spur the overgrowth of yeast, fungi, and parasites. Enzymes like pancreatin and pancrelipase are very efficient in breaking down proteins. Vegetable enzymes from the unripe papaya and pineapple (papain and bromelain) provide enzyme support.

Digestive enzymes not only promote complete digestion but also help supply enzymes to people who have difficulty digesting and assimilating food. The older we get and the more food we consume, the more enzymes we need for complete digestion. Enzymes are essential in unlocking the vitamins, minerals, and amino acids from our food.

Enzymes help digest cooked and processed foods that lack the natural enzymes of fresh foods.

Program:

Maintenance: 2 or 3 tablets 3 times daily. They are best taken before meals.

Eating out: Carry tablets with you or take them when you return home. After a heavy meal at night and before going to bed, make sure to take plenty of tablets to help prevent fermenting.

A, B, and AB blood types: 2-4 tablets

O blood types: 3-6 or more tablets if you feel it necessary

Cancer or other degenerative diseases:

Phase 1: Take 3 tablets 3 times daily. Increase by one tablet every day until you become nauseated or vomit. Then discontinue Megazyme for 24 to 36 hours.

Phase 2: Take 4 tablets 3 times daily. Increase daily by one tablet until you become nauseated or vomit. Rest again 24-36 hours.

Phase 3: Take 5 tablets 3 times daily. Increase daily by one tablet until you become nauseated or vomit. Rest again for 24-36 hours.

Phase 4: Start again with the amount that was being taken before nausea or vomiting occurred the third time. For example: If you were taking 30 tablets when you started to vomit, you would then start Phase 4 with 29 tablets spread out over each day. Continue with this amount for 6 weeks.

Phase 5: In the 7th week, start the enzyme saturation program again. This means that you begin Phase 1 and increase the amount by one each day until nausea or vomiting starts again. Repeat and continue for 6 weeks as previously described.

If your doctor determines that you are in remission, you can maintain with 20-30 tablets daily for one year, 6 days a week.

Maintenance for this situation: 6 Megazyme 2 times daily

Caution: This is a rigorous program so you should consult with your doctor before starting and have you doctor monitor you.

The Liver Cleanse: JuvaTone and JuvaFlex

The liver is one of the most important organs in the body. It is pivotal for purifying our blood and plays a key role in converting carbohydrates to energy, as well as storing energy in the form of glycogen and fats. An overburdened liver can affect our energy, digestion, skin and blood.

Moreover, the fats and bile within the liver can easily become saturated with toxic by-products, chemicals and heavy metals—many of which are oil-soluble. As these toxins accumulate, the liver becomes taxed and stressed. Skin conditions, rashes, fatigue, headaches, muscle aches, digestive disturbances, pallor, dizziness, irritability, mood swings and mental confusion can all become evident.

The "lipotropic agents" choline, inositol and the powerful antioxidant, dl-methionine, have been researched for the ability to defat and remove toxic byproducts from the liver. dl-Methionine is a sulfur-based amino acid that acts as an important liver-protecting antioxidant.

Oregon Grape Root is a source of berberine, a compound researched for its liver-protecting properties, as well as its ability to slow the liver damage and scarring (cirrhosis) associated with alcohol consumption and hepatitis B and C.

Essential oils can also be valuable in increasing the flow of bile from the liver. These oils include blue chamomile, carrot seed, and geranium. Carrot seed oil is well-regarded by herbalists for its role in liver cleansing.

Program:

Week 1: Take 3 tablets 3 times daily for one week.

Week 2: Increase to 4 tablets 3 times daily for one week.

Week 3: Increase to 5 tablets 3 times daily for one week

Week 4: Increase to 6 tablets 3 times daily for 90 days.

Then decrease in the reverse order.

Rest for two weeks after the completed 120 day cycle.

Nausea or vomiting indicates a toxic liver. Stop and rest 2-3 days and then start again with 1/2 tablet per day. Gradually increase amount.

JuvaTone and ComforTone should not be taken together as they might cause a release of too many toxins at the same time creating nausea, vomiting, dizziness or just discomfort. They are best taken and hour apart to allow them to work individually as the body needs.

JuvaFlex may be massaged over the liver once daily and may also be applied in a hot compress application (see compress). A compress may be applied once a week. JuvaFlex may also be applied on the bottom of the feet through the Vita Flex technique over the liver points.

The Parasite Cleanse: ParaFree

Almost everyone has parasites in one form or another. For the most part, they go entirely unnoticed until they begin to cause fatigue and unwellness.

Pure essential oils have some of the strongest antiparasitic properties known. Some of these oils include thyme, clove, anise, nutmeg, fennel, vetiver, wild tansy, black cumin, melaleuca and laurus nobilis.

Program:

Begin: Take 3-6 gelcaps 2 times daily for one week. Rest for one week to allow the larva eggs to hatch and become active.

Continue for a minimum of 3 weeks and then rest for 3 weeks. Repeat for 3 weeks.

The duration of this program depends on the individual.

For maximum benefit, ParaFree should be taken with Collodial Essence. Terri S. Friedmann, M.D. found that by combining these two products, all parasites we killed.

The Heavy Metal Cleanse: Chelex Tincture

Heavy metals such as lead, mercury and cadmium can unleash damage to our bodies—even in tiny amounts. They disrupt normal functions and can lead to allergic reactions, fatigue, headache, muscle pains, digestive disturbance, dizziness, depression and mental confusion.

Of even graver concern is their tendency to accumulate in the brain, kidneys, nerves, immune system and fatty tissues. Some highly poisonous heavy metals, such as cadmium, can remain in the body for up to 30 years.

Herbs such as astragalas, garlic, sarsaparilla, and red clover have the ability to bind heavy metals so they can be expelled from the body. Essential oils also have a natural ability to dissolve insoluble heavy metal salts so that they can be eliminated.

Program:

Begin: Put 3-4 droppers in distilled water and drink 3-4 time daily for up to 120 days. Depending on type of mineral or chemical toxicity it may be necessary to follow this regimen for 1 1/2 years.

Maintenance: 1-2 droppers 2 times daily, 5 days a week. The duration of this program depends on one's own knowledge of exposure and contamination.

Hair analysis may help in determining the duration of this program.

Maintenance Cleansing

Our lifestyle should incorporate cleansing at all times. The extremity of the cleansing depends on the individual. You should always take ComforTone, Megazyme and I.C.P. at the same time.

Program:

ComforTone: 1 tsp. 5-6 days per week.

Megazyme: 3 tablets 3 times daily to continue the digestion of toxic waste in your body from everyday metabolism.

Blood Cleanse: Rehemogen Tincture

Contains herbs which that were traditionally used by Chief Sundance and the native Americans for cleansing and purifying the blood. It builds red blood cells and is recommended for any blood disorders. It works as a strong companion with JuvaTone and Chelex.

Program:

Chelation with Chelex and JuvaTone: 2 droppers (approx. 50 drops) in water 2-3 times daily.

Blood disorders: Put 2-3 droppers (Approx. 50-75 drops) in distilled water every 2-3 hours. JuvaTone with Rehemogen is invaluable.

Royaldophilus: Restores proper flora in bowels

If taking antibiotics, chemotherapy, radiation: Take 3 capsules 3 times daily for one week after finishing with antibiotics or medical intervention.

Maintenance: Take 3 capsules 3 times weekly.

Hering's Four Laws of Healing

Constantine Hering, a German homeopath who emigrated to the United States in the 1830's, is considered the father of American homeopathy. He formulated four fundamental principles of healing:

1. Healing progresses from the deepest part of the organism—the mental and emotional levels and the vital organs—to the external parts, such as the skin and extremities.

2. As healing progresses, symptoms appear and disappear in the reverse of their original chronological order of appearance.

3. Healing progresses from the upper to the lower parts of the body. This means that head symptoms may clear before stomach symptoms. Deep toxins in the colon or liver will be released before the more surface areas.

4. The most recent illnesses will be the first to leave. This means that flu symptoms experienced a month ago will leave earlier in the fast than the bronchitis suffered two years before.

Building the Body

Nutritional supplements enhanced with essential oils can help support and balance body systems. The following products will nourish, strengthen and build your body.

Program:

Power Meal—The ultimate superfood.

Use 2 scoops (4 tbs) in liquid 2-3 times per day. Mix in water, rice or soy milk. It can be mixed in orange or apple juice, but this may make it too sweet and lower the pH. It also may be mixed with cereal, fruits, deserts, and other foods.

Combine equal parts Power Meal and Body Balance for a high-powered protein blend.

Drink as needed.

Master Formula HERS/HIS—Premium multivitamin, mineral and amino acid supplement.

O Blood Type: 8-10 tablets daily

B Blood Type 6-8 tablets daily

A Blood Type 4-6 tablets daily

Megazyme—Enzyme function for mental clarity and physical activity

O Blood Type: 4-8 tablets daily (depending on type of food eaten and time of day)

B Blood Type: 8-10 tablets daily

A Blood Type: 10-12 daily (A types tend to have more digestive needs)

Note: When eating heavy protein foods after 3:00 p.m., it would be very helpful to take more Megazyme before going to bed.

Exodus—Supercharged antioxidant formula for immune supporting.

O Blood Type: 6-8 capsules daily

B Blood Type: 6-7 capsules daily

A Blood Type: 4-6 capsules daily

VitaGreen—Protein-rich chlorophyll formula.

O Blood Type: 8-10 capsules daily

B Blood Type: 6-8 capsules daily

A Blood Type: 4-6 capsules daily

Ultra Young—Supports healthy pituitary and growth hormone secretion.

Apply 3 sprays on the inside of the cheeks to maximize absorption. Avoid swallowing. Inhale the fragrance of the oils if possible.

Age 15-30: Spray (3 squirts) 2 times daily (for immune support).

Age 30-45: Spray (3 squirts) 2-3 times daily.

Age 45-65: Spray (3 squirts) 4-6 times daily.

Juvenile Pituitary Retardation: Take 3 sprays 3-6 times daily.

Spray 6 days a week for 3 weeks and rest for one week and then repeat.

ImmuneTune

O Blood Type: 6-8 capsules daily

B Blood Type: 6 plus capsules daily

A Blood Type: 4 plus capsules daily

Super C

O Blood Type: 8-10 tablets daily

B Blood Type: 6-8 tablets daily

A Blood Type: 6-8 tablets daily

Super Cal

2-6 daily or as needed.

Mineral Essence

3-6 droppers (75 to 150 drops) in water 1-2 times daily.

Sulfurzyme

Start: 1-2 tsp daily for 1-2 days

Increase: 1-2 tbs 2 times daily for maximum results.

Daily Maintenance

The human body has a daily need for nutrients to keep it in peak condition. The nutritional products listed below contain essential oils to help support normal digestive function and nutrient absorption.

Power Meal or Body Balance—Complete protein foods.

Combine or use individually: 1-2 scoops in water, rice milk, oat milk, or other liquid

VitaGreen—Protein-rich chlorophyll formula very beneficial for vegetarians and O blood types.

O Blood Type: 8-10 capsules daily

B Blood Type: 6-8 capsules daily

A Blood Type: 4-6 capsules daily

Master HIS/HERS—**Gender-specific** vitamin, mineral, and amino acid complexes.

O Blood Type: 8-10 tablets daily

B Blood Type 6-8 tablets daily

A Blood Type 4-6 tablets daily

ComforTone—All natural colon cleanser

Essential Manna—Whole food complex can be a fiber- mineral-rich snack.

Fortifying the Immune System

Dietary supplements containing essential oils provide nutritional support for normal immune system function. Many ingredients in these nutritional products are used to reinforce the body's natural defense system. Research has found that micro-organisms do not develop resistance to essential oils as much as they do to many other products.

Exodus II—is blended with oils referenced in the Old and New Testaments.

Massage 3-6 drops on bottom of feet, thymus, throat, or wherever desired.

Exodus—is a strong immune builder.

Maintenance: 2-4 daily, O blood types may increase amount

For weaker system: Take 6-10 capsules 3 times daily for 10 days and then reduce. Type A bloods may want to use less.

Sulfurzyme—contains MSM and Chinese Wolfberry.

Maintenance: 1-2 tsp. daily in water or juice. May increase as needed.

Deficiencies: Begin 1-2 tsp. daily and work up to 3-4 Tbs daily or more if desired.

ImmuneTune—is a strong antioxidant, anti-inflammatory, anti-tumoral properties. Helps maintain electrolyte and pH balance.

Maintenance: 2-4 daily

Radex—contains herbs and essential oils that have been researched for their antioxidant properties and their effects on DNA-damaging free radicals. This blend also contains Super Oxide Dismutase, widely reported to be another powerful free-radical scavenger.

Super C—is a special formula of ascorbic acid, scientifically balanced with rutin, biotin, bioflavonids and trace minerals to balance electrolytes and assist in the absorption of vitamin C. The essential oils Grapefruit, Tangerine, Lemon, and Mandarin may increase the oxygen and bioflavonoid activity.

Thyromin—is an herbal complex with amino acids, minerals, herbs and essential oils to support to the thyroid. This gland regulates body metabolism and temperature and is important for immune function.

Immugel—is a blend of liquid amino acids, ionic trace minerals and herbal extracts with essential oils. Amino acids are the building blocks of protein and form the enzymes used to support immune function.

Protec—is a blend of essential and vegetable oils for the prostate, designed for a night-long retention enema.

Mineral Essence—is a precisely-balanced complex of essential oils and more than 60 trace minerals that are essential to a healthy immune system. It includes well-known antioxidants and immune-supporters such as zinc, selenium and magnesium.

Digestive System

"The gastrointestinal tract is a tube 25 to 32 feet long that begins at the mouth and ends at the anus. It comprises the mouth, pharynx, esophagus, stomach, small intestine (duodenum, jejunum, and ileum), large intestine (cecum, ascending colon, transverse colon, and descending colon), rectum, and anus. Other organs, such as the liver, pancreas, and gallbladder, all play an important role in digestion.

"Digestion begins when food mixes with enzymes in saliva. The process is then carried on in the stomach by hydrochloric acid (HCl) and pepsin. Food is liquefied in the stomach and passes into the small intestine, where it is further broken down by digestive enzymes from the pancreas (the enzyme protease digests proteins, the enzyme amylase digests carbohydrates, and the enzyme lipase digests fats). The gallbladder secretes bile, formed by the liver, to aid absorption of fats and fat-soluble vitamins.

"Most food absorption takes place in the small intestine, while water, electrolytes (essential body chemicals), and some of the final products of digestion (including B vitamins) are absorbed in the large intestine." (Alternative Medicine-The Definitive, p. 680)

Digestive Tract

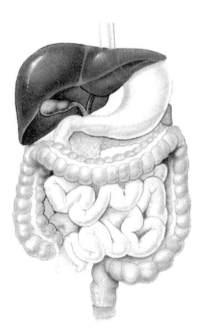

The Clock Diet

The Clock Diet was originated by Dr. Charlotte Holms who maintained a private practice even at 100 years of age in 1989. This diet was based on the fact that stomach acid and enzyme production (pepsin and hydrochloric acid) begins in the morning (about 6 a.m.) and tapers off during the afternoon (between 1:00 and 3:00 p.m.)

This diet mandates that we should schedule our consumption of animal and plant protein to coincide with the highest output of stomach acid and enzymes. Unless our body produces the enzymes to break down protein, high-protein foods will merely ferment in the stomach and lead to fungal and bacterial overgrowth, laying the groundwork not only for indigestion, but also for disease.

Ideally, we should consume all of our high-protein foods once a day during the morning meal. These foods include grains, such as oats, cornmeal, millet, soy milk, and brown rice, and animal products, such as cheese, milk, and meats.

When the stomach's production of acid and enzymes drops during midafternoon, the best foods to eat consist of simple and complex carbohydrates, such as fresh fruits, cooked and raw vegetables. Avoid mixing protein and carbohydrates in the same afternoon or night meal.

Weight Management

Fitness

Power Meal: 2 scoops, 4-6 times daily in water or rice milk or as needed.

Be-Fit: 2 capsules before working out and 2 capsules after working out.

> Capsules may be increased or decreased as needed according to body weight and blood type.

VitaGreen: As desired, anywhere from 4-10 capsules daily

Master HIS/HERS: As desired, anywhere from 4-8 capsules daily.

Pregnancy

Babies and children respond very well to oils and supplements. It is only that the amount and dosage is less.

Babies: Put 1-2 drops in your hand and rub them together until the hands are practically dry. Then hold then over any particular area of the baby. This works very well without direct application.

Direct application: Mix 1-2 drops of an essential oil in V-6 Mixing oil or Massage Oil Base and apply to bottom of feet.

Children: Put 1-2 drops on bottom of feet or anywhere else on the body as long as the oil is diluted in V-6 Mixing oil or any vegetable or massage oil. The dilution is always the important factor in comfortability.

> *"It is a mystery to me why synthetic progestins and estrogen are recommended when the natural progesterone is available, cheaper, and safer."*
>
> —John R. Lee, M.D.
> Author of WHAT YOUR DOCTOR MAY
> NOT TELL YOU ABOUT MENOPAUSE

Hormone Balance: Women

Progesterone Balance Creme

Many women—especially those who are postmenopausal—are estrogen dominant. This means their bodies produce excess estrogen and not enough progesterone. As a result, the following symptoms emerge:

Headaches / Migraines
Mood swings
Depression / Fatigue
Cramps / PMS
Irregular cycles
Breast cancer
Osteoporosis
Breast tenderness
Bloating / Inability to lose weight
Blood sugar imbalance
Reduced sex drive
Facial hair
Hot flashes
Insomnia

A natural transdermally-absorbed progesterone cream can reduce all of these symptom by providing a source of natural progesterone that can counterbalance excessive estrogen levels.

EssPro 7 Progesterone Creme

EssPro 7 contains over 550 mg of highly-purified soy-derived natural progesterone, which is identical to the hormone produced by the human body. This natural progesterone in chemically far different from the synthetic hormones—such as Premarin—which have harmful side effects ranging from weight gain to increased cancer risk. Natural progesterone is readily accepted by the body with few side effects.

In addition to soy-derived progesterone, EssPro 7 includes black cohosh, clary sage, sage, and other natural extracts that balance the effect of progesterone. Clary sage and sage contain sclareol which mimics estrogen action in the body if there is an estrogen deficiency. If there is a progesterone or testosterone deficiency, it can mimic those hormone as well.

- Start: 1/8 tsp. once per day, 5 times weekly.

- Rub into soft or delicate skin areas, such as inside arms or thighs. Rotate sites of application.

- Generally, between the third and fourth day, you should recognize a change.

- With moderate results: Increase to 1/8 tsp. twice daily.

- Extreme deficiency: Increase to 1/2 tsp. per day.

- After the first 3 weeks, a maintenance dosage of 1/8 tsp. 2-3 times weekly should be sufficient.

Cycling women

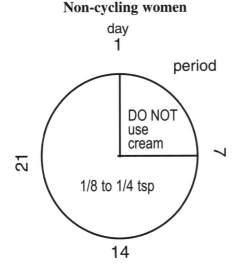

Non-cycling women

What is Progesterone?

For both men and women, natural progesterone is among the most pivotal hormones in the body. Synthesized from cholesterol in the body, progesterone is the precursor from which testosterone, estrogen, estrone, estriadol, and corticosteroids, and a host of other key hormones are made. When progesterone levels drop, a biochemical cascade effect is created which impacts numerous other hormones and affects glands ranging from the pancreas to the thyroid. This can translate into physical effects ranging from mood swings and headaches to reduced sex drive and increased cancer risk.

Using too much you may experience:

- Fuzzy vision

- Depression

- Headache

If EssPro 7 does not produce results after two months—

- Try balancing the entire nutritional profile.

- Because the thyroid function plays a major role in hormonal balance, Thyromin should accompany EssPro 7. Estrogen dominant women usually suffer thyroid function deficiency.

- Use Estro Tincture. In some rare cases, you might be deficient in progesterone and estrogen. By using EssPro 7 together with Estro,

- Consume foods with vitamin B6, magnesium, and potassium. Several studies have shown that these nutrient will not only reduce PMS symptoms, but will also enhance hormonal balance.

- Massage clary sage and/or sage on the feet to help create hormonal balance.

- Massage EndoFlex over the adrenal points through the VitaFlex points on the feet.

SoyPro

This international version of EssPro 7 is a progesterone-only cream. It contains no wild yam extract, clary sage, sage, or fennel.

Estro Tincture

Estro is desgined for women who are estrogen deficient. Numerous studies have researched the benefits of black cohosh for relieving PMS symptoms, without the side effects associated with synthetic estrogen. The German Commission E has approved black cohosh as a natural alternative to estrogen in Europe.

Estro is comforting for cramping and irregular bleeding. In these cases, FemiGen should accompany Estro to help give more balance to the estrogen.

Begin: Drink 2-3 droppers in water, 1-3 times daily.

FemiGen

Food to strengthen the reproductive system, creating better hormonal balance and helping with night-time sweats.

Deficiencies: 3-4 capsules, 2-3 times daily.

Maintenance: 4-8 capsules, 2 times weekly.

Femalin

May help cervical lesions and cysts, ovarian cysts, and endometriosis.

Begin: 2-3 droppers in water, 3 times daily.

Increase if necessary: 3-4 droppers in water, 4 times daily or as necessary to alleviate cramping and irregular bleeding.

Douche: Mix 6 droppers in distilled water, 2-3 times daily.

Dragon Time

Massage: 3-4 drops around inside and outside of ankles, over lower back for premenstrual problems, ovarian imbalance, cramping or irregular flow. Add 2-3 drops of clary sage may also be added for extra strength.

Suppository: 20 drops in a capsule, insert at night for night retention

Bath: Mix 30 drops in bath gel base for a relaxing and soothing bath

Mister

Many women ages 40 plus have found that Mister helps in preventing hot flashes. May be used in bath, on Vita Flex points, rubbed on lower back and over lower abdomen. It is a good companion to Dragon Time.

Hormone Balance: Men

Because progesterone is a natural precursor to testosterone, men also may benefit from progesterone. In this case the use of a progesterone creme, such as EssPro 7, may be highly beneficial.

Rub 1/2 tsp. of EssPro 7 into soft tissues. Use no more than 2 times daily and rotate applications sites each day for four days.

ProGen

Helps feed and nourish the male reproductive system.

Maintenance: Take 2-3 capsules, 2 times daily

Aggressive deterioration: 6 capsules, 3 times daily.

Mister

Supports male reproductive system. May be taken as a dietary supplement 3-10 drops under tongue 2-3 times daily. Take 10-20 drops in water or in a capsule 2 times daily. Use no more than 7 days and then rest 4 days. Massage on Vita Flex points and between scrotum and rectum.

Longevity

Priority: Ultra Young, Essential Manna, Power Meal, VitaGreen, Master Formula, Thyromin. ImmuneTune, Royal Essence.

Scientific Research: Supplement Ingredients

The Chinese Wolfberry: A Breakthrough in Anti-aging and Immunity

In the early 1980s, a group of researchers from the Natural Science Institute began studying a region on the West Elbow Plateau of the Yellow River in Inner Mongolia where people lived to be over 100 years old—10 to 20 years longer than the average person in the region. The inhabitants shared one trait that distinguished them from others. They were predominantly vegetarian and regularly consumed wolfberries. Moreover, the people who consumed this fruit lived free of common diseases like arthritis, cancer, and diabetes.

Both the Chinese wolfberry (also known as *Lycium barbarum* by botanists and as the goji berry by native Chinese) and ginseng *(Panax ginseng)* have been highly regarded for centuries as the foremost nutritional and therapeutic plants in China. In fact, the Chinese hold a strong belief that human life might be extended significantly by using either of these herbs for an extended period. Unfortunately, ginseng is considered too strong for continuous use, and large amounts may not be suitable for people with high blood pressure or heart disease. On the other hand, the wolfberry is much milder, with no known risk from continuous use.

18 Amino Acids and 21 Trace Minerals

In 1988, the Beijing Nutrition Research Institute conducted detailed chemical analyses and nutritional composition studies of the dried wolfberry fruit. What they discovered was stunning! The wolfberry contained over 18 amino acids, 21 trace minerals, more protein than bee pollen, more vitamin C than oranges, and nearly as much beta carotene as carrots.

Perhaps this is why the Chinese have traditionally attributed so many benefits to the wolfberry, claiming it protects liver function, replenishes vital essences, improves visual acuity, and lowers blood pressure and cholesterol. The wolfberry was also said to strengthen muscles and bones, stimulate the

A university in Japan experimented with diffusing different oils in the office. When they diffused lemon, there were 54% fewer errors, with jasmine there were 33% fewer errors, and with lavender there were 20% fewer errors. When oils were diffused while studying and taking a test, test scores increased by as much as 50%.

Diffusing an essential oil while studying may also improve memory while taking a test. By inhaling the same aroma, the smell of the oil may encourage recall of facts or figures learned previously by bringing back the memory of what was studied.

heart, and work as an aid to treat diabetes and impotence. The big question was: Could these results be substantiated in clinical studies?

Since the early 1980s, the Chinese wolfberry has been the subject of a number of important clinical studies—including several published by the State Scientific and Technological Commission in China. These studies have documented the antioxidant and immune-stimulating properties of the Chinese wolfberry.

From July 1982 to January 1984, the Ningxia Institute of Drug Inspection conducted a pharmacological experiment using multi-index screening (Register No. 870303). Their conclusion was:

> The fruits and pedicels of wolfberry were effective in increasing white blood cells, protecting the liver, and relieving hypertension. The alcoholic extract of wolfberry fruits inhibited tumor growth in mice by 58 percent, and the protein of wolfberry displayed an insulin-like action that was effective in promoting fat decomposition and reducing blood sugar.

Another clinical experiment by the Ningxia Institute (Register No. 870306, October 1982 to May 1985) studied the effects of wolfberry on the immune, physiological, and biochemical indexes of the blood of aged volunteers. The results indicated that the wolfberry caused the blood of older people to noticeably revert to a younger state.

Can the Wolfberry Boost Immune Function?

According to a report of the State Scientific and Technological Commission of China, the wolfberry contains compounds known as lycium polysaccharides, which appeared to be highly effective in promoting immunity. These results were supported in a number of clinical trials.

In one study on a group of cancer patients, the wolfberry triggered an increase in both lymphocyte transformation rate and white blood cell count (measures of immune function). In another study involving a group of 50 people with lower-limit white blood cell counts, the wolfberry increased phagocytosis and the titre of serum antibodies (another index of immune function). Unhealthy levels of titre of serum antibodies have long been associated with Chronic Fatigue Syndrome (also known as Epstein-Barr). Does this mean that the wolfberry could be used as a weapon against Epstein-Barr? The possibilities are intriguing.

In another study, consumption of wolfberry led to a strengthening of immunoglobulin A levels (an index of immune function). Because the decline of immunoglobulin A is one of the signs of aging, an increase in these levels suggests that the wolfberry may enable injured DNA to better repair itself and ward off tissue degeneration.

Is the Wolfberry a Powerful Antioxidant?

As we grow older, the levels of lipid peroxide in our blood increase, while levels of health-protecting antioxidants, like superoxide dismutase (SOD), decrease. In a clinical study of people who consumed doses of wolfberry, SOD in the blood increased by a remarkable 48 percent while hemoglobin increased by 12 percent. Even better, lipid peroxide levels dropped by an astonishing 65 percent.

Does the Wolfberry Protect Eyesight?

A test was conducted on the effects of wolfberry on eyesight. Twenty-seven people were tested and showed a dramatic improvement in both dark adaptation and vitamin A and carotene content of their serum (measures of eyesight acuity).

More recent studies in the 1990s have lent additional scientific support.

Use of Wolfberry (*Lycium barbarum polysaccharides*) to Treat Cancer

Conclusion: Lycium barbarum polysaccharides can be used as an adjuvant in the treatment of cancer.

Abstract: Seventy-nine advanced cancer patients were treated with a combination of LAK/IL-2* and *Lycium barbarum* polysaccharides. Patients treated with only LAK/IL-2 showed a response rate of only 16 percent, while those treated with both LAK/IL-2 and *Lycium barbarum* polysaccharides showed a response rate of 40.9 percent. Moreover, the mean remission in the *Lycium barbarum* group lasted significantly longer. *Lymphokine-activated natural killer cells (LAK) and interleukin 2 (IL-2).

Author: G. W. Cao, W. G. Yang, P. Du

Journal: Chunghua Chung Lui Tsa Chih 16 (Nov. 1994): 428-31

Location: Second Military Medical University, Shanghai

The Role of Lycium barbarum Polysaccharide as an Antioxidant

Conclusion: The effects of free radicals on cells can be prevented and reversed by incubation with either *Lycium barbarum* polysaccharide or superoxide dismutase.

Abstract: Researchers incubated cells (Xenopus Oocytes) in a solution containing a free-radical-producing system for 6 hours. The changes in the electrical profile of the cell membranes were determined using a microelectrode electrophysiological technique. The results showed that *Lycium barbarum* polysaccharide prevented and reversed free radical damage to the cells.

Author: X. Zhang

Journal: Chung Kuo Chung Yao Tsa Chih 18 (Feb. 1993): 110-2, 128

Location: Beijing Military Hospital

Protective Action of Lycium barbarum on Hydrogen Peroxide-induced Lipid Peroxidation

Conclusion: *Lycium barbarum* protects red blood cell membranes against lipid peroxidation.

Abstract: Hydrogen peroxide (H2O2), a powerful promoter of oxidative damage, was used to promote lipid peroxidation of the red blood cell membranes of rats. Dried Lycium berries showed the greatest protective effect against H2O2 damage, followed by *Lycium barbarum* polysaccharide.

Author: B. Ren, Y. Ma, Y. Shen, B. Gao

Journal: Chung Kuo Chung Yao Tsa Chih 20 (May 1995): 303-4

Location: Ningxia Medical College, Yinchuan

Effects of Lycium barbarum on the Attachment and Growth of Human Gingival Cells to Root Surfaces

Conclusion: *Lycium barbarum* improved the attachment and growth of human gingival cells to root surfaces.

Abstract: A dose of 1.25 mg/ml *Lycium barbarum* was used to stimulate the in vitro attachment of human gingival fibrobasts to the surfaces of dental roots. In response to *Lycium barbarum* exposure, cells on diseased root surfaces increased in quantity, exhibited better growth and distribution. Drynaria displayed similar effects but was not as potent as the *Lycium barbarum*.

Author: B. Liu

Journal: Chung Kuo Chung Yao Tsa Chih 27 (May 1992): 159-61, 190

Location: College of Stomatology, Fourth Medical University, Xian

HMB: A Natural Immune-booster and Muscle-builder

Beta-hydroxy beta-methylbutyrate (HMB), a natural derivative of the amino acid L-leucine, has been shown to be one of the newest and most powerful supplements for promoting growth in lean muscle tissue. Studies have also documented the ability of HMB to improve immune function and increase life expectancy in animals.

According to noted researcher, Richard Passwater, Ph.D., "HMB showed that it lowered total and LDL cholesterol levels in blood and helped strengthen the immune system while building muscles and burning body fat. This news is certainly of interest to body builders and other athletes, but it may also become of interest to cancer, AIDS, and muscular dystrophy patients."

Other health and fitness professionals agree. "HMB is one of the most exciting natural nutrients for supporting muscle growth and immunity that I've seen in quite some time," stated Dr. Robert Delmonteque, an expert on fitness. "HMB will enable many people to attain new levels of health and fitness—especially when combined with regular exercise and sound nutrition."

Method of Promoting Nitrogen Retention in Humans

Conclusion: HMB promotes protein retention and body fat loss in middle-aged adult males.

Abstract: In a placebo-controlled random-designed crossover study, five adult men received a placebo for 2 weeks, followed by 2 grams of HMB daily for another two weeks. During the control period, body fat content decreased from 12.4 to 12 percent and urinary nitrogen loss (a measure of muscle and protein loss) increased from 14.5 to 16.1 grams per day. However, during the HMB supplementation period, body fat dropped from 12.5 to 11 percent, and urinary nitrogen loss decreased from 16.7 to 15.4 grams per day.

Author: Nissen, S. L., N. N. Abumrad, et al.

Journal: U.S. Patent and Trademark Office, Patent #5,348,979

The Effect of Leucine Metabolite HMB on Muscle Metabolism During Resistance Exercise Training

Conclusion: HMB spares muscle-damaged, physically active adults.

Abstract: Forty volunteers participating in a supervised exercise program were divided into three group. The first group received a placebo, the second group received 1.5 grams of HMB daily, and the third group received 3 grams of HMB daily. Muscle damage was assessed by measuring the amount of creatine phosphokinase (CPK) and lactate dehydrogenase (LDH) in the blood. The group receiving the highest amount of HMB had the lowest blood levels of both CPK and LDH. This indicated that HMB had muscle and protein-sparing effects in humans.

Author: Nissen, S. L., J. C. Fuller, Jr., J. Shell, et al.

Journal: Journal of Applied Physiology 81 (1996): 2095-2104

The Effect of Leucine Metabolite HMB on Muscle Metabolism During Resistance Exercise Training (2)

Conclusion: HMB spares muscle-damaged, physically active adult volunteers.

Abstract: Thirty athletes from the Iowa State University football team were randomly divided into two groups. The first group received a placebo, while the second received 3 grams per day of HMB. After seven weeks the gain in muscle mass and strength of the two groups were assessed. The HMB group gained an average of 13 ounces of lean muscle mass, compared with no gain for the control group. Moreover, the HMB group gained an average of 15 pounds in bench-press strength, compared with a 5.4 pound gain in the control group.

Author: Nissen, S. L., J. C. Fuller, Jr., J. Shell, et al.

Journal: Journal of Applied Physiology 81 (1996): 2095-2104

The Effect of HMB Supplementation on Strength and Body Composition of Trained and Untrained Males Undergoing Intense Resistance Training

Conclusion: HMB promotes muscle gain and body fat declines in both athletes and nonathletes who embark on an exercise program.

Abstract: In a double-blind, placebo-controlled study, 40 volunteers submitted to a four-week strenuous exercise program. Half received a placebo, while the remainder received 3 grams daily of HMB. Following the four week regimen, the HMB group's gain in muscle mass was 57 percent greater than the control group. In addition, the HMB group lost 119 percent more body fat as well.

Author: Nissen, S. L., L. Panton, R. Wilhelm, et al.

Journal: FASEB 10 (1996): A287

Effect of HMB on Body Composition Changes Measured by Computerized Tomography in Older Adults Participating in an Exercise Program

Conclusion: HMB can safely increase muscle mass and reduce body fat in older adults.

Abstract: In a double blind, placebo-controlled study, 15 men and 16 women (average age 70) participated in a three day-a-week walking program and a two-day-a-week strength training program. After 8 weeks body composition analyses were conducted by skinfold measurements and computerized tomography. The HMB group gained significantly more muscle mass (+1.6 percent) than the control group (-.2 percent). The HMB group also shed more body fat (-3.9 percent) than the control group (+.7 percent).

Author: Vukovich, M.D., N. B. Stubbs, et al.

Journal: FASEB 12 (1998): A652

Effect of HMB on Health of Calves

Conclusion: HMB dramatically reduced both morbidity (sickness) and mortality of shipping-stressed calves.

Abstract: Three truckloads of cattle (158 animals) were randomly assigned to either a control diet or a diet supplemented with 4 g of HMB. After 28 days the morbidity and mortality of the HMB-supplemented calves was compared with the control group. The HMB group displayed 15 percent less sickness and 94 percent less mortality than the control group.

Author: Van Koevering, M. T., D. R. Gill, et al.

Journal: Oklahoma State Animal Science Research Report (1993)

Enhancement of Immunity by HMB in Chickens

Conclusion: HMB increases the growth and function of macrophage immune cells in chickens.

Abstract: Macrophages from a chicken cell line were exposed to 0, 10, 20, 40, 80, 100 mcg of HMB per $5 \times 10_4$ cells in a 96 well culture plate. At 100 mcg HMB exposure, macrophages exhibited a 19 percent and 21 percent increase in growth compared with untreated cells.

Author: A. L. Peterson, M. A. Qureshi, et al.

Journal: Poultry Science 75 (1997)

Stevia: A New, Safe, Non-caloric Supplement with Health-giving Properties

For over 1600 years, the natives of Paraguay in South America have used this intensely sweet herb as a health agent and sweetener. Known as *Stevia rebaudiana* by botanists and yerba dulce (honey leaf) by the Guarani Indians, stevia has been incorporated into many native medicines, beverages, and foods for centuries. The Guarani used stevia separately or combined with herbs like yerba mate and lapacho.

Fifteen times sweeter than sugar, stevia was introduced to the West in 1899, when M. S. Bertoni discovered natives using it as a sweetener and medicinal herb. However, stevia never gained popularity in Europe or the United States and only gradually was adopted by several countries throughout Far East Asia.

With Japan's ban on the import of synthetic sweeteners in the 1960's, stevia began to be seriously researched by the Japanese National Institute of Health as a natural sugar substitute. After almost a decade of studies examining the safety and antidiabetic properties of the herb, Japan became a major producer, importer, and user of stevia. Hundreds of food products began including it, and eventually stevia use spread through Asia. Stevioside, the super sweet glycoside derived from stevia that is 300 times sweeter than sugar, was even used to sweeten Diet Coke sold in Japan.

Even though stevia is still relatively unknown in the United States, it has gained widespread popularity as a low-calorie sweetener throughout South America and Asia. Both the stevia leaf and stevioside are used in Taiwan, China, Korea, and Japan, with many of these same countries growing large amounts of the raw herb.

In 1994, the U.S. Food and Drug Administration permitted the importation and use of stevia as a dietary supplement. However, its adoption by American consumers as a noncaloric sweetener has been very slow because the FDA does not currently permit stevia to be marketed as a food additive. This means that stevia cannot be sold as a sweetener (all sweeteners are classified as food additives by the FDA). Moreover, stevia faces fierce opposition by both the artificial sweetener (aspartame) and sugar industry in the U.S.

Stevia, however, is more than just a non-caloric sweetener. Several modern clinical studies have documented the ability of stevia to lower and balance blood sugar levels, support the pancreas and digestive system, protect the liver, and combat infectious microorganisms. (Oviedo et al., 1971; Suzuki et al., 1977; Ishit et al., 1986; Boeckh, 1986; Alvarez, 1986.)

In one study, Oviedo et. al. showed that oral administration of a stevia leaf extract reduced blood sugar levels by over 35 percent. Another study conducted by Suzuki et. al. documented similar results. Clearly, these and other clinical evaluations indicate that stevia holds significant promise for the treatment of diabetes.

MSM: A New Solution for Arthritis, Allergies, and Pain

MSM (Methylsulfonalmethane) is a natural sulfur-bearing nutrient that occurs widely in nature (found in everything from mother's breast milk to fresh vegetables). It is an exceptional source of nutritional sulfur—a mineral that is vital to protein synthesis and sound health.

Why is sulfur so important to the body? Because sulfur is a mineral which, like vitamin C, is constantly being used up and depleted. When we fail to replenish our reserves of nutritional sulfur, we become more vulnerable to disease and degenerative conditions. Some possible signs of sulfur deficiency are:

• Poor nail and hair growth
• Eczema
• Dermatitis
• Poor muscle tone
• Acne / Pimples
• Gout
• Rheumatism
• Arthritis
• Weakening of nervous system
• Constipation
• Impairment of mental faculties
• Lowered libido

MSM is more than just another essential nutrient. According to research compiled by Ronald Lawrence, Ph.D., M.D., and Stanley Jacob, M.D., MSM represents a safe, natural solution for chronic headaches, back pain, tendonitis, fibromyalgia, rheumatism, arthritis, athletic injuries, muscle spasms, asthma, and allergies.

In a book entitled, *The Miracle of MSM,* both Dr. Jacobs and Dr. Lawrence discuss how MSM has benefited hundred of patients. A UCLA neuro-psychiatrist, Dr. Lawrence is convinced that MSM will revolutionize how millions of people deal with inflammatory autoimmune diseases like rheumatism, asthma, bursitis, and tendonitis, as well as auto-immune diseases like arthritis, Lupus, scleroderma, and allergies.

Other doctors have also seen their patients dramatically improve using 2 to 4 grams of MSM daily. According to David Blyweiss, M.D., of the Institute of Advanced Medicine in Lauderhill, Florida, many patients experience a 50 percent improvement in their arthritis symptoms, along with less fatigue, better sleep, and better ability to exercise.

Dr. Lawrence has also used MSM to improve the condition of patients who were virtually crippled with arthritis and back pain. One patient was able to get out of bed for the first time after just two weeks on MSM. And after two months of MSM use, he could walk to the grocery store.

Another of Dr. Lawrence's patients was a 70-year-old woman who was suffering from severe arthritis. In this case, MSM actually postponed the need for double knee replacement. Moreover, after only two months on oral MSM, he was walking again with much less pain and stiffness.

Numerous other MSM users have experienced results equivalent to cortisone—but without side effects like immune suppression, fluid retention, and weakness.

According to Stanley Jacobs, M.D., there may be no pharmaceutical therapy better—or safer—than MSM. "MSM has an important role to play in the nonsurgical treatment of back pain," he said. "I have seen several hundred patients for back pain secondary to osteoarthritis, disc degeneration, spinal misalignments, or accidents. For such pain-related conditions, MSM is usually beneficial."

"I have been recommending MSM for more than six months," said Richard Shaefer, a chiropractor from Wheeling, Illinois. "The results have been excellent. I consistently see major reduction in pain and inflammation in the area of arthritis joints, along with improved range of motion. I can't think of a single individual who isn't getting some kind of positive effect."

MSM may have other benefits aside from its pain and inflammation-reducing properties. Numerous patients have reported a surge in energy levels along with thicker hair, nails, and skin. Some have even reported a softening or disappearance of scar tissue.

One user reported a marked increase in stamina and energy after starting on MSM. "For a long while I have had the blahs," complained Lou Salyer of Tucson, Arizona. "I had no stamina. I had to force myself to get things done around the house. After two days on MSM, it was like a blast of energy. I am amazed at how much I get done now."

MSM may also do much more than relieve pain. "Prior to taking MSM (30 grams a day for 20 years), I would have a cold or flu two or three times a year," stated Dr. Jacobs. "Since I've been taking MSM, I've not had a single cold or the flu. I can't say that MSM prevented my cold or the flu, but it is a fascinating observation."

MSM contains an exceptionally bioavailable source of sulfur, one of the most neglected minerals needed by the human body. Carl Pfeiffer, M.D., Ph.D., a world-renowned expert on nutritional medicine, agreed, "Sulfur is the forgotten essential element."

Found in such foods as garlic and asparagus, the sulfur within MSM is a critical part of the amino acids cysteine and methionine, which form the building blocks of the nails, hair, and skin. Sulfur is also found in therapeutic mineral baths and hot springs that have brought relief to arthritis sufferers for centuries.

MSM is very closely related to DMSO, a powerful pain reliever that was the subject of a *60 Minutes* report in April, 1980. DMSO has been approved by the FDA for interstitial cystitis, a painful urinary tract condition.

The Youth Nutrient

Of particular importance is MSM's ability to equalize water pressure inside the cells—a considerable benefit for those plagued with bursitis, arthritis, and tendonitis. These kinds of inflammatory outbreaks are created when the water pressure inside the cells jumps past the pressure outside the cells, creating pressure and pain. MSM acts as a sort of cellular safety valve, affecting the protein envelope of the cell so that water transfers freely in and out of the cell. The result: rapid relief and less damage to tissues. And because it elasticizes the hold between the cells, MSM can restore flexibility to inflamed tissues.

When our bodies grow older and are chronically shortchanged of key minerals like sulfur and MSM, the bonds between our cells become increasingly rigid and brittle—a condition that can lead to a loss in skin flexibility and contribute to skin wrinkles. The internal manifestations of this cellular brittleness are far less visible but have a far greater negative impact on the body. MSM's ability to reintroduce flexibility into cell structures, therefore, can have widespread restorative affects.

FOS: Supernutrient Documented to Rebuild Intestinal Flora and Combat Candida, Cancer, and Infections

FOS (Fructooligosaccharides) are one of the best-documented, natural nutrients for promoting the growth the Lactobacilli and bifidobacteria bacteria that are the linchpin of sound health. FOS has also been clinically studied for its ability to increase magnesium and calcium absorption, lower blood glucose, cholesterol, and LDL levels, and to inhibit production of the reductase enzymes that can contribute to cancer. Because FOS can increase magnesium absorption, it can also lead to lowered blood pressure and better cardiovascular health.

In addition, FOS also has another benefit: It has a naturally sweet taste. Consisting of undigestible sugars found in fruits, vegetables, and grains, FOS possesses a palate-pleasing sweetness with only a fraction of the calories of refined sugar.

However, gaining beneficial quantities of FOS as part of a normal diet is very difficult, since you would have to consume over 15 tomatoes, a dozen bananas, or over 350 cloves of garlic to obtain just a 1/4 teaspoon of FOS.

The subject of over 40 human studies and 60 animal studies throughout the world, FOS has been intensively researched in Japan, the United States, and Europe for over a decade. FOS provides an outstanding source of nourishment for the beneficial bacteria that are our front-line defense against disease, while at the same time reducing the populations of harmful putrefactive bacteria and pathogenic yeast and fungi that can contribute to candida, Chronic Fatigue Syndrome, and other illnesses.

Herbal Supplements and Vitamins with Essential Oils

These supplements contain both herbs and therapeutic-grade essential oils. The essential oils act as catalysts to help deliver nutrients through the cell membrane while assisting in the removal of cellular wastes.

It is important to remember that these supplements are usually dissolved and assimilated by the body within a couple of hours. Therefore, spacing them throughout the day will provide better assimilation and nutrient value than consuming a handful all at once.

When using supplements, a general guideline is to discontinue use for at least one or two days a week to allow the body to regain homeostasis and permit its natural recuperative powers to engage.

An approximate frequency is indicated for some of the supplements. Please keep in mind that these are only estimates; and that due to the many variables involved in determining frequency, the results may be difficult to duplicate.

AlkaLime

This specially-designed alkaline mineral powder contains an array of high-alkaline salts and other yeast/fungus-fighting elements, such as citric acid and essential oils. Its precisely-balanced, acid-neutralizing mineral formulation helps preserve the body's proper pH balance—the cornerstone of health. By boosting blood alkalinity, yeast and fungus are deprived of the acidic terrain they require to flourish. The effectiveness of other essential oils is enhanced when the body's blood and tissues are alkaline.

AlkaLime may help reduce the following signs of acid-based yeast and fungus dominance: Fatigue/low energy, unexplained aches and pains, overweight conditions, low resistance to illness, allergies, headaches, irritability/mood swings, indigestion, colitis/ulcers, diarrhea/constipation, urinary tract infections, rectal/ vaginal itch.

Contains:

Calcium carbonate provides calcium, which is needed for healthy bones.

Potassium bicarbonate added for electrolyte balance.

Sodium bicarbonate used for electrolyte and pH balance.

Magnesium supports healthy intestinal flora, the first-line defense against fungus overgrowth.

Citric acid is added to help cleanse the digestive system.

Sea salts added to provide trace minerals and regulate pH balance.

Essential Oils:

Lemon (*Citrus limon*) promotes leukocyte formation and increases lymphatic function.

Lime (*Citrus aurantifolia*) decongests the lymphatic system.

Companion Products: Royaldophilus, VitaGreen, Mineral Essence, Megazyme, and Mint Condition

Companion Oils: Di-Tone, peppermint, spearmint, Thieves, and Purification.

Suggested Use: Stir one rounded teaspoon into 6-8 oz. of distilled or purified water and drink immediately. To aid in alkalizing connective tissue, AlkaLime may be taken 1-3 times per day before meals or before eating. As an antacid, AlkaLime may be taken as needed. Otherwise, an ideal time to take AlkaLime would be prior to bedtime.

ArthroTune

An herbal complex that may help arthritis and rheumatoid conditions.

Ingredients:

Alfalfa leaf supports muscles and joints.

Butcher's Broom has anti-inflammatory action.

Yucca improves blood circulation.

Capsicum has been used for pain relief and to help stimulate circulation.

Uncaria tomentosa, known as Cat's Claw, is used as an immune system stimulant and possesses anti-inflammatory properties.

Grade seed proanthocyanidins inhibits swelling and is used as an antioxidant.

Magnesium relaxes muscles.

Essential Oils:

Birch (*Betula alleghaniensis*) helps reduce bone, joint, and muscle pain.

Spruce *(Picea mariana)* helps the respiratory and nervous systems.

Helichrysum (*Helichrysum italicum*) has been studied by European researchers for regenerating tissue and improving circulation.

Pepper (*Piper nigrum*) has been used for soothing deep tissue muscle pain.

Cypress (*Cupressus sempervirens*) can improve circulation.

Fir (*Abies alba*) high in terpenes to soothe and tone the muscles.

Basil (*Ocimum basilicum*) relaxes both striated and smooth muscles.

Marjoram (*Origanum majorana*) is used extensively for soothing the muscles.

Juniper (*Juniperus communis*) has been used to stimulate nerve function.

Companion Products: Arthro Plus, VitaGreen, Megazyme, Royaldophilus, Sulfurzyme (capsules or powder), and Ortho Ease or Ortho Sport massage oils.

Companion Oil Blends: Relieve It and PanAway.

Suggested Use: 2 Capsules, 3 to 4 times daily or as desired. Best taken before meals. If you have sensitive digestion, take with meals.

AuraLight

This spray neutraceutical utilizes a unique, nutrient delivery system through oral mucosa absorption (directly into the bloodstream through the dense network of blood vessels lining the mucus membrane inside the mouth). This type of delivery system is 90 percent efficient, with five times the efficiency of assimilating the nutrients in tablets or supplements. This unique product combines several natural mood-elevating compounds with the essential oils that are effective for reducing stress.

Contents:

Vitamin B6 promotes the production of mood-balancing neurotransmitters in the brain, including serotonin. It requires the presence the magnesium.

Vitamin B12 helps protect against deterioration of mental functioning, neurological damage, and other psychological disturbances.

Magnesium works with Vitamin B6 synergistically with the neurotransmitters in the brain, which regulate mood, attitude, and emotion.

St. John's Wort (*Hypericum perferatum*, standardized to .3 percent hypericin) has been extensively researched for its ability to promote relaxation and uplift attitude.

Humulus lupulus (Hops extract) contains a natural sedative-like compound, which is highly effective in combating stress.

Passiflora incarnata (Passion Flower extract) helps ease nervous tension and enhances feelings of relaxation.

Para aminobenzoic acid (PABA) assists healthy bacteria produce folic acid. It also helps the bones form red blood cells.

L-tyrosine supports the formation of neurotransmitters, such as dopamine and serotonin.

Ginko Biloba *(standardized for flavone glycosides and terpene lactones)* helps improve energy levels, improve memory, helps with oxygenation and blood flow, and increases hormonal balance. It also helps to improve mood and reduce depression by increasing circulation in the brain.

Kava Kava *(Piper methysticum—30 percent kavalactones)* contains natural compounds that exhibit sedative, analgesic, and muscle-relaxant effects.

Essential Oils:

Lavender (*Lavendula officinalis*) is calming and relaxing.

Sandalwood (*Santalum album*) stimulates the pineal gland, which produces melatonin, a hormone associated with deep sleep.

Roman chamomile (*Chamaemelum nobile*) is relaxing and sedating.

Orange (*Citrus sinesis*) is rich in compounds noted for their stress-reducing effects.

Companion Supplements: Mineral Essence, Seagal Power Meal, Super B, and VitaGreen.

Companion Oils: Peace & Calming, Joy, Hope, Surrender, Passion, and Forgiveness.

Suggested Use: Three sprays, three times a day, or as needed. (Vial contains approximately 30 servings, on average, 9 sprays per day). Shake gently before using. For additional benefit, take a deep diaphragmatic breath after each spray.

Be-Fit

A high-powered formula for enhancing strength and endurance and promoting muscle formation. Several ingredients are utilized in this product to help build muscle tissue.

Contents:

Wolfberry powder contains over 15 percent protein by weight. It is rich in amino acids for supporting muscle integrity.

HMB (Betahydroxy beta-methylbutyrate) well-researched nutrients for increasing muscle mass.

Siberian Ginseng extract helps provide energy and reduce stress. It also has the unique ability to stimulate lymphocyte formation (an essential part of the immune system).

Ginko Biloba extract improves energy, memory, mood due to its ability to enhance cerebral and peripheral circulation, and blood flow.

L-arginine is an amino acid that promotes circulation in the small capillaries of our tissues, allowing greater nutrient absorption and cellular metabolism.

L-lysine (HCl) works to enhance the benefits of the amino acid L-leucine found in wolfberry powder.

Creatine monohydrate is a naturally occurring compound of three amino acids, providing high-energy fuel for muscles. It helps to increase muscle mass as well as muscle contraction for improved intensity and endurance.

Cayenne is excellent as a general stimulant and stamina booster.

Essential Oils:

Birch (*Betula alleghaniensis*) has a cortisone-like action for pain relief due to its high concentration of percent methyl salicylate.

Lemongrass (*Cymbopogon flexuosus*) is used for ligament support.

Nutmeg (*Myristica fragrans*) is used for its adrenal cortex-like activity, which helps support the adrenal glands for increased energy.

Rosemary (*Rosmarinus officinalis*) helps overcome mental fatigue.

Companion Supplements: Seagal Power Meal, Ultra Young, Wolfberry Power Bars, Royal Essence, and Master HIS/HERS.

Companion Oils: Brain Power, Envision, En-R-Gee, EndoFlex, Live With Passion, and Valor.

Suggested Use: Two capsules in the morning and two capsules at night.

Body Balance

Body Balance is a milk and soy protein supplement fortified with vitamins, minerals, and essential oils. It helps balance the body at its ideal weight and promotes muscle formation. It contains soy solids that have been studied for their effects against breast and ovarian cancer.

Contents:

Non-fat dry milk supplies calcium and protein.

Fructose is a low glycemic sweetener, raising blood sugar levels only a fraction of table sugar

Calcium and sodium caseinate are the most complete sources of protein. The enzymes in these proteins are left intact, thanks to an advanced low-heat, glass-pack pasteurization technology.

Soy protein isolate is used extensively for protein without harmful side effects of the hormonal system.

Potassium citrate is needed to help prevent cancer, heart disease, strokes, and high blood pressure.

Lecithin is a part of the phospholipid membranes of almost every cell in the body.

Xanthan gum is a natural stabilizer.

Sodium chloride is needed for proper electrolyte balance.

Magnesium is needed for normal muscle contractions and heart rhythm. High intake can reduce high blood pressure, fight arteriosclerosis, and improve insulin action.

Vitamin C (ascorbic acid) helps the body manufacture collagen for connective tissue, cartilage, tendons, etc., and is used for proper immune function. It is also an antioxidant.

Vitamin E protects against cardiovascular disease and is beneficial for acne, allergies, and wound healing.

Vitamin A is an important antioxidant.

Calcium pantothenate is needed for the prevention of AIDS, depression, and tinnitus.

Niacinamide (vitamin B3) is essential for the production of energy, is involved in the regulation of blood sugar, and helps regulate cholesterol.

Zinc is crucial for proper immune function and is needed for proper action of many hormones, including insulin and growth hormone. It helps improve wound healing.

Iron chelation plays a central role in transporting oxygen from the lungs to the body's tissues and carbon dioxide from tissues to lungs.

Copper is necessary for proper red blood cell and immune function.

Vitamin D helps with the absorption of calcium and has many anticancer properties.

Vitamin B6 supports immune function and protects the heart and blood vessels. It inhibits skin cancer growth and helps prevent kidney stones and PMS symptoms. Vitamin B6 requires folic acid and magnesium to maximize its effects.

Vitamin B2 has shown to be crucial in the production of energy and is involved in regenerating glutathione and may help prevent certain esophageal cancers.

Vitamin B1 functions as part of an enzyme essential for energy production, carbohydrate metabolism, and nerve cell function.

Vitamin B12 is critical for red blood cell formation and proper immune and nerve function.

Folic acid plays an important role in cardiovascular health.

Biotin helps convert fats and amino acids into energy. It promotes healthy nails and hair and combats yeast and fungus overgrowth.

Essential Oils:

Lime (*Citrus aurantifolia*) decongests the lymphatic system.

Tangerine (*Citrus nobilis*) is an anticoagulant and helps decongest the lymphatic system.

Orange (*Citrus sinesis*) helps reduce fluid retention and is beneficial to the skin.

Lemon (*Citrus Limon*) promotes leukocyte formation and increases lymphatic function.

Cypress (*Cupressus sempervirens*) helps circulation and decongests the lymphatic system.

Companion Products: Mineral Essence, Royal Essence (tincture), Super B, Be-Fit, Super Cal, Thyromin, and Cel-Lite Magic Massage Oil.

Companion Oil Blends: Citrus Fresh, Live with Passion, Magnify Your Purpose, Envision, and EndoFlex.

Suggested Use: One measuring scoop added to 8-10 oz. purified water, juice, or low fat milk. Blend in blender for 30 seconds. Ice cubes may be added to thicken like a shake. Body Balance works with all juices. It is a predigested protein and may be taken anytime.

For optimum results, take with Master Formula His or Hers and Thyromin food supplements.

Tips for Getting the Most from Body Balance

1. **For fast weight loss:** Enjoy Body Balance as a replacement for breakfast and dinner. Eat a sensible, low-fat, well-balanced lunch, which includes vegetables, fruits, and whole grains. As with any weight loss program, fats, sugars, and high-calorie foods should be omitted from your diet. Raw organic vegetables and fruits are excellent snacks.

2. **For weight gain:** Enjoy Body Balance mixed with whole milk or apple juice. Add a banana or a pear and drink after each meal.

3. **For good health and weight maintenance:** After you have achieved your ideal weight, enjoy a Body Balance shake as a meat alternative daily, possibly for breakfast. Body Balance may also be used as a filling and nutritious snack for the entire family. Drink plenty of distilled or purified water.

Note: Anyone who is pregnant or nursing, has health problems, or wants to lose more than 50 pounds or more than 20 percent of his/her body weight should consult a physician before starting this or any other weight management program.

Frequency: Approximately 87 MHz.

For optimum benefits, Body Balance may be mixed with soy or rice milk.

CardiaCare

Strengthens and supports the heart and cardiovascular system.

Contents:

Rhododendron Caucasicum contains phenyl-propanoids that have been shown in clinical studies to increase the efficiency of the cardiovascular system.

Wolfberry powder contains the amino acids that are vital to supporting cardiovascular function.

Magnesium is needed for normal muscle contractions and heart rhythm. High intake can reduce high blood pressure, fight arteriosclerosis, and improve insulin action.

Hawthorne berry has been used for decades in European cardiac medicine. Active constituents in the berries dilate coronary blood vessels, thereby increasing blood circulation in the heart.

CoQ10 is used by every cell in the body to convert food to energy. Heart cells require more CoQ10 to maintain muscle strength because of their higher demand for energy.

Vitamin E prevents oxidative damage to low-density lipoproteins (LDLs), a primary cause of clogged coronary arteries and heart disease.

Essential Oils:

Helichrysum (*Helichrysum italicum*) helps regulate cholesterol, stimulates liver function, helps regulate blood thickness, allowing for better blood flow between vessels and tissues.

Lemon (*Citrus limon*) helps dissolve cholesterol and cellulite, increases lymphatic function.

Marjoram (*Origanum compactum*) provides support for smooth muscles of the heart, relieves spasms, and may work as a diuretic.

Ylang Ylang (*Cananga odorata*) has been used traditionally to support heart functions.

Companion Products: HRT, Mineral Essence, and A. D. & E.

Companion Oil Blends: Aroma Life, Forgiveness, Live with Passion, Harmony, and Joy.

ComforTone

An herbal complex of bentonite, apple pectin, and herbal extracts that may relieve constipation, enhance colon function, and dispel parasites and toxins.

ComforTone can help eliminate parasites from the body, break up the encrustation along the colon wall, and relax spasms that may occur. If you experience nausea when using ComforTone, use Di-Tone or Peppermint (diluted if necessary); if you experience constipation, increase your water intake and avoid using I.C.P. If you have a history of chronic constipation, do not start I.C.P. and ComforTone at the same time. First use Comfor-Tone until the system is open, and then follow with I.C.P. Drink 10 glasses of water per day.

Contents:

Licorice root cleanses the blood and supports the liver, the most important organ for cleansing.

Psyllium seed helps relieve abdominal pain, constipation, diarrhea, and protects against flatulence (gas) and nausea.

Apple pectin helps with enzyme production and supports proper digestive function.

Bentonite is an intestinal cleansing agent.

Fennel is antiparasitic, antimicrobial, antispasmotic, is a digestive aid, helps regulate intestinal flora, and increases gastric secretions.

Garlic is antifungal, antiparasitic, antiviral, an immune stimulant, works as a digestive aid, and is a catalyst for the oils.

German Chamomile is antimicrobial, anti-inflammatory, suppresses the parasympathetic nervous system that produces excess mucus, and relaxes spasms in the colon wall.

Echinacea is antimicrobial, antiparasitic, lowers bowel transit time, absorbs toxins in the colon, and stimulates the immune system.

Ginger root is anti-inflammatory, antispasmotic, helps lower cholesterol, and cleanses the colon.

Cascara segrada works as an herbal laxative and as a liver cleanser.

Burdock root lowers bowel transit time, balances intestinal flora, and absorbs toxins from the bowels.

Contains therapeutic-grade essential oils of:

Rosemary (*Rosmarinus officinalis*) is antiparasitic and balances the endocrine system.

German chamomile (*Matricaria recutita*) helps prevent acne, rashes, and eczema.

Tarragon (*Artemisia dracunculus*) has been used to reduce flatulence (gas), intestinal spasms, sluggish digestion, and to prevent fermentation.

Peppermint (*Mentha piperita*) reduces candida, nausea, and vomiting.

Ginger (*Zingiber officinale*) combats indigestion, diarrhea, loss of appetite, and congestion.

Anise (*Pimpinella anisum*) helps prevent flatulence, colon spasms, and indigestion.

Mugwort (*Artemisia vulgaris*) has been used traditionally to calm nerves.

Tangerine (*Citrus nobilis*) helps decongest the lymphatic system and is anti-inflammatory.

Companion Products: Megazyme, JuvaTone, ParaFree, Chelex, and I.C.P. Fiber Beverage).

Companion Oil Blends: Purification, Release, JuvaFlex, Di-Tone, and Thieves.

Suggested Use: Start with 2-5 capsules, first thing in the morning and 2-5 capsules, just before going to bed. Drink 8-10 eight-ounce glasses of purified or distilled water per day for best results. If you get cramps, skip the next morning or day and start up again with two capsules in the morning and two in the evening. After starting ComforTone, you may cut back; but do not stop completely because all the toxins that have been pulled out of the system will go back into the system. Take at least one in the morning and one in the evening, but do not stop once you start. For maximum results, use with JuvaTone and Megazyme. ComforTone maybe taken every day without becoming addictive.

Safety Data: ComforTone may be taken during pregnancy, as long as you do not get diarrhea. Diarrhea might cause cramping, which could bring on labor.

Frequency: Approximately 43 MHz.

Essential Manna

This is a nutritionally dense, fiber-rich superfood that has been based on the diet of the Hunza people. The Hunza's longevity has been attributed to their consumption of a high potassium, high magnesium diet of dried fruits (especially apricots), nuts, and a variety of whole grains.

Contents:

Apricots contain high concentrations of carotinoids, a class of high-powered antioxidants that includes beta carotene (provitamin A). Apricots are also rich in rutin, which strengthens blood vessels.

Chinese wolfberry (*Lycium barbarum*) has been studied for its ability to combat cancer and improve the immunity.

Barley is exceptionally rich in soluble fiber and is an ideal food for type II diabetics.

Buckwheat is high in potassium, magnesium, and other essential minerals. It helps improve cholesterol levels and glucose tolerance.

Amaranth is rich in lysine, an amino acid lacking in many traditional grains, such as wheat and corn.

Figs are high in potassium, magnesium, and plant enzymes. They help moderate blood sugar rises.

Almonds contain high amounts of magnesium and vitamin E, which enhance immune support.

Millet contains over 12 percent protein and is a source of 12 essential minerals, including magnesium, potassium, zinc, and iodine.

Brown rice is rich in protein with high concentrations of the muscle-building amino acids, L-leucine, L-isoleucine, and L-valine. Brown rice is packed with a fiber content necessary for proper digestion.

Coconut is rich in potassium and low in sodium.

Dates contain enzymes that helps break down the phytic acid that can block mineral absorption.

Rolled oats contain high amounts of manganese, selenium, and magnesium.

Pineapples are rich in potassium and contain bromelain, a protein-digesting enzyme.

Raisins contain iron and fiber, which is needed for proper digestion.

Sesame seeds are rich in linoleic and oleic acid and contain unusual antioxidant compounds, used to prevent free radical damage.

Stevia is an all-natural supplement. *(See Stevia).*

Use: It comes in three delicious flavors—Apricot, Spice, and Carob. Snacks throughout the day when desired.

Companion Products: Seagal Power Meal, Juva-Tone, Megazyme, Sulfurzyme (capsules or powder), and Mineral Essence.

Companion Oils: En-R-Gee, EndoFlex, Magnify Your Purpose, Envision, JuvaFlex, and Valor.

Exodus

Exodus is the ultimate supercharged antioxidant containing a biblical blend of essential oils and other nutritional herbs that provide important support for the defenses of the body.

Contents:

Uncaria tomentosa (Cat's Claw, Una de Gato) contains alkaloids, such as mitraphylline, that may fortify the immune system. Julian Whittaker, M.D., discusses this herb in an article entitled, "Take Una de Gato for All-around Immunity."

Amino acid complex of alanine, cystine, arginine, glycine, lycine, threonine, and thorine is used as the building block of the enzymes, proteins, and cells of our natural defenses.

Yucca has been used for its blood-cleansing properties.

Echinacea is one of the best-studied immune boosters. Extensive research indicates that it increases the number and activity of white blood cells involved with immunity and boosts the activity of T-cells and natural interferon.

Vitamin A is a powerful antioxidant that supports the eyes, hair, and skin.

Grape seed proanthocyanidin is one of the strongest-known antioxidants.

Ionic minerals contain a specially balanced formula with trace minerals from boron to zinc. *(See Mineral Essence)*

Pantothenic acid supports adrenal function and the formation of antibodies, aids in vitamin utilization, and helps convert fats, carbohydrates, and proteins into energy.

Essential Oils:

Frankincense (*Boswellia carteri*) was well known for its healing properties during the time of Christ because it is antitumoral and immune stimulating.

Hyssop (*Hyssopus officinalis*) has been used for thousands of years for its anti-inflammatory, anti-infectious, and antiparasitic properties. It helps discharge toxins and mucus, and regulates lipid metabolism.

Bay laurel (*Laurus nobilis*) contains antiseptic and antimicrobial properties.

Spikenard (*Nardostachys jatamansi*) is highly regarded in India as a medicinal herb.

Myrrh (*Commiphora myrrha*) is anti-infectious and supports the immune system.

Companion Products: ComforTone, VitaGreen, Seagal Power Meal, Essential Manna, Radex, Super C, and ImmuTune

Companion Oil Blends: Exodus II, Thieves, ImmuPower, and Purification.

Suggested Use: Take 3 capsules, 2 - 3 times daily.

FemiGen

This is an herbal formula with non-animal glandular substances and amino acids, which helps aid and balance the reproductive system to maintain better hormonal balance for developmental years all the way through menopause. When one has experienced mood swings, PMS, and symptoms related to menopause, it is an indication that the body is nutritionally out of balance. FemiGen acts as a natural estrogen and helps balance the hormones.

Contents:

Damiana has been described as a blood purifier, an expectorant, and is used as a diuretic.

Epimedium has been used to help detoxify kidneys and help eliminate lower back pain and frequent urination.

Dong Quai has estrogenic qualities and increases blood flow to the reproductive organs of the female system. It has also been used as a menstrual balancer.

Muira puama has been used for treatment of frigidity, menstrual cramps, impotency, and PMS.

Wild yam root contains compounds that are similar in structure to steroids; but these compounds must be digested, absorbed, and processed by one's own body and then utilized as such. It is also good for muscle spasms and contains anti-inflammatory compounds.

Includes a base of: American ginseng, licorice root, black cohosh, cramp bark, squaw vine, magnesium, L-carnitine, dimethylglycine, L-phenylalinine, L-cystine, L-cysteine, and L-trytophan.

Essential Oils:

Clary sage (*Salvia sclarea*) has been used for regulating cells and balancing hormones.

Fennel (*Foeniculum vulgare*) has hormone-like activity that helps balance hormones.

Sage (*Salvia officinalis*) helps alleviate premenopause symptoms, such as depression.

Ylang Ylang (*Cananga odorato*) has been used for sexual disabilities, frigidity, and relaxation.

Suggested Use: Take two capsules with breakfast and two capsules with lunch. A maintenance dose of 2 capsules may be taken 3 times a day for 10 days before a period.

Companion Products: Femalin, EssPro 7, Aura-Light, and Dragon Time Massage Oil.

Companion Oils: Dragon Time, Relieve It, Mister, PanAway, and Peace & Calming.

Goji Berry Tea

Goji Berry is the colloquial name for the wolfberry, which is grown in China. This delicious, nourishing tea, is made from the Chinese wolfberry, which has been used by the Chinese for centuries to strengthen the liver and reduce the effects of arthritis and other degenerative diseases. Several ingredients from other cultures enhance the immune-building effects of the wolfberry and provide tremendous nourishment to the body. Research at the Beijing Nutrition Research Institute and State Scientific and Technology Commission of China found that those who drank the tea and ate the berries did not experience liver disease, hepatitis, or other degenerative problems and lived 20-30 years longer than the average person in China.

Contents:

Chinese wolfberry (*Lycium barbarum*) has been prized in China to protect the body from degenerative disease by strengthening the body's defense mechanism, working as an antioxidant, and promoting longevity.

Cat's claw (*Uncaria tomentosa*) has been used to fight and prevent degenerative disease.

Nopal is a traditional herb used in Mexico and is harvested from a native cactus. It was tested and found to reduce cholesterol, burn fat, and support the pancreas.

Purple lapacho (also known as Pau D'arco in Brazil and Taheebo in Argentina) is reported to help support the body by cleansing the lymphatic system and building blood cells.

Panax ginseng has been used for thousands of years in the Orient to extend life and invigorate the body.

Essential Oils:

Lemon (*Citrus limon*) has been used to cleanse the lymphatic system and promote well being.

Peppermint (*Mentha piperita*) helps reduce candida, fever, and cools the body.

Spearmint (*Mentha spicata*) is antiparasitic and anti-infectious. Its hormone-like properties help bring about a sense of balance and well being.

Companion Products: Exodus, ImmuneTune, ComforTone, and Seagal Power Meal.

Companion Oil Blends: Exodus II, ImmuPower, Release, Thieves, Valor, and Purification.

Suggested Use: Bring one cup of purified or distilled water to the boiling point. Remove from heat and add one tea bag. Steep 15-30 minutes for desired taste. Add Stevia or honey as a nutritional supplement.

I.C.P.

I.C.P. Multiple Fiber Beverage is a unique source of fiber and bulk for the diet, which helps speed the transit time of waste matter through the intestinal tract. The psyllium, oat bran, flax, and rice bran are specifically balanced to eliminate allergy symptoms that many people experience when taking psyllium alone. Essential oils enhance the flavor and may help dispel gas and pain. This formula is unsurpassed as an aid in enhancing normal bowel function.

Contents:

Psyllium seed powder expands when put with water and is smooth and filling, not abrasive, to the intestinal walls.

Apple pectin slows absorption of food after meals, removes unwanted metals and toxins, is valuable against the effects of radiation therapy, and helps lower cholesterol.

Aloe vera extract is a natural laxative and lubricant, relaxing the colon.

Rice bran is an outstanding source of soluble and semisoluble fiber.

Oat bran binds up fat so it does not enter the blood stream.

Black cumin helps digestion and is an antioxidant.

Guar gum has been used in expanding and cleansing the colon.

Flax seed is an excellent cleanser for intestinal walls and the digestive system. It is also a lubricant, an antioxidant, and is very harmonious with essential oils.

Yucca helps break up obstructions in the digestive system and contains enzymes for digestion.

Fennel seed stimulates the gastrointestinal mucous membrane, which in turn stimulates the pancreas to secrete digestive enzymes to dissolve undigested proteins. It is antiparasitic.

Pepsin is an enzyme to aid digestion.

Essential Oils:

Fennel (*Foeniculum vulgare*) has been used to help reduce symptoms associated with menopause, help with flatulence (gas), and is antibacterial and antiparasitical.

Tarragon (*Artemisia dracunculus*) has been shown to be anti-infectious, antispasmotic, and antiviral.

Ginger (*Zingiber officinale*) improves digestion and helps combat parasites.

Lemongrass (*Cymbopogon flexuosus*) is antifungal and promotes digestion.

Rosemary (*Rosmarinus officinalis*) reduces indigestion and helps regulate cholesterol.

Anise (*Pimpinella anisum*) helps flatulence, colon spasms, and indigestion.

Suggested Use: Take five times a week for maintenance (1/2 cup water, 1/2 cup apple juice, and 1 heaping tsp. of I.C.P.). Take more often for cleansing (start with 1 heaping tsp., 2 to 3 times a day with carrot or other vegetable juices. When things are going well, increase to 3 tsp. 3 times a day). I.C.P. dilutes better in warm water. Drink immediately as this product tends to thicken quickly when added to liquid.

For best results, take ComforTone first, then I.C.P. morning and night. If added to citrus juices, it creates more acid. It is best to use other juices. I.C.P. absorbs toxins and can build and improve the wave-like movement of the intestinal walls.

Frequency: Approximately 56 MHz.

Companion Products: ComforTone, Megazyme, ParaFree (capsules or liquid), and JuvaTone.

Companion Oil Blends: Di-Tone, JuvaFlex, Purification, and Thieves.

ImmuGel

ImmuGel is a unique blend of naturally-occurring liquid amino acids, trace minerals, and herbal extracts with essential oils. This blend creates one of nature's most powerful antioxidant and antimicrobial formulas. It destroys fungi and bacteria, thereby boosting the immune defenses. Amino acids have a unique ability to neutralize and help eliminate free radicals in the system. This formula is used for general maintenance, and use should be increased during times of fatigue, depression, or to help prevent illness. It is also used as a support in eliminating candida.

Contents:

Deionized water helps cleanse and purify the body's tissues and organs.

Hydrolyzed protein (contains alanine, arginine, aspartic acid, glutamic acid, glycine, histidine, hydroxyproline, leucine and isoleucine, lycine, methionine, phenylalanine).

Methylcellulose has been used by parasitologists to slow down single-cell organisms, such as amoebae, flagellates, etc.

German chamomile extract contains elements that are antibacterial and antifungal.

Trace minerals help restore electrolyte balance in the cells.

Essential Oils:

Cinnamon bark (*Cinnamomum verum*) is antifungal, antibacterial, antiviral.

Clove bud (*Syzygium aromaticum*) is anti-infectious, antiviral, antifungal, antiparasitic, and has been used in European hospitals for viral hepatitis, bronchitis, flu, sinusitis, and cholera.

Rosemary (*Rosmarinus officinalis*) supports the heart and helps moderate hypertension.

Lemon (*Citrus limon*) promotes leukocyte formation and increases lymphatic (immune) function.

Thyme (*Thymus vulgaris*) is one of the strongest antibacterial, antifungal, and antiviral essential oils.

Oregano (*Origanum compactum*) has been used for infections, pneumonia, and dysentery.

Suggested Use: Take 1/2-1 tsp. 3 times daily. May be taken with water.

Companion Products: ImmuneTune, Exodus, Super C, and JuvaTone.

Companion Oil Blends: ImmuPower, Thieves, JuvaFlex, Exodus II, Purification, Valor, and Release.

ImmuneTune

A super antioxidant complex that supports the immune system and fights free radicals. The curcuminoid blend in this product has been found to be 60 percent stronger in antioxidant activity than pine bark or grape pit extract. However, synergism is the key to obtaining maximum effect. Through the combining of curcuminoids and grape seed extract, the antioxidant frequency is almost doubled.

Contents:

Curcuminoids (from curcumin and turmeric) are potent antioxidants and immune supporters.

Grape seed extract is one of the strongest antioxidants. .

Magnesium is needed for normal muscle contractions and heart rhythm. High intake can reduce high blood pressure, fight arteriosclerosis, and improve insulin action.

Potassium citrate is needed for prevention of cancer, heart disease, strokes, and high blood pressure.

Calcium pantothenate may serve as protection against high blood pressure and colon cancer.

Alpha lipoic acid is found in many foods. It has produced great results in the prevention and treatment of diabetes, cataracts, heart disease, liver ailments, cancer, and kidney stones.

Chromium improves insulin sensitivity and blood sugar metabolism.

Selenium has been extensively researched for its anticancer and antioxidant properties.

Echinacea increases the white blood cells and stimulates the immune system.

Yucca is an excellent antioxidant that supports the liver and gall bladder.

Essential Oils:

Orange (*Citrus sinesis*) is excellent for flatulence, circulation, and fluid reduction.

Pine (*Pinus mariana*) is used for respiratory infection and bronchitis.

Fir (*Abies alba*) has also been used for different types of respiratory infections and bronchitis.

Cistus (*Cistus ladanifer*) has been used to improve immune function.

Ravensara (*Ravensara aromatica*), known as the "oil that heals," may help activity in the immune system.

Lemon (*Citrus limon*) promotes leukocyte formation and increases lymphatic (immune) function.

Companion Products: Exodus, ImmuGel, ParaFree (capsules or liquid), or Super C.

Companion Oil Blends: Exodus II, ImmuPower, Thieves, Envision, and Release.

Suggested Use: For slow metabolism, 2 to 3 capsules daily. For fast metabolism, 3 to 6 capsules daily. It is best taken on an empty stomach. For stomach sensitivity, take with meals.

Frequency: Approximately 108 MHz.

JuvaTone

JuvaTone is a special herbal complex designed to support the liver. The liver is one of the most important organs of the body. It **purifies the blood** and is a key to **converting carbohydrates to energy**. An overtaxed liver may affect our **energy, digestion, and skin**. Fats and bile within the liver can easily become oversaturated with oil-soluble toxins, synthetic chemicals, and heavy metals. As toxins build, the liver becomes taxed and stressed, resulting in aggravating **skin conditions, rashes, fatigue, headaches, muscle pain, digestive disturbances, pallor, dizziness, irritability, mood swings, and mental confusion**. The liver also plays a major role in helping the body detoxify. The final products of digestion are transported through the portal vein from the colon to the liver to be cleansed.

Contents:

Choline bitartrate has been used in the treatment of many liver disorders, including elevated cholesterol levels, viral hepatitis, and cirrhosis.

Inositol helps the liver rid itself of fat and bile.

Dl-methionine is one of the most powerful antioxidants in the body, and especially important to protect the liver.

Oregon grape root contains berberine, which has been studied as a liver protectant and for its effects against hepatitis.

Dandelion root is used for disturbances in bile flow and liver disorders.

Other Ingredients: Alfalfa sprouts, echinacea root, parsley, sodium, and copper in herbal extracts.

Essential Oils:

Geranium (*Pelargonium graveolens*) has been used for centuries as a liver cleanser and to regenerate tissue and nerves.

German chamomile (*Matricaria recutita*) improves bile flow from the liver.

Rosemary (*Rosmarinus officinalis*) supports the liver and combats cirrhosis.

Lemon (*Citrus limon*) promotes leukocyte formation and increases lymphatic (immune) function.

Blue tansy (*Tanacetum annum*) is anti-inflammatory and is used for hypertension and arthritis.

Myrtle (*Myrtus communis*) helps break up mucus and stimulate the thyroid.

Companion Products: ParaFree (capsules or liquid), ComforTone, I.C.P., Seagal Power Meal, and Megazyme.

Companion Oil Blends: JuvaFlex, Di-Tone, Thieves, Release, Surrender, and Forgiveness.

Suggested Use: For slow metabolism, take 2 tablets, 3 times daily. Increase as needed up to 4 tablets, 4 times daily. For fast metabolism, take 3 tablets 3 times daily and increase to 4 tablets, 4 times daily or as needed. Best taken between meals. Tablets may be chewed, broken, or swallowed whole. For maximum results, use with ComforTone.

Frequency: Approximately 140 MHz.

Master Formula HIS/HERS and CHILDREN'S

This is a high-quality multivitamin, mineral, and amino acid supplement, which is formulated using a special sixteen stage Synergistic Suspension Isolation, which separates the antagonistic vitamins and herbs from the synergistic ones so they do not become abrasive and destroy each other's effectiveness. The Master Formula tablet has a special Zein coating derived from corn and the amino acid L-phenylalaine, enabling the body to recognize this supplement as a food, allowing for a faster conversion and assimilation.

Contents:

Vitamin A and beta carotene are powerful antioxidants that support the eyes, hair, and skin.

Vitamin D (cholecalciferol) is beneficial for the absorption of calcium, and may prevent liver and kidney dysfunctions.

Vitamin E protects the heart and blood and combats free-radical oxidative damage.

Vitamin C supports immune function and blood vessel integrity, and combats free-radical damage associated with premature aging. It has been used to treat cataracts, glaucoma, high blood pressure, periodontal disease, eczema, gingivitis, and infections.

Folic acid plays an important role in cardiovascular health. Helps prevent neural tube defects.

Vitamin B1 is essential for energy production, carbohydrate metabolism, and nerve cell function.

Vitamin B2 is crucial in the production of cellular energy, helps regenerate the liver, protecting antioxidant glutathione, and may help prevent migraine headaches and some esophageal cancers.

Vitamin B3 is essential for turning carbohydrates into energy. It lowers cholesterol and helps regulate blood sugar. At least 4.4 mg is needed for every 1,000 calories consumed to avoid pellagra.

Vitamin B6 supports immune function and protects the heart and blood vessels. It inhibits skin cancer growth and helps prevent kidney stones and PMS symptoms. Vitamin B6 requires folic acid and magnesium to maximize its effects.

Vitamin B12 is critical for red blood cell formation and proper immune and nerve function.

Biotin helps convert fats and amino acids into energy. It promotes healthy nails and hair and combats yeast and fungus overgrowth.

Pantothenic acid (d calcium pantothenate) is needed for the prevention of AIDS, depression, and tinnitus.

Choline bitartrate has been used in the treatment of many liver disorders, including elevated cholesterol levels, Alzheimer's disease, viral hepatitis, and cirrhosis.

Calcium (hydrolyzed protein complex) is used primarily for the treatment of many conditions associated with osteoporosis, such as bone loss. It is also helpful for elevated blood pressure.

Iodine (kelp) helps prevent goiters, reduced thyroid hormones, and estrogen imbalance.

Iron is needed to prevent anemia, fatigue, hemorrhoids, and peptic ulcers.

Magnesium is crucial for proper enzyme function and is needed for normal muscle contractions and heart rhythm. High intake can reduce high blood pressure, fight arteriosclerosis, and improve insulin action.

Copper is necessary for proper red blood cell and immune function.

Zinc is crucial for proper immune function and is needed for proper action of many hormones, including insulin and growth hormone. It helps improve wound healing.

Potassium (citrate) supports cellular fluid balance and healthy muscle, nerve, heart, and adrenal function. It reduces high blood pressure and balances water distribution.

Manganese is needed for blood sugar control, energy metabolism, and proper thyroid function. It is also good for antioxidant activity.

Chromium improves insulin sensitivity and blood sugar metabolism.

Selenium has been extensively researched for its anticancer and antioxidant properties.

Silicon is required for proper functioning of an enzyme that is essential for the formation of collagen in bone, cartilage, and other connective tissues.

In a base of betaine HCl, citrus bioflavonoids, L-cysteine, histidine, tyrosine, lysine, arginine, PABA (para amino benzoic acid), molybdenum, and amino acid complex.

HIS

Master Formula HIS is formulated with more zinc and arginine, especially for men.

Companion Products: Be-Fit, ProGen, Mineral Essence, Power Meal, VitaGreen, Sulfurzyme, Essential Manna, and Wolfberry Power Bars.

Companion Oil Blends: Mister, Envision, Magnify Your Purpose, and Sacred Mountain.

Suggested Use: 3 tablets with breakfast and 3 with lunch (take before meals).

Frequency: Approximately 86 MHz.

HERS

Master Formula HERS is formulated with more magnesium, calcium, and B vitamins to specifically help the special nutritional needs of women.

Companion Products: VitaGreen, Be-Fit, Femi-Gen, AuraLight, Estro, and EssPro 7.

Companion Oil Blends: Mister, Dragon Time, Joy, Magnify Your Purpose, Abundance, and Harmony.

Suggested Use: For slow metabolism: 3-6 tablets daily. For fast metabolism: 6-8 tablets daily. Take 1/2 amount before breakfast and 1/2 before dinner. Best taken before meals.

Free of allergens. Contains no artificial flavors, preservatives, sugar, cornstarch, corn, wheat, yeast or soy products.

Frequency: Approximately 88 MHz.

Master Formula CHILDREN'S

A special chewable multivitamin formulated for children in the early growth years and for adult maintenance in late years. It is made with Chinese Wolfberry *(Lycium barbarum)* and grain proteins for added immune support, with beta carotene, vitamin C, amino acids, and stevia.

Essential Oils:

Lime *(Citrus aurantifolia)* is anti-inflammatory, antispasmotic, supports cardiovascular function.

Mandarin *(Citrus reticulata)* is antifungal, antispasmotic, and promotes digestion.

Orange *(Citrus sinesis)* has been used as an anticoagulant to reduce flatulence and to stimulate circulation.

Companion Products: Mineral Essence, Body Balance, Seagal Power Meal, Essential Manna, and Wolfberry Power Bars.

Companion Oil Blends: Peace & Calming, Gentle Baby, Joy, White Angelica, and Harmony.

Suggested Use: Chew three tablets daily with breakfast as a dietary supplement.

Megazyme

A high-quality enzyme complex that may improve and aid digestion and the elimination of toxic waste from the body. Megazyme was formulated to help supply the enzymes to people who have difficulty digesting or assimilating food. Helps promote and reestablish proper enzyme balance in the digestive system and throughout the body and helps improve intestinal flora. It may also help to retard the aging process. Flavor enhanced with essential oils.

Contents:

Pancrelipase is an enzyme used to help digest foods.

Trypsin is an animal product that has amino acid precursor action, carbohydrate conversion, and assimilation.

Carrot powder has the second highest concentration of natural enzymes in vegetables.

Alfalfa sprouts help improve electrolyte balance for digestion.

Pancreatin is an enzyme complex that has been studied for the treatment of cancer.

Papain is a vegetable enzyme and carbonate (starch) digester.

Bromelain is a natural enzyme and carbohydrate (starch) digester.

Betaine HCl helps with the digestion of protein.

Black cumin assists with the digestion of protein.

Essential Oils:

Tarragon *(Artemisia dracunulus)* is antiviral, antibacterial, and anti-inflammatory.

Peppermint *(Mentha piperita)* has been used for indigestion, ulcers, and gastro-intestinal disorders.

Anise *(Pimpinella anisum)* is excellent in helping alleviate flatulence (gas), and congestion.

Fennel *(Poeniculum vulgare)* has been used for centuries for proper digestion, indigestion, and dyspepsia.

Clove *(Syzygium aromaticum)* is beneficial for its antibacterial, antiviral, antifungal, anti-infectious, and antiparasitic properties.

Suggested Use: 2 or 3 tablets, 3 times daily or as needed. Take Megazyme with meals, especially protein meals, after 3 p.m., as it will help lessen the burden on the digestive system. Megazyme also helps with digestive functions in the liver.

Companion Products: Mint Condition, Comfor-Tone, Seagal Power Meal, Mineral Essence, Royaldophilus, and JuvaTone.

Companion Oil Blends: JuvaFlex, Di-Tone, and Harmony.

Frequency: Approximately 83 MHz.

Mineral Essence

A balanced organic, ionic mineral complex with more than 60 different minerals. Without minerals, vitamins cannot be properly assimilated or absorbed by the body. Mineral Essence has a natural electrolyte balance, which enhances bioavailability, provides antimicrobial protection, and significantly improves oxygenation to the cell, which helps prevent disease and premature aging. Minerals are also necessary for proper immune and metabolism functions.

Mineral essence also includes essential oils to enhance their bioavailability. To demonstrate this, a group of volunteers consumed a teaspoon of liquid trace minerals without any essential oils. Each volunteer experienced diarrhea within 24 hours. Following a washout period of several days, the same volunteers were given double the dosage of the same liquid trace minerals blended with essential oils. None experienced any diarrhea.

In the July 1996 issue of the *Young Living Essential Edge,* an article entitled "Sunburn Relief" contained the following information: "Dr. Alex Schauss, a prominent mineral researcher, has discovered that burns are painful because certain trace minerals are depleted from the skin and surrounding tissue. If the trace minerals are replenished to the affected area, then the pain will subside almost immediately. . . . We have had many who have topically applied Mineral Essence directly on the sunburn or burn and received instant pain relief as the healing process began. . . ."

Contents:

Purified Water is needed to dilute the minerals for liquifying this blend.

Honey is a an emulsifier and natural sweetener.

Royal Jelly is a very rich source of proteins and amino acids. It has been traditionally known to prolong youthfulness and improve skin beauty, increase energy, and reduce anxiety, sleeplessness, moodiness, memory loss, and support the immune system.

Trace minerals include beryllium, bismuth, boron, bromine, calcium, carbon, cesium, chloride, chromium, copper, gallium, germanium, gold, hafnium, indium, iodine, iron, lithium, lutecium, manganese, magnesium, molybdenum, nickel, niobium, nitrogen, oxygen, phosphorus, potassium, rubidium, scandium, selenium, silicon, silver, sodium, strontium, sulfur, tantalum, thallium, tin, titanium, tungsten, vanadium, yttrium, zinc, and zirconium.

Essential Oils:

Lemon (*Citrus limon*) promotes leukocyte formation and increases lymphatic (immune) function.

Cinnamon bark (*Cinnamomum verum*) is anti-infectious, antibacterial, antiviral, antifungal, antiparasitic, anticoagulant, and is used for all types of infections.

Peppermint (*Mentha piperita*) is anti-infectious, antibacterial, antifungal, and used for pancreatic complaints, sinusitis, laryngitis, hypotension.

Companion Products: Master Formula HIS/HERS and CHILDREN'S, Royal Essence, VitaGreen, Sulfurzyme, and Wolfberry Power Bars.

Companion Oil Blends: Citrus Fresh, Harmony, Envision, Gathering, and Valor.

Mint Condition

A vegetarian digestive enzyme complex that combines select herbs and essential oils. It may help soothe irritated digestive systems and reduce inflammation, ulcers, colitis, irritable bowel syndrome, bloating, gas, and acid indigestion. It works well with Megazyme and Di-Tone. Use Megazyme before meals and Mint Condition after meals.

Contents:

Fennel seed powder has been researched for regulation of intestinal flora and as a digestive aid.

Papaya fruit powder is a source of natural fruit enzymes and fiber.

Apple pectin is a source of fiber and may help prevent high cholesterol and cancer and may aid digestion.

Peppermint has many beneficial constituents that have spasmolyctic activity that stimulate the production of digestive fluids. It also has anti-inflammatory and anti-ulcer properties.

Ginger root powder has been used to treat indigestion, flatulence, diarrhea, and stomachache.

Spearmint is used for many digestive disorders and as a remedy for flatulence (gas).

Trace minerals are needed for proper electrolyte balance, and all functions in the body are dependent on these. They are essential for proper digestion and elimination.

Essential Oils:

Peppermint (*Mentha piperita*) has been used for indigestion, ulcers, and gastro-intestinal disorders for centuries. Recent clinical studies have shown it to reduce the intestinal spasms.

Spearmint (*Mentha spicata*) improves digestion.

Ginger (*Zingiber officinale*) improves digestion and combats constipation.

Tarragon (*Artemisia dracunculus*) is antiparasitic, antispasmotic, and antiviral.

Companion Products: Megazyme, ComforTone, Seagal Power Meal, Mineral Essence, Royaldophilus, and JuvaTone.

Companion Oil Blends: JuvaFlex, Di-Tone, and Harmony.

ParaFree

An advanced blend of some of the strongest essential oils that have been studied for their antiparasitic properties.

Base Oils:

Sesame seed and olive oil.

Essential Oils:

Black cumin (*Cuminum cyminum*) has been shown to be antiparasitic and antiviral. It supports immune function.

Anise (*Pimpinella anisum*) is antiparasitic and promotes digestion and protein breakdown.

Fennel (*Foeniculum vulgare*) is antiseptic and antiparasitic and improves digestive and pancreatic functions.

Bay laurel (*Laurus Nobilis*) is antiseptic, antibacterial, antiparasitic, and antiviral. It is also a diuretic, fungicidal, and digestive aid.

Vetiver (*Vetiveria officinalis*) is antiseptic, anti-inflammatory, and immune-supporting.

Nutmeg (*Myristica fragrans*) supports adrenal glands, is antibacterial and anti-inflammatory, and stimulates immune function. It has also been used to reduce diarrhea.

Melaleuca (*Melaleuca alternifolia*) is antifungal, antiparasitic, and antibacterial.

Idaho tansy (*Tanacetum vulgare*) is one of the most potent worm-expelling essential oils.

Clove (*Sygygium aromaticum*) has potent antiparasitic, antibacterial, and antifungal properties.

Companion Products: ComforTone, Megazyme, Rehemogen, VitaGreen, I.C.P., and JuvaTone.

Companion Oil Blends: Di-Tone, Thieves, Purification, Release, and JuvaFlex.

Suggested Use: Take 2-4 droppers, 3 times daily for 21 consecutive days for liquid. Take 2-4 gelcaps, 2-3 times a day for 21 consecutive days out of each month for gelcaps. Repeat for three cycles or as needed. Use ParaFree with ComforTone and I.C.P. for cleansing. The I.C.P. will help break up the plaque along the intestinal walls.

Note: Use in moderation during pregnancy, possibly 2 capsules daily, If diarrhea occurs, discontinue. A good parasite cleanse is recommended before conception. Consult your health care provider before starting a cleansing program.

For additional information, review the book, *Essential Oil Safety—A Guide for Health Care Professionals* by Robert Tisserand and Tony Balacs.

ProGen

ProGen is an all-vegetable and herbal support for the prostrate and male glandular system. Saw palmetto is one of the most widely used herbs to combat the prostrate enlargement that effects most men over 45. *Pygeum Africanum* has been used for years to prevent prostate atrophy and malfunction.

Contents:

Seronoa serrulata (saw palmetto) has been used to help reduce enlarged prostrate and relieve the inflammation and pain of benign prostatic hypertrophy.

Dioscorea villosa is another name for wild yam and is antispasmodic and helps supports the reproductive organs.

Pygeum africanum is used to prevent prostate atrophy and malfunction.

L-glutathione is a sulfur-bearing liver antioxidant.

Di-methylglycine (DMG) is excellent for heart muscle and tissue support.

L-carnitine supports the heart and helps convert calories into energy. It has been used to help lower cholesterol and improve memory.

Siberian ginseng is used for invigoration or concentration in times of fatigue.

Zinc is important for prostate health. It also may help restore sexual potency.

Essential Oils:

Yarrow (*Achillea millefolium*) is supportive to the prostrate and nerves.

Sage (*Salvia officinalis*) has estrogen-like properties and may help balance hormones.

Myrtle (*Myrtus communis*) helps prevent candida and helps prevent an inflamed prostate.

Myrrh (*Commiphora myrrha*) has hormone-like properties and is anti-inflammatory.

Peppermint (*Mentha piperita*) helps decongest the prostate and urinary tract.

Fennel (*Foeniculum vulgare*) has estrogen-like properties and helps balance the hormones.

Lavender (*Lavendula officinalis*) is calming and balancing.

Companion Products: Protec, Goji Berry Tea, Seagal Power Meal, Exodus, Be-Fit, Master His, Sulfurzyme (capsules or powder), or VitaGreen.

Companion Oil Blends: Mister, Exodus, Magnify Your Purpose, Live with Passion, or Valor.

Radex

Radex is an antioxidant complex that helps prevent the build-up of free radicals from air pollution and radiation while detoxifying, cleansing, and building the systems of the body.

Contents:

Vitamin E (d alpha tocopherol acid succinate) quenches free radical damage that can contribute to premature aging. It also affords protection against cardiovascular diseases, diabetes, menopausal conditions, and is beneficial for acne, allergies, and wound healing.

Vitamin C (ascorbic acid) helps the body to manufacture collagen for connective tissue, cartilage, tendons, etc., and is used for proper immune function. It is also an antioxidant.

Pantothenic acid supports adrenal function and the formation of antibodies, aids in vitamin utilization, and helps convert fats, carbohydrates, and proteins into energy.

Selenium has been extensively researched for its anticancer and antioxidant properties.

Wheat germ extract supports the body's ability to regenerate cells and tissue.

Black cumin helps digest protein and is an excellent antioxidant.

Essential Oils:

Melaleuca (*Melaleuca quinquenervia*) is anti-infectious and antibacterial.

Melaleuca (*Melaleuca alternifolia*) protects the body against radioactive materials and is anti-infectious and antibacterial.

Thyme (*Thymus vulgaris*) is one of the strongest antibacterial, antifungal, and antiviral essential oils.

Clove (*Syzygium aromaticum*) is antibacterial, antifungal, and antiviral.

Chamomile mixta (*Chamaemelum mixtum*) is a hybrid that supports skin and tissues.

Suggested Use: 2 tablets in the morning and 2 tablets in the evening.

Frequency: Approximately 89 MHz.

Royaldophilus

Royaldophilus is an outstanding source of *Lactobacillus acidophilus* and *bifidus* cultures required for optimum health. Derived from whole milk, these friendly bacteria are our first-line defense against disease and fungus overgrowth.

Excessive use of antibiotics and drugs, chlorinated water, and processed foods reduce the number of friendly bacteria in our intestines, which can lead to systemic yeast infection (candida). Currently about 70 percent of females and 30 percent of males suffer some form of candida.

Acidophilus may remain potent for several weeks without refrigeration; however, it is recommended that it be refrigerated before opening the bottle and kept refrigerated at less than 40 degrees. It is unwise to freeze acidophilus as this may affect its potency.

Acidophilus works with the enzymes to digest our food. It also aids the growth of intestinal flora. When we have a good enzyme base, acidophilus will complement enzyme production. It is extremely important for acidophilus to implant on the intestinal wall for the returning of intestinal flora. Milk is the only true acidophilus lactobacillus bifidus that the human body recognizes and accepts. The whole milk acidophilus used in Royaldophilus provides greater culture and inhibits allergy reaction.

Plantain reduces digestive problems and is very smooth to irritable bowel problems where intestinal flora is absent. This formula has proven to be superior to all forms of acidophilus.

Contents:

Lactobacillus and bifidus cultures contain the best natural digestive aid, acidophilus, which has many benefits, including correcting lactose intolerance, eliminating bad breath and acne, reducing cholesterol, inhibiting candida, and preventing yeast infection.

Plantain has been used for bleeding of the lungs and stomach, consumption, and dysentery.

Companion Products: Megazyme, I.C.P., ComforTone, and VitaGreen.

Companion Oil Blends: Di-Tone, Thieves, JuvaFlex, Harmony, Release, and Forgiveness.

Seagal Power Meal

A complete vegetarian protein drink mix powder containing Chinese wolfberry and rice protein with a large spectrum of antioxidant herbs, vitamins, enzymes, and minerals. Whether used as a meal alternative or snack, the Seagal Power Meal can serve as an excellent weight management tool. Free of fats and synthetic ingredients, Seagal Power Meal provides most of the building blocks the body requires for regeneration and maintenance.

The protein-rich formula of Seagal Power Meal, when combined with exercise and proper nutrition, can help the body build lean muscle tissue, which is the foundation of a lean physique and an important element in weight management. Because muscle burns 22 times as many calories as fat, the addition of muscle tissue can significantly accelerate metabolism and contribute to a more slender body. Because muscle tissue weighs more than adipose (fat) tissue, the addition of muscle mass to the body may not always be accompanied by weight loss, even though body fat may have dropped substantially.

Contents:

Chinese wolfberry (*Lycium barbarum*) has 18 amino acids, 21 trace minerals, beta carotene, and vitamins B1, B2, B6, and E. It is an excellent whole food and has many functions in the body.

Rice protein concentrate is high in branched chain amino acids required for building muscles.

Siberian ginseng root strengthens the adrenal glands, enhances immune function, normalizes blood pressure, improves mental alertness, and promotes hormonal balance.

Stevia leaf extract supports pancreas function.

Ginkgo biloba extract increases energy, improves memory and is excellent for cerebral circulation, oxygenation, and blood flow.

Bee pollen is high in protein and low in fat and sodium. It contains many minerals and vitamins. including potassium, calcium, magnesium, zinc, manganese, copper, and B vitamins.

Guar Gum is promotes healthy colon function.

Calcium carbonate is needed for healthy bones, teeth, and joints.

Lecithin (food for the brain) is excellent for liver disorders and helps to balance cholesterol.

Choline bitartrate has been used in the treatment of many liver disorders (including elevated cholesterol levels), Alzheimer's disease, viral hepatitis, and cirrhosis.

Silicon is required for skin, ligaments, bones, and tendons.

Magnesium is also crucial for proper enzyme function, muscle contractions, and heart rhythm. High intake can reduce high blood pressure, fight arteriosclerosis, and improve insulin action.

Potassium is important for proper muscle and nerve cell function.

MSM supports healthy hair, skin, liver, and immune function.

Inositol helps the liver rid itself of fat and bile.

Betaine HCl promotes protein digestion.

Amylase promotes fat digestion.

Kelp contains iodine, which is necessary to prevent goiters.

PABA (para amino benzoic acid) assists healthy bacteria in producing folic acid and helps form red blood cells.

L-carnitine helps convert fatty acids into energy.

Zinc is crucial for proper immune function and is needed for proper action of many hormones, including insulin and growth hormone. It helps improve wound healing.

Boron promotes the absorption and utilization of calcium.

Betatane is a mixed carotenoid complex containing lycopene, lutein, zeaxanthin, and alpha carotene.

Copper is necessary for proper red blood cell and immune function.

Manganese citrate is an antioxidant that regulates blood sugar levels and increases cellular energy

Vitamin E protects the heart and blood and combats free-radical oxidative damage.

Vitamin B3 is essential for turning carbohydrates into energy. It lowers cholesterol and helps regulate blood sugar.

Pantothenic acid supports antibody formation, aids in vitamin utilization, and helps convert fats, carbohydrates, and proteins into energy

Vitamin D3 stimulates the absorption of calcium and exerts many anticancerous properties, especially against breast and colon cancer.

Vitamin B6 supports immune function and protects the heart and blood vessels. It inhibits skin cancer growth and helps prevent kidney stones and PMS symptoms. Vitamin B6 requires folic acid and magnesium to maximize its effects.

Selenium has been extensively researched for its anticancer and antioxidant properties.

Riboflavin has shown to be crucial in the production of energy and is involved in regenerating glutathione and may help prevent certain esophageal cancers.

Thiamine HCl functions as part of an enzyme essential for energy production, carbohydrate metabolism, and nerve cell function.

Chromium improves insulin sensitivity and blood sugar metabolism.

Folic acid plays an important role in cardiovascular health. Helps prevent neural tube defects.

Biotin helps convert fats and amino acids into energy. It promotes healthy nails and hair and combats yeast and fungus overgrowth.

Vitamin B12 is critical for red blood cell formation and proper immune and nerve function.

Essential Oils:

Grapefruit (*Citrus paradisi*) has been used for disinfection and cellulite elimination.

Orange (*Citrus sinesis*) is anti-inflammatory, antispasmotic, and anticoagulant.

Lemon (*Citrus limon*) promotes leukocyte formation and increases lymphatic (immune) function.

Cypress (*Cupressus sempervirens*) helps improve circulation and improve lymph flow.

Anise (*Pimpinella anisum*) promotes digestion and helps eliminate parasites.

Fennel (*Foeniculum vulgare*) is antiparasitic, antimicrobial, antispasmotic, helps regulate intestinal flora, is a digestive aid, and increases gastric secretions.

Nutmeg (*Myristica fragrans*) helps support the adrenal glands for increased energy.

Companion Products: Be-Fit, Master Formula HERS/HIS, ComforTone, I.C.P., Megazyme, Thyromin, Wolfberry Power Bars, Essential Manna, and VitaGreen.

Companion Oil Blends: EndoFlex, Citrus Fresh, Envision, Live with Passion, Magnify Your Purpose, and Abundance.

Stevia Extract

Stevia extract is a super-sweet, low-calorie dietary supplement that helps regulate blood sugar and supports the pancreas. It is valuable for anyone with diabetes and hypoglycemia.

It is a wonderful aid to weight loss and weight management because it contains no calories. In addition, research indicates that it significantly increases glucose tolerance and inhibits glucose absorption. People who ingest stevia daily often report a decrease in their desire for sweets and fatty foods. It may also improve digestion and gastrointestinal function, soothe upset stomachs, and help speed recovery from minor illnesses.

Stevia also inhibits the growth of some bacteria and infectious organisms, including those that cause tooth decay and gum disease. Many individuals using stevia have reported a lower incidence of colds and flu. Many who have used stevia as a mouthwash have experienced a significant decrease in gum disease.

When topically applied, it softens the skin and smooths out wrinkles while healing various skin blemishes, acne, seborrhea, dermatitis, and eczema. When used on cuts and wounds, it promotes rapid healing without scarring.

Contents:

Stevia Leaf Extract—intensely sweet with a mild licorice-like aftertaste.

Companion Products: Thyromin, Megazyme, VitaGreen, AuraLight (oral spray), and Mineral Essence.

Companion Oil Blends: JuvaFlex and Thieves.

Suggested Use: As a dietary supplement and for skin care.

Stevia Select

Stevia Select is the powdered form of a popular South American food supplement and fructooligosaccharides that may balance blood sugar levels and support a healthy pancreas. This product is an excellent supplement for diabetics.

Contents:

Fructooligosaccharides (FOS) are one of the best-documented natural nutrients for promoting the growth the lactobacilli and bifidobacteria that are the linchpin of sound health. FOS has also been clinically studied for its ability to increase magnesium and calcium absorption, lower blood glucose, cholesterol, and LDL levels, and to inhibit production of the reductase enzymes that can contribute to cancer. Because FOS may increase magnesium absorption, it may also lead to lowered blood pressure and better cardiovascular health.

In addition, FOS also has another benefit: It has a naturally sweet taste.

Stevia leaf extract is an all-natural supplement. *(See Stevia for further nutritional information about this wonderful extract).*

Companion Products: Thyromin, Megazyme, VitaGreen, Stevia, Power Meal, and Mineral Essence.

Companion Oil Blends: JuvaFlex and Thieves.

Sulfurzyme

Sulfurzyme is a unique combination of methyl-sulfonalmethane (MSM), the protein-building compound found in breast milk, fresh fruits and vegetables, and Chinese wolfberry (*Lycium barbarum*). Together, they create a new concept in balancing the immune system and supporting almost every major function of the body. Of particular importance is the ability of MSM to equalize water pressure inside of the cells—a considerable benefit for those plagued with bursitis, arthritis, and tendonitis.

Chinese wolfberry is contained in this product to supply the necessary nutrients for the proper assimilation and metabolism of sulfur.

Contents:

Methylsulfonolmethane (MSM)—a natural form of sulfur found in all living organisms, combats rheumatism, asthma, bursitis, and tendonitis, as well as autoimmune diseases, like arthritis, Lupus, scleroderma, and allergies. One of the best sources of nutritional sulfur, MSM is critical to proper skin health, hair and nail growth, and liver function. MSM is the subject of a bestselling book, THE MIRACLE OF MSM, authored by UCLA neuropsychiatrist Ronald Lawrence M.D., Ph.D., and Stanley Jacob, M.D.

Chinese wolfberry (*Lycium barbarum*) contains minerals and coenzymes to support sulfur metabolism.

Companion Products: ArthroTune, Arthro Plus, Master HIS/HERS and CHILDREN'S, Megazyme, ComforTone, I.C.P., Ultra Young, Ortho Ease and Ortho Sport massage oils, and Seagal Power Meal.

Companion Oil Blends: En-R-Gee, PanAway, Envision, Valor, and Magnify Your Purpose.

Super B

Super B is a comprehensive source of the B vitamins essential for good health, including, thiamine (vitamin B1), Riboflavin (vitamin B2), niacin (vitamin B3), pantothenic acid (vitamin B5) complex, pyridoxine (vitamin B6), vitamin B12, bioin, folic acid. and PABA. It also includes minerals that aid the assimilation and metabolism of B vitamins.

B vitamins are particularly important during times of stress when reserves are depleted. Although research has shown that megadoses of B vitamins are not healthy, it has been known that the diets of many Americans do not provide the recommended amount of B vitamins that are essential for normal functions of immune response.

When many B vitamins are combined at once in the stomach, it can cause a fermentation resulting in stomach upset. To avoid this, Super B uses a synergistic suspension isolation process to isolate the various vitamins so they are released at different times.

Contents:

Folic acid is important in lowering homocysteine levels and protecting the heart and blood vessels. It also aids osteoporosis, candidiasis, epilepsy, gout, and periodontal disease.

Vitamin B1 is essential for energy production, carbohydrate metabolism, and nerve cell function.

Vitamin B2 is crucial in the production of cellular energy, helps regenerate the liver-protecting antioxidant glutathione, and may help prevent migraine headaches and some esophageal cancers.

Vitamin B3 is essential for turning carbo-hydrates into energy. It lowers cholesterol and helps regulate blood sugar. At least 4.4 mg is needed for every 1,000 calories consumed to avoid pellagra.

Vitamin B6 supports immune function and protects the heart and blood vessels. It inhibits skin cancer growth and helps prevent kidney stones and PMS symptoms. Vitamin B6 requires folic acid and magnesium to maximize its effects.

Vitamin B12 helps prevent deterioration of mental functioning, neurological damage, and to a number of psychological disturbances. Vegetarians often lack adequate B12, since this nutrient is not found in non-animal products.

Biotin helps convert fats and amino acids into energy. It promotes healthy nails and hair and combats yeast and fungus overgrowth.

Magnesium is crucial for proper enzyme function and is needed for normal muscle contractions and heart rhythm. High intake can reduce high blood pressure, fight arteriosclerosis, and improve insulin action.

Para amino benzoic acid (PABA) assists healthy bacteria in producing folic acid. It also helps the bones form red blood cells.

Zinc is crucial for proper immune function and is needed for proper action of many hormones, including insulin and growth hormone. It helps improve wound healing.

Selenium has been extensively researched for its anticancer and antioxidant properties.

Suggested Use: 1/2 to 1 tablet daily, preferably with a meal and not on an empty stomach.

Note: If taken on an empty stomach, one may experience a niacin flush, which may last up to an hour.

Frequency: Approximately 63 MHz.

Super C

Research has shown that physical stress, alcohol, smoking, and using certain medications may lower the blood levels of this essential vitamin. When citrus fruits are not readily available, diets may not contain enough vitamin C. Super C is properly balanced with rutin, biotin, bioflavonoids, and trace minerals to work synergistically, balancing the electrolytes and increasing the absorption rate of vitamin C. Without bioflavonoids, vitamin C has a hard time getting inside the cell; and without proper electrolyte balance and trace minerals, it will not stay there for long.

Contents:

Vitamin C helps the body manufacture collagen for connective tissue, cartilage, tendons, etc., and is used for proper immune function, as well as an antioxidant.

Citrus bioflavonoids are anti-inflammatory, antiallergic, antiviral, and anticarcinogenic. They have been used to prevent heart disease.

Rutin helps prevent capillary fragility, easy bruising, swelling, and nosebleeds.

Calcium carbonate is needed for healthy bones, teeth, and joints.

Zinc is crucial for proper immune function and is needed for proper action of many hormones, including insulin and growth hormone. It helps improve wound healing.

Potassium is required for proper electrolyte balance and to prevent high blood pressure.

Essential Oils:

Orange (*Citrus sinesis*) helps reduce fluid retention.

Tangerine (*Citrus nobilis)* is an anticoagulant and helps decongest the lymphatic system.

Lemon (*Citrus limon*) promotes leukocyte formation and increases lymphatic function.

Grapefruit (*Citrus paradisi*) has been used for disinfection and cellulite elimination.

Lemongrass (*Cymbopogon flexuosus*) is antiparasitic, antifungal, and promotes digestion.

Companion Products: ImmuneTune, Exodus, VitaGreen, Rehemogen, and ImmuGel.

Companion Oil Blends: Citrus Fresh, ImmuPower, Exodus II, Motivation, Thieves, or Valor.

Suggested Use: For reinforcing immune strength, 6 to 10 tablets daily. For maintenance, 2 to 3 tablets daily. Best taken before meals.

Frequency: Approximately 80 MHz.

Super Cal

Formulated with calcium, potassium, and magnesium citrate (which is easier for the body to utilize) specifically for proper electrolyte balance, hormonal balance, and muscle and bone development.

Contents:

Calcium supports healthy bones and teeth and helps prevent kidney stones.

Magnesium works side by side with calcium to build strong bones. It is also crucial for proper enzyme function, muscle contractions, and heart rhythm. High intake can reduce high blood pressure, fight arteriosclerosis, and improve insulin action.

Potassium is crucial for proper cellular fluid balance. It plays a role in reducing high blood pressure, increasing insulin sensitivity, and improving bone density.

Boron helps with the absorption and utilization of calcium.

Stearic Acid is a manufacturing aid used for lubrication of the formula.

Essential Oils:

Birch (*Betula alleghaniensis*) assists with bone, joint, and muscle pain.

Marjoram (*Origanum majorana*) supports muscles and nerves.

Lemongrass (*Cymbopogon flexuosus*) is used for ligament support.

Myrtle (*Myrtus communis*) has been researched for its effects in soothing the respiratory system.

Companion Products: ArthroTune, Arthro Plus, Sulfurzyme, Seagal Power Meal, Megazyme, EssPro 7, and Ortho Sport and Ortho Ease massage oils.

Companion Oil Blends: PanAway, Valor, Grounding, and Harmony.

Suggested Use: 1 to 2 capsules before each meal.

Frequency: Approximately 78 MHz.

Thyromin

This product was developed to nourish the thyroid, balance metabolism, and reduce fatigue. It contains a combination of specially selected glandular nutrients, herbs, amino acids, minerals, and essential oils. All of the oils are therapeutic-grade quality and are perfectly balanced to bring about the most beneficial, biological, and nutritional support to the thyroid.

Contents:

Vitamin E (d alpha tocopheryl acid succinate) is a potent antioxidant that protects against cardiovascular disease, diabetes, and menopausal conditions.

Iodine (kelp) is a key component of the T3 and T4 thyroid hormones that are pivotal for increasing energy levels and metabolism.

Potassium supports healthy thyroid function.

CoQ10 is used by cells in the body to convert food to energy. Heart cells require more CoQ10 to maintain muscle strength because of their higher demand for energy. CoQ10 helps in the prevention of heart disease and cancer and may help protect against blood cholesterol.

L-cysteine is an amino acid that supports proper liver function and healthy hair.

L-cystine is an amino acid that supports healthy liver function and hair.

In a base of: Irish moss and adrenal and pituitary substances.

Essential Oils:

Peppermint (*Mentha piperita*) supports digestion and pancreatic function.

Spearmint (*Mentha spicata*) has hormone-like properties that support the thyroid.

Myrtle (*Myrtus communis*) may help increase thyroid function.

Myrrh (*Commiphora myrrha*) has hormone-like properties and is anti-inflammatory.

Companion Products: FemiGen, JuvaTone, Megazyme, Mineral Essence, VitaGreen, and Ultra Young (oral spray).

Companion Oil Blends: EndoFlex, JuvaFlex, Clarity, En-R-Gee, and Magnify Your Purpose.

Suggested Use: 1 to 2 capsules daily before going to sleep (NOT BED).

Frequency: Approximately 52 MHz.

Ultra Young

Ultra Young is a revolutionary spray supplement that supports healthy pituitary and growth hormone secretion. It contains Vicia faba, which contains L-dopa. A 1976 the National Institute of Aging study found that administration of L-dopa to patients over 60 years of age resulted in a dramatic increase in growth hormone levels. A study conducted by Dr. George Cotzias showed that mice, fed small doses of L-dopa, lived twice as long as the control group not receiving L-dopa.

Contents:

Vicia faba major contains unusually high concentrations of L-dopa, an amino acid that has been shown in several studies to restore the sensitivity of the hypothalamus, which can lead to dramatic increases in both GHRH and GH levels.

Chinese wolfberry (*Lycium barbarum*) is rich in polysaccharides, which have potent immune-stimulating effects. These polysaccharides appear to be highly effective in raising levels of immunoglobulin A (IgA), an immune protein that steadily declines with age.

L-arginine is an amino acid that helps increase natural growth hormone production.

L-glutamine is an amino acid that has been researched for its hGH-promoting effects.

Zinc complex plays a pivotal part in maintaining optimal pituitary function.

GABA (Gamma-aminobutyric acid) is a nutrient that can amplify growth hormone production.

Vitamin B3 provides nutritional support for the hypothalamus and pituitary.

Vitamin B6 supports glandular and cognitive function.

Vitamin E protects the heart and blood and combats free-radical oxidative damage.

Selenium has been extensively researched for its anticancer and antioxidant properties.

Stevia is a super sweet supplement.

Contains therapeutic-grade essential oils of:

Sandalwood (*Santalum album*) is high in sesquiterpenes, which stimulate the hypothalamus and pituitary glands.

Conyza (*Canadensis fleabane*) overcomes retarded puberty, according to Dr. Daniel Penoël.

Companion Products: Seagal Power Meal, Be-Fit, Mineral Essence, Vitagreen, JuvaTone, Wolfberry Power Bars, Essential Manna, Sulfurzyme, and A. D. & E. liquid vitamin.

Companion Oil Blends: Envision, Magnify Your Purpose, JuvaFlex, Release, Joy, Live with Passion, En-R-Gee, Abundance, EndoFlex, and Valor.

Suggested Use: Spray Ultra Young directly inside cheeks and on the roof of the mouth. Avoid swallowing for 1 to 2 minutes. Spray upon waking, between meals, and just before retiring. Avoid spraying on the tongue because this reduces its effectiveness. It is best used 1 to 2 hours before or after meals, with no snacking in between because high blood sugar levels also reduce its effectiveness.

VitaGreen

This supplement is a high protein, high-energy chlorophyll formula that invigorates and revitalizes the body. It contains ingredients that help cleanse the blood and support the immune system, as well as support the thyroid and digestive systems.

Contents:

Spirulina (blue-green algae) is a source of concentrated protein and chlorophyll, a magnesium-rich pigment that has been linked to improved energy and metabolism.

Barley grass juice concentrate is an antioxidant that is rich in minerals.

Bee pollen is high in protein and low in fat and sodium. It is loaded with vitamins and minerals, including potassium, calcium, magnesium, zinc, manganese, copper, and B vitamins.

Panax Ginseng boosts energy and reduces stress. It also has the unique ability to stimulate lymphocyte formation (an essential part of the immune system).

L-arginine is an amino acid that promotes circulation in the small capillaries of our tissues, allowing greater nutrient absorption and cellular metabolism.

L-cystine is an amino acid that supports healthy liver function and hair.

L-tyrosine supports the formation of neurotransmitters, such as dopamine and serotonin.

Choline bitartrate has been used in the treatment of many liver disorders, including elevated cholesterol levels, Alzheimer's disease, viral hepatitis, and cirrhosis.

Kelp contains iodine that helps prevent goiters, thyroid hormonal imbalance, and estrogen imbalance.

Essential Oils:

Melissa (*Melissa officinalis*) is anti-inflammatory and energizing.

Lemon (*Citrus limon*) helps dissolve cholesterol and increase lymphatic (immune) function.

Lemongrass (*Cymbopogon flexuosus*) is antiparasitic, antifungal, and promotes digestion.

Rosemary (*Rosmarinus officinalis*) helps fight candida and balance the endocrine system.

Companion Products: Thyromin, JuvaTone, AuraLight, Royal Essence, Seagal Power Meal, Be-Fit, Sulfurzyme (powder or liquid), and Wolfberry Power Bars.

Companion Oil Blends: JuvaFlex, En-R-Gee, Envision, Magnify Your Purpose, Live with Passion, Release, Abundance, Awaken, Motivation, and Valor.

Suggested Use: Take three capsules three times daily.

Frequency: Approximately 76 MHz.

Experience has shown that before putting oils in VitaGreen, there was 42 percent blood absorption in 24 hours. After adding essential oils to VitaGreen, blood absorption increased to 64 percent in 30 minutes and 86 percent in an hour. The conclusion was that the cells were now receiving nutrients that they had previously not been able to assimilate.

Wolfberry Power Bar (Almond)

Wolfberry Power Bars are rich in the essential amino acids and minerals for building muscle and supporting immunity. These power bars combine Chinese wolfberries (over 15% protein) with amaranth (over 16% protein). Amaranth is rich in L-lysine, an essential amino acid lacking in traditional cereal grains, such as wheat and oats. The Power bars also include dried cranberries and essential oils of orange and cinnamon. These essential oils are high in phenylpropanes and may activate the amino acid conversion of L-leucine in the body. L-leucine is converted into HMB, a powerful muscle builder.

Contents:

Rice protein concentrate is high in branched chain amino acids (valine, leucine, and isoleucine), which are crucial for muscle building.

Chinese wolfberry (*Lycium barbarum*) has been used for many years to help combat cancer and improve the immune system.

Honey is a an emulsifier and natural sweetener.

Puffed amaranth is an South American grain rich in the amino acid L-lysine. Many traditional cereals, such as wheat and corn, lack sufficient amounts of L-lysine for optimum health.

Coconut is added for flavoring.

Cranberries have been proven effective for treatment of urinary tract infections in a number of clinical trials. Its action may be due to an antibacterial compound, hippuric acid, as well as other compounds that reduce the ability of bacteria to adhere to the lining of the bladder and urethra.

Soy protein is a complete source of amino acids, the building blocks of muscles and immunity. The FDA recently recognized soy's ability to combat cardiovascular disease and protect the heart.

Contains therapeutic-grade essential oils of:

Orange (*Citrus sinesis*) helps reduce fluid retention.

Cinnamon (*Cinnamomum verum*) is anti-infectious, antibacterial, antiviral, antifungal, antiparasitic, anticoagulant, and is used for all types of infections. It is used in the Wolfberry Power Bars as a natural preservative.

Companion Products: Be-Fit, Master Formula HERS/HIS and CHILDREN'S, ComforTone, I.C.P., Megazyme, Thyromin, Essential Manna, and VitaGreen.

Companion Oil Blends: EndoFlex, Citrus Fresh, Envision, Live with Passion, Magnify Your Purpose, and Abundance.

Food "Ash" pH

The following is a list of common foods with an approximate, relative potential of acidity (-) or alkalinity (+), as present in 1 ounce of food.

Alfalfa Grass	+29.3	Cheese, Hard	-18.1	Lecithin, pure (soy)	+38.0
Almond	+3.6	Cherry, Sour	+3.5	Leeks (bulbs)	+7.2
Apricot	-9.5	Cherry, Sweet	-3.6	Lemon, fresh	+9.9
Artichokes	+1.3	Chia, sprouted	+28.5	Lentils	+0.6
Asparagus	+1.1	Chicken	-18.0 to -22.0	Lettuce	+2.2
Avocado (protein)	+15.6	Chives	+8.3	Lettuce, Fresh cabbage	+14.1
Banana, Ripe	-10.1	Coconut, fresh	+0.5	Lettuce, Lamb's	+4.8
Banana, Unripe	+4.8	Coffee	-25.1	Limes	+8.2
Barley Grass	+28.7	Comfrey	+1.5	Liquor	-28.6 to -38.7
Barley malt syrup	-9.3	Corn oil	-6.5	Liver	-3.0
Beans, French cut	+11.2	Cranberry	-7.0	Macadamia Nuts	-11.7
Beans, Lima	+12.0	Cream	-3.9	Mandarin Orange	-11.5
Beans, White	+12.1	Cucumber, fresh	+31.5	Mango	-8.7
Beef	-34.5	Cumin	+1.1	Margarine	-7.5
Beer	-26.8	Currant	-8.2	Marine Lipids	+4.7
Beet sugar	-15.1	Currant, Black	-6.1	Mayonnaise	-12.5
Beet, fresh red	+11.3	Currant, Red	-2.4	Meats, Organ	-3.0
Biscuit, White	-6.5	Dandelion	+22.7	Milk sugar	-9.4
Blueberry	-5.3	Date	-4.7	Milk, Homogenized	-1.0
Borage	+3.2	Dog grass	+22.6	Millet	+0.5
Brazil Nuts	-0.5	Eggs	-18.0 to -22.0	Molasses	-14.6
Bread, Rye	-2.5	Endive, fresh	+14.5	Mustard	-19.2
Bread, White	-10.0	Fennel	+1.3	Nut soy (Soaked,	
Bread, whole-grain	-4.5	Fig juice powder	-2.4	then air dried)	+26.5
Bread, whole-meal	-6.5	Filbert	-2.0	Olive Oil	+1.0
Brussels Sprouts	-1.5	Fish, Fresh Water	-11.8	Onion	+3.0
Buckwheat groats	+0.5	Fish, Ocean	-20.0	Orange	-9.2
Butter	-3.9	Flax seed oil	-1.3	Oysters	-5.0
Buttermilk	+1.3	Flax seed	+3.5	Papaya	-9.4
Cabbage, Green,		Fructose	-9.5	Peach	-9.7
December harvest	+4.0	Garlic	+13.2	Peanuts	-12.8
Cabbage, Green,		Gooseberry, Ripe	-7.7	Pear	-9.9
March harvest	+2.0	Grapefruit	-1.7	Peas, fresh	+5.1
Cabbage, Red	+6.3	Grapes, Ripe	-7.6	Peas, ripe	+0.5
Cabbage, Savoy	+4.5	Hazelnut	-2.0	Pineapple	-12.6
Cabbage, White	+3.3	Honey	-7.6	Pistachios	-16.6
Cantaloupe	-2.5	Horseradish	+6.8	Plum, Italian	-4.9
Caraway	+2.3	Juice, natural fruit	-8.7	Plum, yellow	-4.9
Carrot	+9.5	Juice, white sugar		Pork	-38.0
Cashews	-9.3	sweetened fruit	-33.4	Potatoes, stored	+2.0
Cauliflower	+3.1	Kamut Grass	+27.6	Primrose	+4.1
Cayenne Pepper	+18.8	Ketchup	-12.4	Pumpkin	-5.6
Celery	+13.3	Kohlrabi	+5.1	Quark	-17.3

Radish, Sprouted	+28.4	Soybeans, fresh	+12.0	Tomato	+13.6
Radish, Summer black	+39.4	Spelt	+0.5	Turbinado	-9.5
Radish, White (spring)	+3.1	Spinach		Turnip	+8.0
Raspberry	-5.1	(other than March)	+13.1	Veal	-35.0
Red radish	+16.7	Spinach, March harvest	+8.0	Walnuts	-8.0
Rhubarb stalks	+6.3	Straw grass	+21.4	Watercress	+7.7
Rice syrup, brown	-8.7	Strawberry	-5.4	Watermelon	-1.0
Rice, brown	-12.5	Sugar cane juice, dried		Wheat Germ	-11.4
Rose Hips	-15.5	(Sucanat)	-9.6	Wheat Grass	+33.8
Rutabaga	+3.1	Sugar Cane, Refined		Wheat	-10.1
Sesame seeds	+.5	(white)	-17.6	Wine	-16.4
Shave grass	+21.7	Sunflower Oil	-6.7	Zucchini	+5.7
Sorrel	+11.5	Sunflower Seeds	-5.4		
Soy beans, (cooked,		Sweeteners, artificial	-26.5		
then ground)	+12.8	Tangerine	-8.5		
Soy Flour	+2.5	Tea (Black)	-27.1		
Soy Sprouts	+29.5	Tofu	+3.2		

Reference:
Young, Robert O. Sick and Tired.
Alpine, UT, 1977.

Herbal Tinctures

Arthro Plus

Arthro Plus is an herbal tincture that, when combined with essential oils, may be taken orally or topically. It works well with ArthroTune. Take 1 to 3 droppers (25-75 drops) 3 to 6 times daily in distilled or purified water with meals as a dietary supplement.

Contents:

Yucca—is popular in the southwest U.S. as a folklore medicine. Known as the Joshua-tree

Alfalfa—high in chlorophyll, beta carotene, calcium, and the vitamins D, E and K.

Chaparral—used by Native American healers as a tonic for cancer, snake bite, infection, arthritis, and tuberculosis treatments.

Cayenne—traditionally an aid to digestion, this red pepper also possesses fibrinolytic activity (able to break down blood clots).

Dandelion Root—traditionally used arthritis and rheumatism.

Burdock Bark—a diuretic and believed to be useful in treating impotence and sterility.

Cascara Sagrada—a safe and natural laxative, it is often prescribed by herbalists to stimulate the liver, pancreas, gallbladder, and stomach and to support the digestive system.

Licorice Root—traditionally used for rheumatism and arthritis.

Juniper Berry (*Juniperus communis*)—acts as a detoxifier and is used to stimulate nerve function.

Birch (*Betula alleghaniensis*)—contains an active principle similar to cortisone and is beneficial for massage associated with bone, muscle, and joint discomfort.

Marjoram (*Origanum majorana*)—used for soothing the muscles and the respiratory system. It also assists in calming the nerves. It is antimicrobial and antiseptic.

Cypress (*Cupressus sempervirens*)—used to improve the circulatory system. It is antimicrobial.

Chelex

Chelex contains herbs that have been traditionally used to chelate and neutralize heavy metals and and disarm free radicals. Take 1-3 droppers 3 times a day.

Contents:

Astragalus—used as a diuretic, a vasodilator, and respiratory infection treatment, this herb reputedly has immune-stimulating effects and increases energy.

Garlic—demonstrated by Louis Pasteur to have anti-bacterial properties in 1858. Albert Schweitzer used garlic to treat amoebic dysentery. Later, researchers found that garlic can protect against heart disease and cancer. Garlic juice halts the growth of more than 60 types of fungi and 20 types of bacteria.

Sarsaparilla—contains saponins, steroid-like molecules that neutralize endotoxins, poisons secreted by fungi and bacteria in the human body that contribute to many kinds of disease.

Siberian Ginseng—energizes the body and boosts the immune system.

Red Clover—used to treat asthma, bronchitis, skin ailments, ulcers, and arthritis. Used in some cultures to prevent recurrence of cancer.

Royal Jelly—a viscous, milky white secretion produced by the worker bee upon which future queens are continually nourished. Royal jelly's chemistry has been extensively studied and contains all the essential amino acids, unsaturated fats, natural sugars, minerals, and the B-vitamins (B-5 and B-6). Tests have shown that royal jelly can have an effect on the adrenal cortex, stimulating the adrenal glands to produce a positive reaction on increased metabolism and enhanced energy.

Roman Chamomile (*Chamaemelum nobile*)—promotes bile flow and liver function.

Eucalyptus (*Eucalyptus globulus*)—is a powerful antimicrobial agent, rich in eucalyptol (a key ingredient in many antiseptic mouth rinses).

PEOPLE'S DESK REFERENCE FOR ESSENTIAL OILS

Helichrysum (*Helichrysum italicum*)—has been studied by European researchers for regenerating tissue and improving circulation. This oil has also been studied for its natural chelating action.

Estro

Estro is an herbal tincture containing plant-derived phytoestrogens, such as black cohosh, that which are widely used in Europe as a safe alternative to synthetic estrogen. Phytoestrogens have been researched for their ability to support the body during PMS without many of the side effects associated with estrogen-replacement therapies. Contains the therapeutic-grade essential oil of clary sage (Salvia sclarea), which contains natural sclareol, a plant-based estrogen. Start with 1 dropper 2 to 3 times daily. Increase as needed to as much as 3 droppers daily. Estro may take as much as four weeks to reach maximum effectiveness.

Contents:

Black Cohosh—approved by the German Commission E for combating PMS symptoms. Its constituents have been found to mimic those of estrogen.

Blue Cohosh—the main ingredient brewed in a tea used by Native American women to relieve menstrual and labor cramping, now recommended by modern herbalists to induce menstruation and as uterine stimulant and antispasmodic.

Royal Jelly—a secretion produced by the worker bee upon which all bee larvae feed during the first three days of life. Because queen larvae continue to feed on this substance (and live thirty to forty times longer), various herbalists claim that royal jelly is especially effective in halting or controlling the aging process, nourishing the skin, and erasing facial blemishes and wrinkles.

Fennel (*Foeniculum vulgare*)—antiseptic and stimulating to the circulatory and respiratory systems.

Lavender (*Lavandula angustifolia*)—is calming, relaxing, and balancing, both physically and emotionally.

Clary Sage (*Salvia sclarea*)—is a source of natural estrogen.

Femalin

Femalin is an herbal and oil tincture formulated to help protect the female reproductive system. Store in a cool place, out of sunlight. Take 1 dropper (approximately 25 drops) 3 to 6 times daily in distilled water as a dietary supplement. Keep in a cool place and avoid direct sunlight for longer life.

Contents:

Goldenseal Root—a native American medicinal plant used for gastric and urinary disorders.

Blessed Thistle—a popular folk remedy used by by European monks to aid digestion and circulation.

Cayenne—traditionally used to aid digestion, it possesses fibrinolytic activity (able to break down blood clots)

Cramp Bark—used traditionally to combat endo-metriosis, osteoporosis, uterine cysts, and irregular menstruation. Also used as a labor tonic and to remedy cramping of the stomach, intestines, and uterus, from which its name is derived.

False Unicorn—medicinal use is based in Native American tradition, especially in the regulation of menstruation, and to prevent miscarriages.

Ginger Root—especially useful in calming nausea and stimulating appetite. It was also found in 1982 to alleviate motion sickness.

Red Raspberry—especially helpful to women, this herb nourishes the reproductive organs, helping to strengthen and prepare the body for childbirth. It is also an effective remedy for digestive ailments and upset stomach.

Squaw Vine—traditionally used for PMS symptoms: anxiety, edema, fibrocystic disease of the breast, postpartum depression, pregnancy, sore nipples (with olive oil and beeswax), and varicose veins.

Uva Ursi—a mild diuretic, astringent, and urinary tract infection remedy.

Royal Jelly—a secretion produced by the worker bee upon which all bee larvae feed during the first three days of life. Because queen larvae continue to feed on this substance (and live thirty to forty times longer), various herbalists claim that royal jelly is especially effective in halting or controlling the aging process, nourishing the skin, and erasing facial blemishes and wrinkles.

Rosemary (*Rosmarinus officinalis*)—researched for its antiseptic and antimicrobial properties. It may be beneficial for the skin. It helps overcome mental fatigue.

Fennel (*Foeniculum vulgare*)—antiseptic and stimulating to the circulatory and respiratory systems.

Melaleuca (*Melaleuca alternifolia*)—highly regarded as an antimicrobial and antiseptic essential oil. Pure melaleuca has high levels of terpinenol, which is the key active constituent.

Clary Sage (*Salvia sclarea*)—is a source of natural estrogen.

Bergamot (*Citrus bergamia*)—used in the Middle East for hundreds of years for skin conditions associated with an oily complexion.

HRT

HRT tincture combines some of the best-studied herbs for supporting normal heart function, including hawthorn berry, garlic, and cayenne. Hawthorn berry's role in supporting the heart has been gaining increasing notice among both authors and physicians. According to Varro Tyler, Ph.D., one of the most highly esteemed herbalists in the U.S., "Studies are urgently needed for [an herb] as potentially valuable as this one." Take 1 to 3 droppers 3 times daily in distilled water or as desired.

Contents:

Hawthorn berries—used since the time of Dioscorides in the first century A.D., they are one of the best studied herbs to support the heart, protecting against heart muscle weakness, angina, and mild arrhythmia. J. L. Rodale published an entire book on the subject, The Hawthorn Berry for the Heart.

Garlic—demonstrated by Louis Pasteur to have antibacterial properties in 1858. Albert Schweitzer used garlic to treat amoebic dysentery. Later researchers found that garlic can protect against heart disease and cancer.

Garlic juice halts the growth of more than 60 types of fungi and 20 types of bacteria.

Lobelia—a mild sedative and helpful for allergies, coughs, colds and headaches. Evaluated to be one of the most valuable herbs, due its dual properties of stimulation and relaxation.

Cayenne—traditionally an aid to digestion, this red pepper also possesses fibrinolytic activity (able to break down blood clots).

Royal Jelly—a viscous, milky white secretion produced by the worker bee upon which future queens are continually nourished. Royal jelly's chemistry has been extensively studied and contains all the essential amino acids, unsaturated fats, natural sugars, minerals, and the B-vitamins (B-5 and B-6). Tests have shown that royal jelly can have an effect on the adrenal cortex, stimulating the adrenal glands to produce a positive reaction on increased metabolism and enhanced energy.

Lemon (*Citrus limon*)—has antiseptic-like properties and contains compounds that have been studied for their effects on immune function.

Rosewood (*Aniba rosaeodora*)—soothing and nourishing to the skin. It has been researched at Weber State University for its inhibition rate against gram positive and gram negative bacterial growth.

Ylang ylang (*Cananga odorata*)—traditionally used to support heart function and circulation.

Cypress (*Cupressus sempervirens*)—one of the oils most used for the circulatory system.

K&B

K&B tincture contains herbs that support kidney and bladder function. Take 1-3 droppers 3 times daily in distilled water or as desired.

Contents:

Juniper Berries—long used by Greek, Arabic, and Native American peoples as a kidney stimulant to encourage cleansing and increased filtration.

Parsley—widely used to purify the urinary tract.

Uva Ursi—a mild diuretic, astringent, and urinary tract infection remedy.

Dandelion Root—traditionally used for a host of disorders, including anemia, cirrhosis, colitis, constipation, cystitis, dermatitis, digestive complaints, edema, gallbladder disorders, liver disorders.

Roman Chamomile—increases bile flow and liver function.

Royal Jelly—a viscous, milky white secretion produced by the worker bee upon which future queens are continually nourished. Royal jelly's chemistry has been extensively studied and contains all the essential amino acids, unsaturated fats, natural sugars, minerals, and the B-vitamins (B-5 and B-6). Tests have shown that royal jelly can have an effect on the adrenal cortex, stimulating the adrenal glands to produce a positive reaction on increased metabolism and enhanced energy.

Clove (*Syzygium aromaticum*)—one of the most antimicrobial and antiseptic essential oils.

Juniper Berry (*Juniperus communis*)—a strong diuretic.

Sage (*Salvia officinalis*)—strengthens the vital centers and supports metabolism.

Fennel (*Foeniculum vulgare*) is antiseptic to the digestive tract. Supports digestion.

Geranium (*Pelargonium graveolens*)—opens the bile duct.

Roman Chamomile (*Chamaemelum nobile*)—promotes the flow of bile to and from the liver, a key aspect of cleansing and detoxification.

Rehemogen

Rehemogen tincture contains herbs that were used by Chief Sundance and the native American Indians as a blood cleanser and builder. How to use: 1-3 droppers 3 times daily in distilled water or as desired.

Contents:

Red Clover Blossom—used to treat asthma, bronchitis, skin ailments, ulcers, and arthritis. Used in some cultures to prevent recurrence of cancer. Its combined properties act as a diuretic, sedative, and antitussive for whooping cough.

Chaparral—used by Native American healers as a tonic for cancer, snake bite, infection, arthritis, and tuberculosis treatments.

Licorice Root—traditionally used to defeat a host of degenerative ailments, including arthritis, asthma, bronchial ailments, cancer, catarrh, circulatory dysfunction, colitis, dyspepsia, irritable bowel syndrome, liver disorders, rheumatism, stress, and vertigo

Oregon Grape Root—contains berberine, a powerful liver protectant.

Sarsaparilla—contains saponins, steroid-like molecules that neutralize endotoxins, poisons secreted by fungi and bacteria in the human body that contribute to many kinds of disease.

Cascara Sagrada—used to support the liver, pancreas, gallbladder, and stomach.

Burdock Root—eaten as a vegetable in Japan, this root has been used to treat ulcers and arthritis, cleanse the blood, and cure skin diseases.

Rosemary (*Rosmarinus officinalis*)—researched for its antiseptic and antimicrobial properties. It may be beneficial for the skin. It helps overcome mental fatigue.

Thyme (*Thymus vulgaris*)—one of the most antimicrobial and antiseptic essential oils.

Melaleuca (*Melaleuca alternifolia*)—highly regarded as an antimicrobial and antiseptic essential oil.

Roman Chamomile (*Chamaemelum nobile*)—promotes the flow of bile to and from the liver, a key aspect of cleansing and detoxification.

Also contains: Buckthorn bark, stillingia, and prickly ash bark.

Essential Oils in Oral Hygiene

Antibacterial and Antiseptic

Essential oils are ideal for use in oral care products because they are both antiseptic and non-toxic—a rare combination. Jean Valnet, M.D., who used essential oils for decades in his clinical practice emphasized this: "Essential oils are especially valuable as antiseptics because their aggression toward microbial germs is matched by their total harmlessness toward tissue."

Dentarome, Dentarome Plus, and Fresh Essence Mouthwash use therapeutic-grade essential oils at the heart of their formulas. These oils include peppermint, birch, eucalyptus, thyme and a proprietary blend of therapeutic-grade essential oils, which includes clove, lemon, cinnamon, and rosemary. This blend was tested at Weber State University and found to dramatically inhibit the growth of many types of bacteria (both gram negative and gram positive), including Micrococcus luteus and Staphylococcus aureus. Even more remarkably, this blend exhibited a 99.96% kill rate against tough gram negative bacteria, like Pseudonoma auruginosa. These bacteria, because of their thicker cell walls, tend to be far more resistant to antiseptics.

Dentarome Toothpaste

Dentarome is formulated with pure, natural ingredients, such as vegetable glycerine, sodium bicarbonate, ionic minerals, and steviocide (a natural, intensely sweet extract from a tropical plant native to South America). In addition, Dentarome uses an exclusive formula of uniquely antiseptic and antimicrobial therapeutic-grade essential oils to combat plaque-causing microorganisms. Together with other breath-freshening essential oils, like spearmint, Dentarome leaves the mouth fresh, fragrant, and clean.

Dentarome was tested at Weber State University and found to have potent antimicrobial properties against a wide range of oral microbes, including Streptococcus oralis, Streptoccus pneumoniae, Bramunella catarrhalis, and candida albicans. Dentarome Plus includes a higher concentration of thymol and eugenol for extra antiseptic action. Thymol is derived from thyme oil (thymus vulgaris) and eugenol is derived from clove oil (Eugenia caryophyllata).

Fresh Essence Mouthwash

Free of dyes, alcohol, preservatives, another other synthetic ingredients, Fresh Essence uses medicinal-grade essential oils, such as thyme, eucalyptus, birch, peppermint, and Thieves that naturally contain compounds clinically proven to kill the bacteria that can cause bad breath, plaque, and gum diseases, such as gingivitis. By using the entire essential oil rather than isolated active ingredients, Fresh Essence gains significant advantages in safety and antiseptic power. A complete oil exhibits far stronger antimicrobial power than its active constituents alone. The whole oil is also safer because it contains a natural balance of elements that make it nondamaging to human tissue.

Fresh Essence is also formulated with a patented liposome technology (using soy-derived lecithin) that binds the essential oils to the mucus membrane inside the mouth. This enables the essential oils to remain in the mouth longer so that they can provide long-lasting, germ-killing, and breath-freshening effects.

Comparing Toothpastes

	Dentarome & Dentarome Plus	Common Brand
Active Ingredients	Thieves*	Sodium Fluoride
	Thymol	Sodium Monofluorophosphate
	Eugenol	
	Birch oil	
Foaming Agent	None	Sodium Laurel Sulfate (SLS) **
Tooth Health Agent	Ionic Minerals	Pentasodium triphosphate
	Birch Oil	Tetrasodium pyrophosphate
Moisturizer	Vegetable Glycerine	Glycerine, sorbitol
Sweetener	Steviocide	Sodium saccharin
Coloring	None	Titanium Dioxide
		FD&C Blue #1
Cleansing Agent	Baking Soda	Abrasive Silica
		Synthetic Glycerine
Flavoring	Spearmint Oil	Artificial Sources
		Natural Sources
Thickener	Xanthum Gum	Xanthum Gum, Cellulose Gum

* A proprietary blend of clove, lemon, cinnamon, eucalyptus radiata, rosemary.
** Also known as sodium laureth sulfate and sodium laurel sulfate.

Comparing Mouthwashes

	Fresh Essence Mouthwash	Common Brand
Active Ingredients	Thieves*	Thymol
	Thyme oil	1,8 cineol
	Eucalyptus oil	Menthol
	Birch oil	Methyl Salicylate
	Peppermint oil	
Base	Water	Alcohol, SD Alcohol
Sweetener	Steviocide	Sodium saccharin
	Sorbitol	
Coloring	None	D&C Yellow #10
		FD&C Green #3
		FD&C Blue #1
		FD&C Yellow #5
Flavoring	Peppermint	Artificial Sources
Preservatives	None	Benzoic Acid
		Polysorbate 80
Dispersant	Natural Lecithin	Poloxamer 403
		Sodium Hydroxide (Lye)
		Synthetic Glycerine

*A proprietary blend of clove, lemon, cinnamon, eucalyptus radiata, rosemary.

Benefits of Liposomes

The two primary benefits of using liposome technology are:

1. **Controlled release of active ingredients**

2. **Ingredient protection.**

The controlled release aspect of liposome technology used by Young Living is enhanced through the use of a patented "liposome anchoring" system. This technology involves increasing the substantivity of liposomes to specific substrates (e.g., skin and mucin coated tissues for nutriceutical products.) This enables the liposomes to slowly release their cargo at the "site of action." This technology is particularly advantageous for delivering lipophilic actives.

Liposomes that adhere to dental enamel can be used to improve dental health. Dental liposomes contain active materials to prevent plaque formation, treat periodontal disease, and prevent dental caries. Molecules on the surface of the liposome adhere to the tooth's enamel. The liposome slowly releases its therapeutic cargo onto the enamel surface.

The ability of the dental liposomes to release their therapeutic cargo slowly is demonstrated in Fig. 1. A saliva-coated tooth is dipped into a solution containing dental liposomes. The liposomes contain a test material. The tooth is sequentially washed with 1.0 ml. of buffer 30 times. The test material is removed slowly with the washes. Even after 30 washes, some active material is retained on the tooth, and it is removed for demonstration purposes with chloroform, which dissolves the liposomal matrix, releasing the active material from the tooth surface.

Slow Release Systems for Oral Soft Tissues

Liposomal systems that adhere to mucus membranes are designed to slowly release beneficial chemicals in the mouth, nose, and other tissues coated with mucin. This is useful in the slow release of flavors. For example, a breath lozenge containing menthol that is contained in a mucin-binding system can provide extended oral freshness longer than a standard menthol lozenge (Fig. 2).

In another experiment, two thymol-based mouthwashes were compared side by side. The first was a standard commercial product with no liposome-based delivery; the second used a lipsomal delivery system. The results of the experiment are illustrated in Fig. 3.

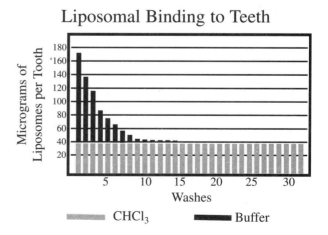

Liposomal Binding to Teeth

Microgrms of Liposomes per Tooth

CHCl₃   Buffer

Figure 1. A saliva-coated human tooth was dipped in a solution of dental liposomes and rinsed repeatedly with 1.0 ml of water. The final rinse was with 1.0 ml chloroform to remove residual, tightly bound liposomes.

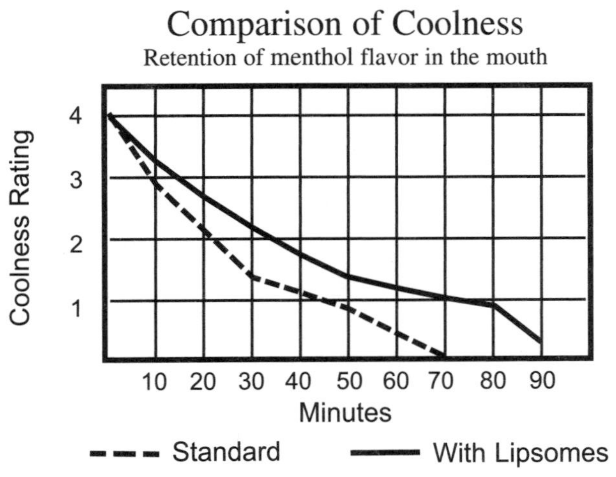

Comparison of Coolness
Retention of menthol flavor in the mouth

--- Standard   —— With Lipsomes

Figure 2. Lozenges made with mucin-binding system to release menthol flavor slowly are compared to control menthol lozenges. Timing began when the lozenge was completely dissolved in the mouth.

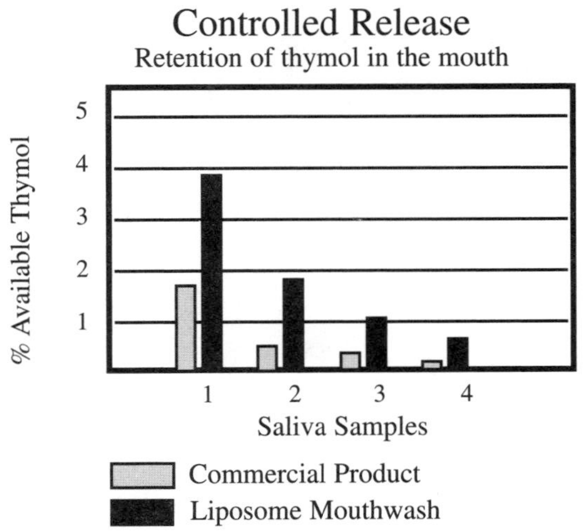

Controlled Release
Retention of thymol in the mouth

☐ Commercial Product
■ Liposome Mouthwash

Figure 3. The retention of thymol was measured over a period of five minutes in various saliva samples. The level of thymol remaining in the saliva dropped off rapidly following usage of the commercial product. However, following usage of the liposome-based mouthwash, there was a significantly higher level of thymol in each saliva sample analyzed.

Massage Oils

Massage, or therapeutic touch, has always been part of healing, both physical and emotional. When essential oils are combined with massage, the benefits are numerous. Massage improves circulation, lymphatic drainage, and aids in the elimination of tissue wastes. The oils bring peace and tranquility as well as keen mental awareness. Massage opens and increases the flow of energy, balancing the entire nervous system and helping to release physical and emotional disharmony. The unrefined carrier vegetable oils are rich in fat-soluble nutrients and essential fatty acids, easily absorbed through the skin and used in the body.

Cel-Lite Magic Massage Oil

Cel-Lite Magic combines vegetable oils and vitamin E with essential oils that tone and nourish the skin. Orange *(Citrus sinesis)* and grapefruit *(Citrus paradisi)* oils are beneficial in improving skin texture. Massage on location.

Contents:

Grapeseed Oil—light-textured and odorless on its own, it is nourishing to the skin and makes an excellent carrier for essential oils.

Olive Oil—a moisturizing agent in many organic cosmetics, this unsurpassed natural preservative also will not clog pores.

Wheatgerm Oil—a rich and lush oil high in lecithin, vitamin E, and B vitamins.

Sweet Almond Oil—this nourishing oil is well suited for massage. It aids the smooth application of the base, reducing negative friction.

Vitamin E—also known as alpha-tocopherol, it protects skin and cell membranes against oxidative damage.

Cedarwood *(Cedrus atlantica)*—historically is recognized for its calming, purifying properties and is used to benefit the skin and tissues near the surface of the skin.

Cypress *(Cupressus sempervirens)*—one of the oils most used for the circulatory system. It is also antimicrobial.

Juniper Berry *(Juniperus communis)*—may work as a detoxifier and cleanser, as well as being beneficial for the skin.

Grapefruit *(Citrus paradisi)*—works as a mild disinfectant. Diffuse for a refreshing, uplifting aroma. Like many cold-pressed citrus oils, it has unique fat-dissolving characteristics.

Clary Sage *(Salvia sclarea)*—supports the cells and hormones. It contains natural estriol, a phytoestrogen.

Pepper *(Piper nigrum)*—a stimulating, energizing essential oil that has been studied for its effects on cellular oxygenation. It has been used for soothing deep tissue muscle aches.

Honeysuckle Fragrance Oil—adds the wonderful fragrance of honeysuckle to this massage oil.

Desert Breeze Massage Oil

Desert Breeze is a relaxing blend of oils designed to soothe muscles and promote calming and tension relief. Makes an excellent all-purpose massage oil.

Contents:

Grapeseed Oil—light-textured and odorless on its own, it is nourishing to the skin and makes an excellent carrier for essential oils.

Sweet Almond Oil—reduces friction and promotes smooth application during massage.

Olive Oil—is a moisturizing agent in many organic cosmetics and will not clog pores.

Wheatgerm Oil—is a rich and lush oil rich in lecithin, vitamin E, and B vitamins.

Vitamin E—protects skin and cell membranes against oxidative damage.

Bergamot *(Citrus bergamia)*—used in the Middle East for hundreds of years for skin conditions associated with an oily complexion. It soothes insect bites and may serve as an insect repellent.

Blue Tansy (*Tanacetum annuum*)—contains azulene, responsible for the rich blue color of the oil. Its extremely powerful anti-inflammatory properties make it perfectly suited to treat sprains, carpal tunnel syndrome, and sports injuries and to balance the emotions after traumatic emotional experiences.

German Chamomile (*Matricaria recutita*)—contains azulene, a powerful anti-inflammatory compound.

Roman Chamomile (*Chamaemelum nobile*)—may help calm and relieve restlessness and tension. Its anti-infectious properties benefit cuts, scrapes, and bruises. It is used extensively in Europe for the skin.

Lavender (*Lavandula angustifolia*)—is highly regarded for the skin and is outstanding for cleansing burns, cuts, bruises, and skin irritations. Combats lice (*Pediculus humanis*).

Melissa (*Melissa officinalis*)—is antiviral and antimicrobial, yet gentle and delicate.

Rose (*Rosa damascena*)—one of the oldest oils for treating skin conditions, including psoriasis and dermatitis. It has an exquisite fragrance that is both intoxicating and aphrodisiac-like. Daniel Penoël, M.D., used this oil for numerous skin conditions in his clinical practice.

Ylang ylang (*Cananga odorata*)—instills relaxation and combats stress.

Also includes Joy and Valor blends

Dragon Time Massage Oil

Dragon Time combines essential oils that have been researched in Europe for their balancing effects on hormones. Can be used in massage or added to bathwater.

Contents:

Grapeseed Oil—light-textured and odorless on its own, it is nourishing to the skin and makes an excellent carrier for essential oils.

Sweet Almond Oil—this nourishing oil is well suited for massage. It aids the smooth application of the base, reducing negative friction.

Olive Oil—a moisturizing agent in many organic cosmetics, this unsurpassed natural preservative does not clog pores.

Wheatgerm Oil—a rich and lush oil high in lecithin, vitamin E, and B vitamins.

Vitamin E—protects skin and cell membranes against oxidative damage.

Clary Sage (*Salvia sclarea*)—contains estrogen-like compounds.

Fennel (*Foeniculum vulgare*)—antiseptic and stimulating to the circulatory and respiratory systems.

Lavender (*Lavandula angustifolia*)—is highly regarded for the skin. Excellent for burns and for cleansing cuts, bruises, and skin irritations. It is uniquely calming and relaxing.

Jasmine (*Jasminum officinale*)—beneficial for dry, greasy, irritated, or sensitive skin. It can also be uplifting and stimulating in times of hopelessness and nervous exhaustion.

Sage (*Salvia officinalis*)—used in Europe for numerous skin conditions and is recognized for its benefits of strengthening the vital centers and supporting metabolism. Containing sclareol, which stimulates the body to produce its own estrogen, it may nutritionally support the body during PMS and menopause. It may also help in coping with despair and mental fatigue.

Ylang ylang (*Cananga odorata*)—may be extremely effective in calming and bringing about a sense of relaxation.

Massage Oil Base

The Massage Oil Base allows you the freedom to custom-blend your favorite oils to your personal specifications.

Contents:

Wheatgerm Oil—a rich and lush oil high in lecithin, vitamin E, and B vitamins.

Grapeseed Oil—light-textured and odorless, it is nourishing to the skin and makes an excellent carrier for essential oils.

Sweet Almond Oil—reduces friction and promotes smooth application during massage.

Olive Oil—a moisturizing agent in many organic cosmetics, this unsurpassed natural preservative does not clog pores.

Vitamin E—also known as alpha-tocopherol, it protects skin and cell membranes against oxidative damage.

Ortho Ease Massage Oil

Ortho Ease is designed to soothe muscle aches, sports injuries, sprains, and minor swelling. It was created after extensive testing and has been used in European hospitals.

Contents:

Wheatgerm Oil—a rich and lush oil rich in lecithin, vitamin E, and B vitamins.

Grapeseed Oil—light-textured and odorless, it is nourishing to the skin and is an excellent carrier for essential oils.

Sweet Almond Oil—reduces friction and promotes smooth application during massage.

Olive Oil—a moisturizing agent in many organic cosmetics, this unsurpassed natural preservative does not clog pores.

Vitamin E—protects skin and cell membranes against oxidative damage.

Birch (*Betula alleghaniensis*)—contains an active principle similar to cortisone and is beneficial for massage associated with bone, muscle, and joint discomfort.

Juniper Berry (*Juniperus communis*)—is stimulating to the nerves and beneficial for the skin. Works as a detoxifier and cleanser.

Marjoram (*Origanum majorana*)—exceptionally soothing to muscles. It is antimicrobial and antiseptic.

Red Thyme (*Thymus serpyllum*)—is one of the most antiviral, antimicrobial, and antibacterial essential oils. It is rubefacient or "warming to the skin."

Vetiver (*Vetiveria zizanioides*)—is well-known for its anti-inflammatory properties and traditionally used for arthritic symptoms. It is psychologically grounding, calming, and stabilizing.

Peppermint (*Mentha piperita*)—has been researched for its ability to block pain, counteract itching, and combat headaches (Dvorshak et. al., 1996). Jean Valnet, M.D., studied peppermint's effect on the liver and respiratory systems. Antifungal and antibacterial.

Eucalyptus ericifolia—antibacterial and antifungal.

Lemongrass (*Cymbopogon flexuosus*)—has powerful antifungal properties that were documented in **Phytotherapy** *Research*.

Ortho Sport Massage Oil

Ortho Sport is designed for soothing strained muscles and ligaments for both professional athletes and amateur sportsmen. It is a stronger version of Ortho Ease, with a higher phenol content, which may produce a greater warming sensation.

Contents:

Wheatgerm Oil—a rich and lush oil rich in lecithin, vitamin E, and B vitamins.

Grapeseed Oil—is a light, nourishing oil that is quickly absorbed into the skin. It makes an excellent carrier for essential oils.

Olive Oil—a moisturizing agent in many organic cosmetics, the properties of olive oil also lend themselves to homeopathic applications. This unsurpassed natural preservative also will not clog pores.

Sweet Almond Oil—reduces friction and promotes smooth application during massage.

Vitamin E—protects skin and cell membranes against oxidative damage.

Birch (*Betula alleghaniensis*)—contains an active principle similar to cortisone and is beneficial for massage associated with bone, muscle, and joint discomfort.

Oregano (*Origanum vulgare*)—one of the most powerful antimicrobial essential oils. Highly damaging to many kinds of viruses, oregano was recently shown in laboratory research conducted at Weber State University to have a 99% kill rate against *in vitro* colonies of *S. pneumoniae*, even when used in one percent concentration. (*S. pneumoniae* causes many kinds of lung and throat infections).

Marjoram (*Origanum majorana*)—used for soothing the muscles and the respiratory system. It also assists in calming the nerves. It is antimicrobial and antiseptic.

Red Thyme (*Thymus serpyllum*)—similar to its cousin, common thyme (or Thymus vulgaris). This oil is powerfully antiviral, antimicrobial, and antibacterial. It is also rubefacient or "warming to the skin."

Peppermint (*Mentha piperita*)—cooling and invigorating, it blocks the sensation of pain, counteracts itching, and combats headaches (Dvorshak et. al., 1996). Antifungal and antibacterial.

Eucalyptus (*Eucalyptus globulus*)—is a powerful antimicrobial agent, rich in eucalyptol (a key ingredient in many antiseptic mouth rinses). Often used for the respiratory system, eucalyptus also repels insects.

Lemongrass (*Cymbopogon flexuosus*)—is a strong antifungal oil.

Vetiver (*Vetiveria zizanioides*)—is well-known for its anti-inflammatory properties and traditionally used for arthritic symptoms. It is psychologically grounding, calming, and stabilizing.

Elemi (*Canarium luzonicum*)—has been used in Europe for hundreds of years in salves for skin and was used in celebrated healing ointments, such as *baume paralytique*. Elemi belongs to the same botanical family as frankincense and myrrh. Antiseptic and antimicrobial, it is widely regarded today for soothing sore muscles, protecting skin, and stimulating nerves.

Protec

Protec is designed to be used in a night-long retention enema or douche. Suitable for both men and women. Use 1/2 to 1 oz. added to a fleet enema or douche.

Contents:

Olive Oil—a moisturizing agent in many organic cosmetics, the properties of olive oil also lend themselves to homeopathic applications.

Grapeseed Oil—makes an excellent carrier for essential oils.

Sweet Almond Oil—this nourishing oil is gentle, emollient, and an excellent essential oil carrier.

Wheatgerm Oil—a rich and lush oil high in lecithin, vitamin E, and B vitamins.

Vitamin E—protects skin and cell membranes against oxidative damage.

Frankincense (*Boswellia carteri*)—is considered the "holy anointing oil" in the Middle East and has been used in religious ceremonies for thousands of years. It is stimulating and elevating to the mind and helps overcome stress and despair as well as supporting the immune system.

Myrrh (*Commiphora myrrha*)—is an antimicrobial oil referenced throughout the Old and New Testaments (*A bundle of **myrrh** [is] my wellbeloved unto me.* Song of Solomon 1:13). Antibacterial, it is widely used in oral hygiene products.

Sage (*Salvia officinalis*)—used in Europe for numerous types of skin conditions.

Black Cumin (*Cuminum cyminum*)—studied for its anticancer properties in "The Anticarcinogenic Effects of the Essential Oils from Cumin, Poppy, and Basil" (Aruna et al., 1996). Rarer and more expensive than the commonly used white cumin. Antiseptic, calming, and a powerful support to the immune system, cumin seeds have been retrieved from the tombs of the pharoahs of Egypt.

Relaxation Massage Oil

Promotes relaxation and easing of tension.

Contents:

Grapeseed Oil—is nourishing to the skin and is an excellent carrier for essential oils.

Sweet Almond Oil—this nourishing oil is well suited for massage. It aids the smooth application of the base, reducing negative friction.

Wheatgerm Oil—a rich and lush-textured oil high in lecithin, vitamin E, and B vitamins.

Olive Oil—a moisturizing agent in many organic cosmetics, the properties of olive oil also lend themselves to homeopathic applications.

Vitamin E—protects skin and cell membranes against oxidative damage.

Tangerine (*Citrus nobilis*)—soothing for anxiety and nervousness.

Rosewood (*Aniba rosaeodora*)—soothing and nourishing to the skin. It has been researched at Weber State University for its inhibition rate against gram positive and gram negative bacterial growth.

Spearmint (*Mentha spicata*)—oil helps support the respiratory and nervous systems. Its hormone-like activity may help open and release emotional blocks and bring about a feeling of balance.

Peppermint (*Mentha piperita*)—cooling and invigorating, it blocks the sensation of pain, counteracts itching, and combats headaches (Dvorshak et. al., 1996). Jean Valnet, M.D., studied peppermint's effect on the liver and respiratory systems. Antifungal and antibacterial.

Ylang ylang (*Cananga odorata*)—extremely effective in calming and bringing about a sense of relaxation.

Lavender (*Lavandula angustifolia*)—is highly recommended for the skin and has been researched for its relaxing effects. It can be used to cleanse burns, cuts, bruises, and skin irritations.

Sensation Massage Oil

Sensation leaves skin feeling silky and youthful. The increased chemicals in our environment, air, food, water, and stressful lifestyles all contribute to glandular and hormonal imbalance. Its beautiful fragrance may stimulate feelings of romance.

Contents:

Grapeseed Oil—light-textured and odorless, it is nourishing to the skin and is an excellent carrier for essential oils.

Sweet Almond Oil—reduces friction and promotes smooth application during massage.

Wheatgerm Oil—a rich and lush-textured oil high in lecithin, vitamin E, and B vitamins.

Vitamin E—protects skin and cell membranes against oxidative damage.

Olive Oil—a moisturizing agent in many organic cosmetics, the properties of olive oil also lend themselves to homeopathic applications.

Rosewood (*Aniba rosaeodora*)—soothing and nourishing to the skin. It has been researched at Weber State University for its inhibition rate against gram positive and gram negative bacterial growth.

Ylang ylang (*Cananga odorata*)—induces a sense of relaxation.

Jasmine (*Jasminum officinale*)—beneficial for dry, greasy, irritated, or sensitive skin. It can also be uplifting and stimulating in times of hopelessness and nervous exhaustion.

V-6 Mixing Oil

V-6 Mixing Oil is a mixture of nourishing, antioxidant vegetable oils that make an ideal carrier for essential oils. It facilitates the penetration of essential oils into the skin.

Contents:

Olive Oil—a moisturizing agent in many organic cosmetics, the properties of olive oil also lend themselves to homeopathic applications.

Sesame Seed Oil—contains vitamins, minerals, amino acids, lecithin, and natural vegetable proteins that soothe skin conditions, such as psoriasis and eczema.

Grapeseed Oil—light-textured and odorless, it is nourishing to the skin and is an excellent carrier for essential oils.

Sweet Almond Oil—this nourishing oil is well suited for massage. It aids the smooth application of the base, reducing negative friction.

Sunflower Seed Oil—compatible with the skin's natural oils and sebum, it is suitable to a variety of skin types.

Wheatgerm Oil—a rich and lush-textured oil high in lecithin, vitamin E, and B vitamins.

Vitamin E—protects skin and cell membranes against oxidative damage.

Skin and Hair Care Products

Skin Care Products

Use Facial Wash, Toner, and Moisturizer Creme together to promote younger and healthier-looking skin.

AromaSilk Pure Essential Oils Orange Blossom Facial Wash

Ingredients: Deionized water, calendula extract, rosebud extract, orange blossom extract, St. John's wort extract, aloe vera extract, MSM, coconut oil, olive oil, alpha hydroxy acids, hydrolyzed wheat protein, citric acid, essential oils of lavender, lemon, melaleuca, rosemary verbonone, and patchouly.

Instructions: For best results, use Orange Blossom Facial Wash twice daily. Follow up with Sandalwood Toner & Moisture Creme to promote younger and healthier looking skin.

AromaSilk Pure Essential Oils Sandalwood Toner

Ingredients: Deionized water, MSM, glycerin, sorbitol, sodium PCA, allantoin, aloe vera gel, cucumber extract, chamomile extract, rosemary extract, echinacea extract, gotu kola extract, arnica extract, witch hazel extract, horse chestnut extract, essential oils of sandalwood, Roman chamomile, rosewood, and myrrh.

Instructions: Lightly mist face and neck with Sandalwood Toner. For best results follow up with Sandalwood Moisture Creme.

AromaSilk Pure Essential Oils Sandalwood Moisturizer Creme

Ingredients: Deionized water, MSM, caprylic/capric triglyceride, sorbitol, shea butter, glyceryl stearate, rosehip seed oil, hypericum extract, calendula extract, matricaria extract, orange flower extract, kelp extract, grape seed extract, aloe vera gel, algae extract, locust bean gum, tocopheryl linnolleate, hydrolyzed soy protein, allantoin, lecithin, retinyl palmitate (vitamin A), tocopheryl acetate (vitamin E), ascorbic acid (vitamin C), wolfberry oil, essential oils of myrrh, sandalwood, rosewood, lavender, and rosemary verbonone.

Instructions: For best results, use Sandalwood Moisture Creme after cleansing and toning the face and neck to promote younger, healthier skin. Put small amount in hand, emulsify, and apply to face and neck using upward strokes.

AromaSilk Pure Essential Oils Boswellia Wrinkle Creme

Ingredients: Deionized water, MSM, ASC 111, serum complex (vitamin C), caprylic/capric triglyceride, sorbitol, shea butter, glycerol stearate (vegetable based), rosehip seed oil, Hypericum extract, calendula extract, orange flower extract, kelp extract, Ginkgo biloba extract, grape seed extract, aloe vera, locust bean gum, tocopheryl linolleate, hydrolyzed soy protein, allantoin, lecithin, retinyl palmitate (vitamin A in liposome form), tocopheryl acetate (vitamin E in liposome form). ascorbic acid (vitamin C in liposome form), wolfberry oil, ocnothera blennis c, essential oils of frankincense, sandalwood, myrrh, geranium, and ylang ylang.

Instructions: Boswellia Wrinkle Creme is a collagen builder. Used daily, it will help minimize and prevent wrinkles. Put small amount in hand, emulsify, and apply to face and neck using upward strokes.

AromaSilk Pure Essential Oils Wolfberry Eye Creme

Eases eye puffiness, and dark circles and promotes skin tightening. Can be used before bed and in the morning.

Ingredients: Deionized water, aloe vera gel, MSM, sorbitol, glyceryl stearate, shea butter, kukui nut oil, rose hip seed oil, centella extract, echinacea extract, sodium PCA, jojoba oil, hydrocotyl cone flower extract, mango butter, sodium hyaluronate, cucumber extract, green tea extract, vitamins A, C, and E in liposome bound form, soy protein, wheat protein, allantoin, wolfberry oil, essential oils of lavender, rosewood, Roman chamomile, frankincense, and geranium.

Instructions: Apply a tiny amount of Wolfberry Eye Creme under eye area and on the eyelid before bed. Repeat in morning if desired.

AromaSilk Pure Essential Oils MSM Night Serum C

Nourishes and protects the skin with antioxidants.

Ingredients: Deionized water, MSM, L-ascorbic acid, L-tyrosine, sorbitol, glycerin, hyaluronic acid, green tea extract, aloe vera gel, urea, bioflavonoids, centella, meadowsweet extract, phospholipids, hydroxymethyl glycinate, pyridoxine HCl (vitamin B6), sodium meta bi-sulfite, zinc sulfite, esssential oils of lemongrass, eucalyptus, cypress.

Instructions: Apply this nourishing serum at night, 15-20 minutes before bedtime, allowing MSM to absorb into the skin. Use fingertips to apply sparingly, covering the entire face and neck. A slight tingling may be felt with the first few applications.

AromaSilk Pure Essential Oils Satin Body Lotion

Nourishes and moisturizes skin. Contains herbal extracts, essential oils, and vitamin C.

Ingredients: Deionized water, MSM, glyceryl stearate (vegetable based), stearic acid, sorbitol, tea tree oil, apricot oil, almond oil, jojoba oil, sesame oil, calendula extract, chamomile extract, orange blossom extract, St. John's wort extract, algae extract, aloe vera gel, ginkgo biloba extract, grape seed extract, tocopheryl acetate (vitamin E), retinyl palmitate (vitamin A), ascorbic acid (vitamin C), sodium hyaluronate, of wolfberry oil, geranium, essential oils rosewood, ylang ylang, jasmine, sandalwood, peppermint, and Roman chamomile.

Instructions: To moisturize the skin, promote healing, and leave the skin feeling soft, silky and smooth, apply Satin Body Lotion to hands, body, and feet. Also good for scars, burns, rashes, itching and sunburns.

AromaSilk Pure Essential Oils Cinnamint Lip Balm

Is a natural lip balm enriched with essential oils and vitamins to soothe and prevent chapping.

Ingredients: Sweet almond oil, beeswax, MSM, hemp seed oil, orange wax, orange oil, tocopherol palmitate (vitamin E), ascorbyl palmitate (vitamin A), ascorbic acid (vitamin C), citric acid, and essential oils of peppermint, and spearmint.

Instructions: To soften and moisturize lips, apply Cinnamint Lip Balm as often as needed.

LavaDerm Cooling Mist

This cooling mist is soothing to any burn from the slightest sunburn to the burn of a fire. Aloe Vera has been a household remedy for years, and lavender made its re-entry into the therapeutic realm through healing the laboratory burn of Dr. Gattfossé. LavaDerm Cooling Mist will certainly become a must in every home.

How to use: Mist as often as needed to keep the skin cool and promote regeneration.

Ingredients: Re-structured water, aloe vera, and lavender essential oil.

Mint Facial Scrub

Eliminates layers of dead skin cells. Oatmeal and corn flour provide a mild abrasive texture that helps stimulate the pores, bringing oxygen to the surface. It is excellent for skin prone to acne. This scrub can be used as a drying face mask to draw impurities from the skin. If the texture is too abrasive, it can be mixed with the Orange Blossom Facial Wash.

How to use: Apply warm water to the face to moisten skin. Apply scrub directly to the face and gently massage in a gentle circular motion, creating a lather. Rinse thoroughly and gently pat dry. May also be mixed with Orange Blossom Facial Wash for a milder scrub. Mix 1/2 tsp. of both in palm of hand before applying. Use four or five times weekly, depending on need.

Ingredients: Floral water, corn flour, glycerin water, kaolin, almond meal, oatmeal, zinc oxide, vegetable oils, lecithin, magnesium silicate, chlorophyllin-complex, and essential oils of Calophyllum, lavender, melaleuca alternifolia, palmarosa, peppermint, rosewood and rosemary.

Rose Ointment

Is a skin ointment that protects and nourishes the skin and is outstanding when applied over essential oils to lock in their benefits. Note: Not recommended for burns initially, but is very helpful to maintain, protect, and keep the the scab soft.

How to use: Apply directly to skin.

Ingredients: Lecithin, lanolin, beeswax, mink oil, sesame seed oil, vitamin E oil, rose hip seed oil, and essential oils of carrot seed, melaleuca alternifolia, myrrh, palmarosa, patchouly, rose hip seed, rose, and rosewood.

Genesis Hand and Body Lotion with MSM

This beautiful blend of coconut oil, lecithin, and essential oils moisturizes, softens and protects the skin from harsh weather, rough work, chemicals, cleaners and other undesirable substances. MSM (sulfur) is one of the nutrients necessary for building and maintaining healthy skin.

How to use: Apply as desired.

Ingredients: Distilled water, cocoa butter, glyceryl stearate, cetyl alcohol, landin oil, tocopheryl acetate, floral water, vitamin E, sesame oil, lecithin castile, and essential oils of palmarosa, rosewood, rose, gardenia, jasmine, fragrance of honesycukle and MSM.

Sensation Hand and Body Lotion

Is delightful to wear with its intoxicating blend of exotic essential oils. It leaves the skin soft and moist as it protects it from harsh weather, chemicals, and dry air.

How to use: Dispense in hand and apply directly to skin.

Ingredients: Deionized water, cocoa butter, glyceryl stearate, cetyl alcohol, lanolin oil, floral water, vitamin E, and essential oils of rosewood, ylang ylang, and jasmine.

Hair Care Products

AromaSilk Pure Essential Oils Lavender Volume Hair & Scalp Wash

Contains all natural ingredients for gently cleansing and volumizing fine hair. Horsetail and coltsfoot extract provide silica, and MSM provides sulfur to help build and strengthen hair. Fortified with vitamin complex, including panthenol, and vitamins A, C, and E. Contains essential oils for a beautiful fragrance.

Ingredients: Coconut oil, decyl polyglucose (natural surfactant), MSM, vegetable protein (wheat, oat, soya), deionized water, rosemary extract, sage extract, nettle extract, coltsfoot extract, horsetail extract, fennel extract, essential oils, aloe vera gel, retinyl palmitate (vitamin A), ascorbic acid (vitamin C), tocopheryl acetate (vitamin E), panthenol (vitamin B5), grape seed extract, inositol, niacin, and essential oils of spruce, rosewood, blue tansy, frankincense, and almond oil.

Instructions: Wet hair thoroughly. Apply small amount of Lavender Volume Hair & Scalp Wash. Massage thoroughly into hair and scalp. Rinse well. Repeat if desired.

AromaSilk Pure Essential Oils Lavender Volume Nourishing Rinse

Conditions and volumizes fine hair with MSM, amino acids, and a multi-vitamin complex. Essential oils enhance and provide essential components for healthy hair.

Ingredients: Natural vegetable fatty acid base, msm, milk protein, phospholipids, amino acids cysteine and cystein 8 methionine, glyco protein (glycogen and mucopolysaccharides, rosemary extract, sage extract, horsetail extract, coltsfoot extract, hydrolyzed wheat protein, hydrolyzed soya protein, retinyl palmitate (vitamin A), ascorbic acid (vitamin C), tocopheryl acetate (vitamin E), panthenol (vitamin B5), grape seed extract, essential oils of spruce, rosewood, blue tansy, frankincense, and almond oil.

Instructions: Apply Lavender Volume Nourishing Rinse through the hair. Leave on hair for just a few seconds for light conditioning or for several minutes for deep conditioning. Rinse well.

AromaSilk Pure Essential Oils Lavender Volume Sealer

Maintains volume and luster while it seals the hair shaft, preventing split ends and other damage.

Ingredients: Water, hydrolyzed glycosaminoglycans, panthenol sorbitol, acetamide MEA, tocopherol, hydrolyzed soy protein, linoleic acid, linoleic acid, arachidonic acid, jojoba oil, wheat germ oil, soluble sulfur, hydroxymethyl glycinate, rosemary essential oil, citric acid, essential oils of lemon, sandalwood, juniper, frankincense, spruce, myrrh, and almond oil.

Instructions: Apply Lavender Volume Sealer evenly to towel-dried hair, leave in, then style.

AromaSilk Pure Essential Oils Rosewood Moisturings Hair & Scalp Wash

Contains natural ingredients to moisturize dry hair while gently cleansing. Contains herbal extracts, vitamins, and essential oils for nourishing the hair.

Ingredients: Coconut oil, olive oil, decyl polyglucose (natural surfactant), MSM, vegetable protein (wheat, oat, soya), deionized water, quinoa extract, rosemary extract, coltsfoot extract, horsetail extract, fennel extract, aloe vera gel, retinyl palmitate (vitamin A), ascorbic acid (vitamin C), tocopheryl acetate (vitamin E), panthenol (vitamin B5), grape seed extract, inositol, niacin, essential oils of sandalwood, juniper, frankincense, spruce, and myrrh, and almond oil.

Instructions: Wet hair thoroughly. Apply small amount of Rosewood Moisturizing Hair & Scalp Wash. Massage thoroughly into hair and scalp. Rinse well. Repeat if desired.

AromaSilk Pure Essential Oils Rosewood Moisturizing Nourishing Rinse

Conditions and moisturizes dry hair with natural vegetable fatty acids, MSM, milk protein, vitamins, and essential oils.

Ingredients: Natural vegetable fatty acid base, MSM, milk protein, phospholipids, amino acids cysteine and cystein 8 methionine, glyco protein (glycogen and mucopolysaccharides), quinoa extract, rosemary extract, sage extract, horsetail extract, coltsfoot extract, hydrolyzed wheat protein, hydrolyzed soya protein, retinyl palmitate (vitamin A), ascorbic acid (vitamin C), tocopheryl acetate (vitamin E), panthenol (vitamin B5), grape seed extract, essential oils of sandalwood, juniper, frankincense, spruce, and myrrh, and almond oil.

Instructions: Apply Rosewood Moisturizing Nourishing Rinse to hair from roots to ends. Leave on hair for a few seconds for light conditioning or for several minutes for deep conditioning. Rinse well.

AromaSilk Pure Essential Oils Rosewood Moisturizing Sealer

Seals the hair cuticle while maintaining moisture and volume in dry hair.

Ingredients: Water, hydrolyzed glycosaminoglycans, panthenol sorbitol, acetamide MEA, tocopherol, hydrolyzed soy protein, linoleic acid, linoleic acid, arachidonic acid, jojoba oil, wheat germ oil, soluble sulfur, hydroxymethyl glycinate, almond oil, citric acid, essential oils of lemon, sandalwood, juniper, frankincense, spruce myrrh, and rosemary.

Instructions: Apply Rosewood Moisturizing Sealer evenly to towel-dried hair, leave in, then style.

AromaSilk Pure Essential Oils Lemon Sage Clarifying Hair & Scalp Wash

Removes buildup of styling products, leaving hair feeling naturally clean and healthy. Contains herbal extracts, vitamins, and essential oils to enhance the hair.

Ingredients: Coconut oil, decyl polyglucose (natural surfactant), MSM, vegetable protein (wheat, oat, soya), deionized water, rosemary extract, sage extract, nettles extract, coltsfoot extract, horsetail extract, fennel extract, aloe vera gel, retinyl palmitate (vitamin A), ascorbic acid (vitamin C), tocopheryl acetate (vitamin E), panthenol (vitamin B5), grape seed extract, inositol, niacin, essential oils of hyssop, spruce, lavender, frankincense, rose geranium fragrance oil, rose, ylang ylang, sandalwood, geranium, angelica, orange, and sage.

Instructions: Wet hair thoroughly. Apply small amount of Lemon Sage Clarifying Hair & Scalp Wash. Massage thoroughly into hair and scalp. Rinse well. Repeat if desired.

AromaSilk Pure Essential Oils Lemon Sage Clarifying Nourishing Rinse

Conditions hair of all types without building up on hair. Herbal extracts, vitamins, and essential oils work together to improve hair condition.

Ingredients: Natural vegetable fatty acid base, MSM, milk protein phospholipids, amino acids cysteine and cystein 8 methionine, glyco protein (glycogen and mucopolysaccharides, rosemary extract, sage extract, horsetail extract, coltsfoot extract, hydrolyzed wheat protein, hydrolyzed soya protein, retinyl palmitate (vitamin A), ascorbic acid (vitamin C), tocopheryl acetate (vitamin E), panthenol (vitamin B5), grape seed extract, essential oils of hyssop, spruce, lavender, frankincense, rose geranium fragrance oil, rose, ylang ylang, sandalwood, angelica, geranium, orange, and sage lavender.

Instructions: Apply Lemon Sage Clarifying Nourishing Rinse to hair from roots to ends. Leave on hair for just a few seconds for light conditioning or for several minutes for deep conditioning. Rinse well.

AromaSilk Pure Essential Oils Lemon Sage Clarifying Sealer

Seals the hair shaft, protecting it from damage without adding buildup.

Ingredients: Water, hydrolyzed glycosamino-glycans, panthenol sorbitol, acetamide MEA, tocopherol, hydrolyzed soy protein, linoleic acid, linoleic acid, arachidonic acid, jojoba oil, citric acid, wheat germ oil, soluble sulfur, hydroxymethyl glycinate, essential oils of rosemary, hyssop, spruce, lavender, frankincense, rose geranium, fragrance oil, ylang ylang, geranium, orange, sandalwood, angelica, sage, and lemon.

Instructions: Apply Lemon Sage Clarifying Sealer evenly to towel-dried hair, leave in, then style.

AromaSilk Pure Essential Oils Boswellia ThairAgain Hair & Scalp Wash

Contains natural herbal extracts. and vitamins for maintaining strong hair growth.

Ingredients: Coconut oil, olive oil, decyl polyglucose (natural surfactant), MSM, vegetable protein (wheat, oat, soy), deionized water, nettle extract, *Ganoderma lucidum* mushroom extract, *Trametes veriscolor* mushroom extract, bilberry (*Vaccinium myrtillus*) extract, sugarcane (*Saccharum officinarum*) extract, aloe vera gel, retinyl palmitate (vitamin A), ascorbic acid (vitamin C), tocopheryl acetate (vitamin E), panthenol (vitamin B5), inositol, and niacin, sugar maple (*Acer saccharinum*) extract, orange, essential oils of spruce, ylang ylang, fir, and cedarwood.

Instructions: Wet hair thoroughly. Apply small amount of Boswellia ThairAgain Hair & Scalp Wash. Massage thoroughly into hair and scalp. Rinse well. Repeat if desired.

AromaSilk Pure Essential Oils Boswellia ThairAgain Hair, Scalp & Root Therapy

Conditions hair with herbal extracts, vitamins, and essential oils to encourage proper hair growth.

Ingredients: Natural vegetable fatty acid base, MSM, milk protein, phospholipids, amino acids cysteine and cystein 8 methionine, glyco protein (glycogen and mucopolysaccharides), nettles extract, *Prunus africana* extract, saw palmetto (*Serenoa serrulata*) extract, *Pueraria thunbergiana* extract, alfalfa (*Medicago sativa*). licorice (*Glycyrrhiza glabra*), sarsaparilla (*Smilax aristolochiaefolia*) extract, wild yam (*Dioscorea villosa*) extract, hydrolyzed wheat protein, hydrolyzed soya protein, retinyl palmitate (vitamin A), ascorbic acid (vitamin C), tocopheryl acetate (vitamin E), panthenol (vitamin B5), and essential oils of spruce, ylang ylang, fir, and cedarwood.

Instructions: Apply Boswellia ThairAgain Scalp, Hair & Root Therapy to hair from scalp to ends. For intensified scalp therapy, allow to remain on scalp for 3-5 minutes before rinsing thoroughly.

AromaSilk Pure Essential Oils Boswellia ThairAgain Sealant Treatment

Ingredients: Natural vegetable fatty acid base, MSM, milk protein, phospholipids, amino acids cysteine (and) cystein 8 methionine, glyco protein (glycogen and mucopolysacchrides), nettles extract, prunus africana extract, alfalfa (medicago) sativa, licorice (glycyrrhiza glabra), sarsaparill (smilax aristolochiaefolia) extract, wild yam (discoria vilosa) extract, hydrolyzed wheat protein, hydrolyzed soya protein, retinyl palmitate (vitamin A), Ascorbic acid (vitamin C), tocopheryl acetate (vitamin E), panthenol (vitamin B5), essential oils of spruce, ylang ylang, fir, and cedarwood.

AromaSilk Pure Essential Oils Citrus Fresh Kinderzoo Hair & Scalp Wash

Is an all-natural shampoo for children, containing natural extracts and essential oils.

Ingredients: Aloe vera, decyle polyglouse, coconut extract, corn extract, palm extract, vitamin E, kiwi nut oil, jojoba oil, citrus seed extract, babassu oil, vitamin B5, hydroxymethyl glycinate, essential oils of rosemary, orange, tangerine, grapefruit, lemon, mandarin, and spearmint.

Instructions: Wet hair thoroughly. Apply small amount of Citrus Fresh Kinderzoo Hair & Scalp Wash. Massage thoroughly into hair and scalp. Rinse well. Repeat if desired.

AromaSilk Pure Essential Oils Citrus Fresh Kinderzoo Nourishing Rinse

Is a gentle, natural conditioner for kids of all ages. Contains herbal extracts and essential oils.

Ingredients: Purified water, plant waxes, jojoba oil, safflower oil, cetyl alcohol, vegetable glycerin, vitamin B-5 (panthenol) herbal complex (yucca, aloe vera, comfrey, rose water, cactus, chamomile, acacia, irish moss, citric acid (natural preservative), hydroxymethyl glycinate, and essential oils of rosemary, orange, tangerine, grapefruit, lemon, mandarin, and spearmint.

Instructions: Apply Citrus Fresh Kinderzoo Nourishing Rinse to hair from root to ends. Leave on hair for just a few seconds for light conditioning or for several minutes for deep conditioning. Rinse well.

AromaSilk Pure Essential Oils Citrus Fresh Kinderzoo Detangling Protectant Spray

Protects children's hair and makes it easier to detangle.

Ingredients: Water, hydrolyzed glycosaminoglycans, panthenol sorbitol, acetamide MEA, tocopherol, hydrolyzed soy protein, linoleic acid, linoleic acid, arachidonic acid, jojoba oil, wheat germ oil, soluble sulfur, hydroxymethyl glycinate, citric acid, essential oils of rosemary, orange, tangerine, grapefruit, lemon, manderin, spearmint, and lemon.

Instructions: Apply Kinderzoo Essential Oils Detangling Protectant Spray evenly to towel-dried hair, leave in, then style.

Lavender Shampoo

May help prevent hair loss, promote normal, healthy hair growth, and reduce dandruff and scalp rashes. The beautiful essential oils make this a favorite shampoo for everyone.

How to use: Wet hair, apply, and lather. For maximum benefit, leave on 2 to 5 minutes. Rinse thoroughly.

Ingredients: Deionized water, castile, coco-diethanolamine, algenic acid, panthenol, vegetable glycerine, aloe vera, nettle extract, pantethine, birch bark extract, biotin, floral water, jojoba oil, safflower oil, and essential oils of lavender, rosemary, juniper, rosewood, clary sage, ylang ylang, and the fragrance of apple blossom.

Pharaoh Aftershave

Pharaoh is rich, refreshing and exotic with the essential oil of cedarwood and the fragrances of orange blossom and musk, creating a unique and regal aroma.

Ingredients: The essential oil of cedarwood with the fragrances of orange blossom and musk.

Rawhide Aftershave

Rawhide combines the essential oil of ylang ylang with fragrances that create the wild, fresh scent of the mountains and the desert.

Ingredients: The essential oil of ylang ylang combined with the fragrances of lilac and honeysuckle.

Bath and Shower Gels

Bath Gel Base

Is a dispersing agent to help unlock the full effects of your aromatherapy bath. Contains natural botanical ingredients for cleansing the pores. You may add single essential oils and blends to create your own fragrance or a specific therapeutic action.

How to use: Add several drops of an essential oil single or blend (depending on the strength of the oil) to the Bath Gel Base. Shake before using.

Ingredients: Olive oil, vegetable glycerine, floral water, algin, vitamin E, lecithin, and wheat germ oil.

Dragon Time Bath & Shower Gel

Was blended for women's stressful time of the month. This custom-formulated blend of essential oils and vegetable oils is exceptionally balancing and uplifting, both physically and emotionally.

Ingredients: Deionized water, sodium dioctyl sulfosuccinate, cocodiethylanolamine, panthenol, sodium chloride, carrageenan, jojoba oil, aloe vera gel, sodium hydroxymethylglycinate, imidazolidinyl urea, citric acid, tetrasodium EDTA, with olive oil, vegetable glycerine, floral water, algin, vitamin E, lecithin, wheat germ oil, and the essential oils of clary sage, rosewood, rose, sandalwood, and ylang ylang.

Evening Peace Bath and Shower Gel

Blends the most natural botanical ingredients with therapeutic-grade essential oils to relax tired, fatigued muscles and help dampen stress and tension.

Ingredients: Olive oil, vegetable glycerin, floral water, algin, vitamin E, lecithin, wheat germ oil, and essential oils of German chamomile, clary sage, rosewood, rose, sandalwood, ylang ylang and the fragrance oil of rose geranium.

Morning Start Bath & Shower Gel

Is an invigorating gel that combines uplifting, energizing essential oils to jumpstart your vigor and energy.

Ingredients: Olive oil, vegetable glycerin, floral water, algin, vitamin E, lecithin, wheat germ, and essential oils lemongrass, rosemary, juniper, and peppermint.

Sensation Bath & Shower Gel

Contains an enchantingly fragrant mix of oils used by Cleopatra to enhance love and increase desire to be close to someone special.

Ingredients: Olive oil, vegetable glycerin, floral water, algin, vitamin E, lecithin, wheat germ oil, and essential oils of rosewood, ylang ylang, and jasmine.

Veterinarian Medicine

Essential oils have been used very successfully on many different kinds of animals from tiny kittens to 2,000 lb. draft horses. Animals respond to essential oils similarly to humans. Animals are not as sensitive to the phenol and sesquiterpene constituents so the oils can be applied "neat," or full strength. A determination must be made which oils are applicable to the situation. For long term treatments or health regimens, a few drops of oil can be applied 3-4 times daily.

General Guidelines:

For small animals (cats and small dogs) apply 3-4 drops per application.

For larger animals, (large dogs) apply 6-7 drops per application.

For horses, apply 15-20 drops per application.

Helpful Tips:

For open wounds or hard-to-reach areas, oils can be put in a spray bottle sprayed directly on location.

After applying the oils locally, cover the open wound with Rose Ointment. It seals the wound and protects it from further infection. It also prevents the essential oils from evaporating.

There is no right or wrong way to apply essential oils. Use common sense and good judgement as you experiment with different methods.

Take care not to get essential oils in the animal's eye.

When treating animals with essential oils internally, make sure that the oils are pure and free of chemicals, solvents, and adulterants.

How to Apply Essential Oils:

For non-ungulate animals (not having hooves), oils can be applied to paws for fast absorption.

For hoofed animals, apply oils on the spine or auricular points of the ears.

Apply on the gums, tongue, or underneath the top lip.

Sprinkle a few drops on the spine or flanks and massage them in.

For a dog or cat, apply on the pads of their feet.

Examples of Applications:

When treating animals for viral or bacterial infection, arthritis, virus, bone injury, use the same oil and protocol recommended for humans.

EXAMPLE: If you have a high-spirited, jittery horse that is tough to saddle, apply Peace & Calming and Valor on yourself. As you approach him, he will have a tendency to bow his head or flare his nostrils when he perceives the aroma. Kneel down or squat beside him and remain still so that the animal can become accustomed to the smell. As he breathes in the fragrances, he will become calmer and easier to manage.

Animal Treatment A to Z

Arthritis: (common in older animals and pure-breeds). To prevent: Power Meal and Sulfurzyme.

Arthritis: Ortho Ease or PanAway (massage on location or put several drops in animal feed).

Use Raindrop-like application of PanAway, birch, pine, or spruce and massage the location. For larger animals use at least 2 times more oil than a normal raindrop would call for on humans.

Put Power Meal and Sulfurzyme in feed or fodder. Small animals: 1/8 to 1/4 serving per day. Large animals 2-4 servings per day.

Birthing: Gentle Baby.

Bleeding: geranium, helichrysum.

Bones (pain, spurs) (all animals): PanAway, birch, lemongrass, and spruce.

Bones (fractured or broken) Mix PanAway with 20-30 drops of birch and spruce. Cover the area. After 15 minutes rub in 10-15 more drops of birch and spruce. Cover with Ortho Sport Massage Oil.

Calming: Peace & Calming, Trauma Life, lavender (domestic animals respond very quickly to the smell).

Colds and flu: Small animals put 1-3 drops Exodus II, ImmuPower, or Di-Tone in feed or fodder. For large animals, use 10-20 drops.

Colic: For large animals (cows) put 10-20 drops of Di-Tone in feed or fodder. For small animals, use 1-3 drops.

Inflammation: Apply Ortho Ease, PanAway, pine, birch, or spruce on location. Put Sulfurzyme in feed.

Insect Repellent: Put 10 drops each of citronella, Purification, eucalyptus, and peppermint in 8 ounce spray bottle with water. Alternate formula: Put 2 drops pine, 2 drops Eucalyptus (*globulus*), 5-10 drops citronella in a spray bottle of water. Shake vigorously and spray over area. Floral waters, such as peppermint and Idaho tansy, can also be used.

Ligaments/tendons (torn or sprained): Apply lemongrass and lavender (equal parts) on location and cover area. For small animals or birds, dilute essential oils with V-6 Mixing Oil (2 parts mixing oil to 1 part essential oil).

Mineral deficiencies: Mineral Essence. (In one case, an animal stopped chewing on furniture once his mineral deficiency was met).

Mites (ear mites): Apply Purification and peppermint to a Q-Tip and swab the inside of the ear.

Nervous anxiety: Valor, Trauma Life, geranium, lavender, and valerian.

Pain: Helichrysum

Saddle sores: Melrose and Rose Ointment.

Shiny coats: Rosemary and sandalwood.

Sinus problems: Diffuse Raven, R.C., pine, myrtle, and Eucalyptus (*radiata*) in animal's sleeping quarters or sprinkle on bed.

Strangle in horses: Mix 4 parts Exodus II and with 1 part Melrose.

Ticks: To remove ticks, apply 1 drop cinnamon or peppermint on Q-Tip and swab on tick.

Trauma: Trauma Life, Valor, Peace & Calming, melissa, rosewood, lavender, valerian, and chamomile.

Tumors or cancers: Mix frankincense with lavender or clove and apply on area of tumor.

Worms and parasites: ParaFree and Di-Tone.

Wounds (open or abrasions): Melrose, helichrysum, and Rose Ointment.

Personal Usage Reference

Symptomology-Application Or Uses

The fragrance of an essential oil has a direct influence on various aspects of the body beginning with the limbic system (a group of subcortical structures, such as the hypothalamus, the hippocampus, and the amygdala of the brain that deal especially with emotion and motivation). When an oil is inhaled, the body's electrical frequency increases through the olfactory and limbic systems. Disease and emotional trauma create a frequency link with the body. Essential oils disrupt or break the link of the frequency range. That is when one begins to experience or notice a change in the structure of the problem.

In the following material, single oils listed are the oils of choice and may also act in a synergistic manner when added to the suggested blends for the same application. Blends are particularly good in achieving a synergistic effect. Synergism is the simultaneous action of separate agencies, which together have a greater total effect than the sum of their individual action.

When the oil suggested is not available or not desired, single oils or blends may be used separately with beneficial results. However, one must realize that the same synergistic effect may not be achieved.

The oils are not listed in any preferential or suggested sequence. This is because an oil might be more synergistic with one person's chemistry than another person. The oils listed have been found to help and should be viewed as a general rule or starting point. Other oils not listed may also give desired results. One may have to experiment to find the most effective oils.

If results are not felt within 1 to 3 minutes, the oil chosen is probably not the most specific to the need. Try another oil, blend, or combination until positive results are felt.

Alternating singles, blends, or combinations is very beneficial because of the different chemical constituents within the oils with their different healing properties.

Essential oils are not harmful when used sensibly either topically or internally. There are toxic oils available, but they are not used here. However, essential oils are generally not recommended for ingestion. The exceptions to this rule are the GRAS oils (Generally Regarded As Safe and approved by the FDA as a digestive supplement), such as peppermint, grapefruit, lime, and others that are listed in the Appendix. Cautionary notes regarding the use of certain oils have been listed under the "Caution" headings.

CAUTION: The oils and supplements listed increase the overall results experienced with essential oils through nutritional assistance. This prepares the body's receptivity to oil inhalation and oil massage. When using supplements in addition to prescription medications, it is best to take them at least one hour apart in order to avoid drug-supplement interactions.

You should always address the overall health improvement of the body when considering a health product solution. For instance, parasite removal is important to overall health, but by itself, parasite removal is not a total solution. Many other problems should be considered at the same time. Researchers have linked most degenerative diseases to lack of nutrients in the body, and trace mineral deficiencies often account for most of these imbalances. Essential oils assist in the utilization of trace minerals to the body.

The cure for disease begins with prevention. The essential oils, blends, and supplements described here are fundamental tools for disease prevention.

Abscess

Single oils: Melaleuca, frankincense, helichrysum, lavender, lemon, chamomile, eucalyptus, rosemary, thyme, mountain savory, patchouly, rosewood, and ravensara with oregano.

Blends: Melrose, Purification, Exodus II, and ImmuPower.

Supplements: Dentarome or Dentarome Plus toothpaste, Fresh Essence, Thieves, and Power Meal.

Fresh Essence Mouthwash: Gargle, add 2-3 drops of Thieves, Exodus II, or clove and gargle.

Single oils and blends may help reduce swelling and inflammation and draw out infection.

Oils may also be applied with a hot compress. This strengthens gums and reduces plaque.

Cause: Diet, congested liver.

Supplements: Cleansing Trio, JuvaTone.

Lymphatic Cleansing: Goji Berry Tea and Cel-Lite Magic.

Bring to head: Lavender, Thieves, frankincense, helichrysum, lemon, chamomile, and rosemary.

For drying and closing open abscess: Thyme, myrrh, frankincense, and birch.

Single oils: 1-2 drops each oregano, mountain savory, melaleuca, and rosemary cineol.

Blends: Purification, Melrose, Thieves, Immu-Power, and Sacred Mountain.

Bone Condition: 5 drops Oregano, 6-8 drops mountain savory, and 1 drop lemon.

Absent Minded

Single oils: Peppermint, cardamom, frankincense, sandalwood, rosemary, and basil.

Blends: Clarity, Brain Power, and M-Grain

Supplements: Power Meal, Ultra Young, Sulfurzyme, VitaGreen, and Mineral Essence.

Abuse

Single oils: Geranium, sandalwood, and melissa.

Blends: SARA, Trauma Life, Release, Acceptance, Forgiveness, Surrender, Humility, Joy, White Angelica, Inner Child, Release, Harmony, Hope, Brain Power, Citrus Fresh, Christmas Spirit, and Valor.

Supplements: Power Meal, Super C, AuraLight, and Super B.

Sexual: Forgiveness, Trauma Life, SARA, Release, and Joy.

Spousal: Forgiveness, Trauma Life, Acceptance, Release, Valor, Joy, and Envision

For Spiritual, Ritual, and Physical Abuse: Begin with Forgiveness, unless suicidal. It is most effective around the naval. Follow with Release over the Vita Flex points, on liver points of feet, and under the nose.

Anorexic: Citrus Fresh, Christmas Spirit, Ultra Young, Motivation, and Brain Power.

Parental, Spousal, Ritual, or Sexual Abuse: SARA over the area where abuse took place; then Forgiveness, Release, Joy, and Present Time.

Feelings of Revenge: 1-2 drops of Surrender on the sternum over the heart, 2-3 drops of Present Time on the thymus, and Forgiveness over navel.

Suicidal: 2 drops Hope on rim of ears, Melissa, Brain Power, and Present Time.

Protection/Balance: 1-2 drops of White Angelica on shoulders, Harmony over thymus and on energy centers of the body.

Acidosis

Single oils: Peppermint

Blends: Di-Tone

Supplements: Royaldolphilus, AlkaLime, Megazyme, Mint Condition, and VitaGreen.

Monitor diet, saliva (6.4-6.5), urine (5.5-5.6), and pH to keep an alkaline acid balance. If acidic: Take Royaldolphilus and Mint Condition with peppermint until acid level is balanced, then add Megazyme.

Stimulate enzymatic action in the digestive tract: Raw carrot juice, alfalfa, trace minerals, and papaya.

AlkaLime: 1 tsp. in water one hour before or after meal.

VitaGreen: 2-6 capsules 3 times daily depending on blood type.

Barley Grass Juice.

A Blood Type: Drink plenty of water, monitor diet.

AlkaLime: 1 tsp. in water before bedtime reduces acid indigestion and distresses in the gastrointestinal tract, and prevents fermentation and gases in the blood that cause bad dreams, restless legs, and constant waking up.

Maintenance: AlkaLime: 1 tsp. once per week in water an hour before or after mealtime.

Drink alkaline water.

Acne

Monitor diet: Eliminate dairy products, fried foods, chemicals, and sugar.

Cleansing Trio (see COLON and LIVER CLEANSE), and Sulfurzyme.

Topical Application: Vetiver, lavender, and patchouly (digests toxic bacteria). Alternate every other night.

Acne caused by hormonal imbalance: EssPro 7 and Ultra Young.

(See SKIN DISORDERS.)

Aches and Pains

Bones

Single oils: Birch, spruce, pine, and helichrysum.

Growing: Birch, spruce, Super Cal, ArthroTune, PanAway, and Sulfurzyme.

Joints: PanAway

Muscle: Aroma Siez, Ortho Sport, Ortho Ease, marjoram, lavender, and elemi.

Ligaments: Lemongrass, lavender, Ortho Ease, Essential Manna, and Sulfurzyme.

General: Poor bone and muscle development can be hGH and potassium deficient – Ultra Young, Essential Manna, Power Meal, Super Cal, and Sulfurzyme. Acid pH: Too much acid in the body can create pain (see regimen for Acidosis). AlkaLime: 1 Tbs. 1 hour before or after meals.

ADD

(See ATTENTION DEFICIT DISORDER.)

Addictions

The blueprint for food and chemical addictions, such as smoking, caffeine containing drinks, drugs, alcohol, sugar, chocolate, and social drugs, is stored in the liver.

Blends: Harmony, Peace & Calming, and JuvaFlex.

Supplements: JuvaTone, Rehemogen, and Stevia.

Cleanse: (see COLON and LIVER CLEANSE).

Rehemogen helps detoxify, purify, and cleanse the blood. JuvaTone helps erase the addiction blueprint (RNA) in the liver and helps rebuild the liver. Stevia has been reported to decrease cravings for sweets, fatty foods, tobacco, and alcohol.

(See LIVER AILMENTS, DETOXIFICATION, and SMOKING.)

Adenitis

(See LYMPHATIC SYSTEM.)

Adrenal Glands

Adrenal glands are about the size of a grape, with one located on top of each kidney. They produce hormones that help control heart rate, blood pressure, and the chemical balance in the body. These glands also help regulate the process of converting carbohydrates to energy that produces glycogen for the liver in addition to androgens (male hormones), estrogen, and progesterone (female hormones).

Single oils: Sage with nutmeg, clove, rosemary, or basil.

Use: Add 1-3 drops of each oil to the corresponding oil above (according to your sensitivity).

Sage may help regulate sweating. Nutmeg has adrenal-like activity, which supports the adrenal glands for increased energy.

Blends: EndoFlex, Joy, and En-R-Gee.

Use: Add 1-3 drops of each single oil to the corresponding blends above (according to your sensitivity).

Hot compress:
- 3 drops clove
- 3 drops nutmeg
- 7 drops rosemary
- 20 drops massage oil or V-6 Mixing Oil or Massage Oil Base

Apply over the adrenal glands, located on top of the kidneys, found on the back, about 2 inches above a line through the elbows (see Compress).

Flavonoids, which are present in citrus oils, stimulate the pituitary and adrenal glands.

Supplements: Thyromin, VitaGreen, Royal Essence, Super B, Master HIS/HERS, Master CHILDREN'S, and Mineral Essence.

Take Thyromin in the morning. Take 1 Super B tablet after meals. If there is a strong niacin flush (skin becoming red and itchy, which lasts for about 15 minutes, then the next time, take 1/2 of the tablet).

Master HIS/HERS: 2-6 tablets 3 times daily according to blood type and need.

Master CHILDREN'S Chewable: 2-4 tablets daily. Many adults eat these because they are so tasty.

Agent Orange Exposure

Blends: JuvaFlex and EndoFlex.

Rub JuvaFlex over liver area or apply in a hot compress. Apply 2-4 drops of EndoFlex over adrenal gland area.

Supplements: Radex, ImmuneTune, Cleansing Trio, JuvaTone, and Thyromin.

Colon and liver cleanse:

- Megazyme - 3 times/day.

- ImmuneTune- 4 times/day.

- Rub 3 drops EndoFlex on the thyroid (hollow at base-front of neck) and 3 drops over kidneys - 3 times/day.

- Rub 3 drops EndoFlex on thyroid reflex points on bottom of feet (base of big toes) and kidney reflex points on bottom of feet - 3 times/day.

- After 90 days on the above program, gradually reduce the above amounts but stay on the program for a full year.

- Add 1 cup Epsom salts plus 4 ounces of 35% food-grade hydrogen peroxide to bath water – once daily.

Epson Salt Baths with six cups of Epson Salts per tub of water for adult for 30 minutes and drink 3 glasses of lemonade while in the tub.

Agitation

Single oils: Lavender, orange, and Roman chamomile.

Blends: Peace & Calming, Forgiveness, Surrender, and Joy.

Supplements: Super B, Super C, and Super Cal.

AIDS (Acquired Immune Deficiency Syndrome)

Single oils: Cistus

Blends: Brain Power, Exodus, Valor, Thieves, and ImmuPower.

Exodus II: 6-8 drops on spine alternating days with Rain Drop Therapy.

Valor and Thieves: 4-6 drops on feet for 3 weeks.

ImmuPower: 6 drops daily in water and drink.

Rain Drop Therapy: 3 times weekly for virus.

Supplements: Cleansing Trio, JuvaTone, Immu-Gel, Thyromin, ImmuneTune, VitaGreen, Sulfurzyme, Exodus, Super B, Ultra Young, Goji Berry Tea, and Vita Life Juice.

Cleansing Trio for 120 days with JuvaTone.

ImmuGel: 1/2 tsp. 3 times daily. Hold in mouth for better absorption.

Thyromin: Start by taking 2 at night and 1 in morning.

ImmuneTune: 6-8 capsules daily.

VitaGreen: 6-10 capsules daily.

Sulfurzyme: 1 tablespoon.

Exodus: Up to 18 capsules daily.

Super B: 1 tablet daily with a meal.

Ultra Young: 3 Squirts on each inside of each cheek, 4-5 times daily.

Eat 5-6 mini-meals per day, primarily Power Meal (3 times daily) and fish for protein. Do not eat chicken for first 3-6 weeks to allow more energy for immune building.

Vita Life Juice: Drink 8 oz. throughout day (see CLEANSING).

Goji Berry (wolfberry) Tea: 10-12 cups daily.

Anti-Aging

Single oils: Frankincense, sandalwood, myrrh, cypress, and patchouly.

Blends: Brain Power, Di-Tone, EndoFlex, Clarity, Harmony, Live With Passion, and Valor.

Body massage weekly with the oils.

Supplements: Power Meal, Ultra Young, Be-Fit, Master Formula, Goji Berry Tea, Sulfurzyme, VitaGreen, Super C, A.D. & E., and AlkaLime.

- Power Meal: 2 scoops 2-3 times daily as desired.

- Ultra Young: 3-4 sprays inside each cheek 3-4 times daily.

- Be-Fit: 3-4 capsules 2 times daily

- Master Formula: 3-6 tablets 2 times daily, depending on blood type

- Goji Berry (wolfberry) Tea: 1-3 cups daily

- Sulfurzyme: 1-2 Tbs. daily or as desired. For some 2 times weekly is sufficient.

- VitaGreen: O blood types 6-12 capsules daily, A and AB blood types: 2-4 capsules daily.

- Super C: 1-3 capsules daily.

- A. D. & E.: 1 dropper full daily. Mix Power Meal, Body Balance, I.C.P., or any thicker liquid and drop in A. D. & E. It will stay as a drop and will be easy to drink and not stick to sides of glass. Others simply squirt into mouth and swallow.

- AlkaLime: 1 teaspoon in water once daily or even once weekly, depending on need to create proper pH balance.

Hydrate the skin with AromaSilk Satin Body Lotion.

Exercise regularly and stay physically fit (see EXERCISE PROGRAM).

Eat a properly balanced diet.

Air Purification (Airborne Bacteria, Air Pollution)

Single oils: Lemon, peppermint, lavender, rosemary, melaleuca, frankincense, ravensara, eucalyptus, oregano, thyme, cinnamon, bergamot, lime, and grapefruit.

Blends: Purification, R.C., Peace & Calming, Citrus Fresh, Melrose, Exodus II, Sacred Mountain, Inspiration, Christmas Spirit, ImmuneTune, Ravensara, Thieves, and Raven.

Oils alter the structure of molecules that create odors, rather than just masking them. They also increase oxygen availability and negative ions. Harmful bacteria cannot live in ion-charged air.

Diffuse Purification: Removes formaldehydes from substances, such as paint and cleaning substances, allergens from cat and dog hair, chemicals, smoke, mold, fungus, etc.

Set the diffuser high in the room so that the oil mist falls through the air and removes the odor-causing substances.

To eliminate and destroy airborne germs and bacteria, diffuse any of the following: Lemon, Purification, Citrus Fresh, Thieves, or any favorite oil or blend.

Diffuse Thieves in moderation, not over 15 minutes at a time as the cinnamon may irritate the nasal passages.

Do not mix blends in a diffuser as they are already blended. Mixing blends will alter the smell and the therapeutic benefit desired.

However, a single oil may be added to a blend. Always wash diffuser before using a different oil blend.

You can also add a couple of drops of a favorite oil to water in a spray bottle and shake vigorously. Spray the solution in closets, on objects that will not be damaged by water, and on the filter of vacuum cleaners (water bath vacuums and rug cleaners, add oil directly to the water), on furnace or air conditioner filters to purify air and add pleasant fragrance.

Refreshen air:
- 20 drops lavender
- 10 drops lemon
- 6 drops bergamot
- 5 drops Lime
- 5 drops grapefruit

Diffuse or put in 1/2 oz. (3 Tbs.) of distilled water in a spray bottle; shake well.

Alcoholism

Single oils: Lavender, Roman chamomile, orange, helichrysum, elemi, and rosemary verbonon.

Blends: JuvaFlex, Forgiveness, Acceptance, Surrender, Motivation, and Joy.

Supplements: JuvaTone, Cleansing Trio, Thyromin, Power Meal, and Mineral Essence.

Alertness

Single oils: Pepper, peppermint, rosemary cineol, basil, spearmint, and pine.

Blends: Clarity, En-R-Gee, Sacred Mountain, Live With Passion, Motivation, and Valor.

Supplements: Ultra Young, VitaGreen, Super B, Royal Essence, Mineral Essence, and Thyromin.

Alkalosis

Single oils: Ginger, tarragon, and anise seed.

Blends: Di-Tone

Supplements: Megazyme, Sulfurzyme, and Body Balance.

Allergies

Single oils: Lavender and Roman chamomile.

Blends: Harmony and Valor.

Supplements: Royaldophilus, Megazyme, Mineral Essence, Power Meal, Master Formula, and VitaGreen.

Dairy products: Allergies are often created by the inability of the body to digest milk and other diary products. Pasteurization of these products kills the enzymes, creating a lactose intolerance.

Allergies are the body's way of screaming "Help, I am over-toxic!" It is necessary to rid the body of toxins. Hay fever (allergic rhinitis) is inflammation of the fragile lining of the nasal passages, sinuses, eye lids, and surface layer of the eyes, causing sneezing, runny nose, watery red itchy eyes, dry throat, and wheezing. Generally triggered by airborne allergens (pollen, animal hair, feathers, dust mites), which cause the release of histamines and subsequent inflammation of nasal passages and sinus-related areas. Allergies are somewhat like asthma, which manifests in the chest and lungs.

Cleanse: Cleansing Trio and JuvaTone (see COLON and LIVER CLEANSE).

Aluminum Toxicity

Single oils: Helichrysum

Blends: PanAway

Supplements: Chelex, JuvaTone, and Comfor-Tone.

Alzheimers

(See NEUROLOGICAL DISEASE.)

Anemia

Single oils: Lemon

Supplements: Chelex, Rehemogen, JuvaTone, and VitaGreen.

Lemon stimulates red blood cell formation and helps anemia. Use Rehemogen, which helps elevate blood cell count and is excellent for treating anemia.

Anesthesia

Single oils: Elemi, birch, lavender, lemongrass, and tansy.

- Helichrysum with clove, melaleuca with rosemary.

- Birch, spruce, and pepper.

- Combine equal parts of helichrysum and clove.

- Combine 3 parts melaleuca to 5 parts rosemary.

Blends: PanAway

Use: Add 1-3 drops to the corresponding oils above (according to your sensitivity).

Aneurysm

Single oils: Helichrysum, sandalwood, tansy, and cypress.

Blends: Aroma Life and Brain Power.

Supplements: Ultra Young and Rehemogen.

Anorexia

(See EATING DISORDERS.)

Single oils: Tarragon

Blends: Christmas Spirit

Anthrax

Single oils: Thyme, oregano, rosewood.

Blends: Thieves and Exodus II.

Supplements: Exodus, Radex, and Super C.

Antibiotics

Single oils: Oregano, thyme, cinnamon, mountain savory, lemon, rosewood, melaleuca, clove, ravensara, and eucalyptus radiata.

Blends: Thieves, Exodus II, ImmuPower, Melrose, Inspiration, and Sacred Mountain.

Supplements: Royaldophilus, ImmuGel, Exodus, Super C, Radex, and ImmuneTune.

Antibiotic drugs diminish all bacteria and intestinal flora indiscriminantly, both the disease-causing pathogenic and friendly digestion-promoting varieties. This diminishing of intestinal flora disrupts the digestive process, reduces the assimilation of nutrients, and allows candida and fungi to flourish, since the friendly bacteria tend to keep candida in check.

The average adult has between 3 and 4 pounds of beneficial bacteria permanently residing in the intestines. These beneficial flora make the first line of defense against foreign invaders, control mucus and debris, produce B vitamins, vitamin K, and maintain pH balance, thus opposing yeast and fungus overgrowth.

While a person is on antibiotics, he/she might need 2 or 3 servings of acidophilus per day. Take on an empty stomach, before meals, and for at least 10 to 15 days after finishing the antibiotics.

Antioxidants

Antioxidants prevent mutations, are free radical scavengers, prevent fungus, help oxygenate the cells, and prevent oxidation of cells.

Single oils: Thyme, clove, cumin, chamomile, cinnamon bark, frankincense, helichrysum, melaleuca (alternifolia), oregano, ravensara, and rosemary.

Blends: Aroma Life, Di-Tone, JuvaFlex, Melrose, PanAway, Purification, R.C., and Thieves

Supplements: Radex, Super C, Super B, ComforTone, JuvaTone, Vitagreen, Megazyme, ImmuGel, ImmuneTune, Master HIS/HERS, and CHILDREN'S, Mineral Essence, Colloidal Essence, and Goji Berry Tea.

Thyme, clove or cumin added to pure (cold pressed) vegetable oil works as an antioxidant and stabilizes the oil. These oils can also be used as antioxidants to make foods keep longer.

Antiseptic

Single oils:

- Birch with lavender, mountain savory, lavendin, peppermint, spearmint, ravensara, sage, clove, bergamot, cinnamon, juniper, or nutmeg.

- Frankincense with lavender, cedarwood, rosemary, melaleuca, lemon, oregano, thyme, myrrh, geranium, rose, black cumin, angelica, eucalyptus (globulus and radiata), or sandalwood.

- Lemongrass with melaleuca, lavendin, cedarwood, lemon, rosemary, citronella, basil, cypress, fennel, fir, pine, mandarin, neroli, tarragon, patchouly, rosewood, ylang ylang, laurus nobilis, or vetiver.

Use: Add 1-3 drops to the corresponding oils above (according to your sensitivity).

Blends: Birch, frankincense, or lemongrass (single oils) with Purification, Melrose, Christmas Spirit, Citrus Fresh, Thieves, ImmuPower, R.C., or Raven.

Use: Add 1-3 drops of each single oil to the corresponding blends above (according to your sensitivity).

Supplements: Rose Ointment and A. D. & E.

Melrose plus Rose Ointment and essential oils make a potent combination as a disinfectant and fast healing agent.

Aneurysm

(See CARDIOVASCULAR SYSTEM.)

Apnea

Temporary cessation of breathing, asphyxia

Blends: Clarity, Surrender, and Valor.

Supplements: Royal Essence, VitaGreen, Super B, AuraLight, and Thyromin.

- Diffuse Clarity in bedroom.

- Rub Valor on bottom of feet.

- Take 3 droppers of Royal Essence, 4 times per day.

- Take VitaGreen, 2 times per day.

- Take Super B 3 times per day with meals.

- Take Thyromin at bedtime.

Appetite, Loss of

Single oils: Bergamot, ginger, spearmint, orange, and nutmeg

Ginger stimulates digestion and helps with loss of appetite (see DIGESTION and STOMACH).

Blends: Inner Child, Citrus Fresh, and Christmas Spirit.

Supplements: Megazyme, Mint Condition, and ComforTone.

Arteriosclerosis

Single oils: Helichrysum, cypress, and frankincense.

Blends: Aroma Life

Supplements: HRT, Chelex, JuvaTone, and Rehemogen.

Arthritis

Microbes and toxins, which react within the bone joint spaces, can produce inflammation of joints. Researchers have linked most degenerative diseases to lack of nutrients in the body. Minerals and trace minerals account for most of the nutritional deficiencies.

Single oils:

- Birch with helichrysum, spruce, fir, pine, cypress, peppermint, vetiver, marjoram, rosemary cineol, eucalyptus citridona, basil, oregano, lemongrass, Idaho tansy, black pepper, elemi, or peppermint.

- Idaho tansy with birch, basil, rosemary, peppermint, marjoram, mountain savory, cypress, ginger, black pepper, or tarragon.

- Elemi with spruce, fir, pine, cedarwood, juniper, rosemary, peppermint, helichrysum, birch, basil, wild Idaho tansy, lemon, nutmeg, or oregano.

- Juniper, rosemary, Roman chamomile, lemon, or melaleuca.

Use: Add 1-3 drops to the corresponding single oils above (according to your sensitivity).

Blends:

- Birch (single oil) with Aroma Siez, PanAway, Relieve It, or Peace & Calming.

- Lavender (single oil) with PanAway, Relieve It, or Aroma Siez.

- 1-2 drops cypress (single oil) with one of the following: Aroma Life, PanAway, Purification, Aroma Siez, or Sacred Mountain. Apply on location as desired and then follow with massage oil.

Use: Add 1-3 drops of each single oil to the corresponding blends above (according to your sensitivity).

Supplements: Super Cal, Super C, Mineral Essence, Goji Berry Tea, ArthroTune, Rehemogen, ImmuneTune, Exodus, AlkaLime, EssPro 7, Ortho Ease, Ortho Sport, and Relaxation Massage Oils.

- Super Cal: 2-3 capsules 2 times daily.

- Super C: 3-4 tablets 3 time daily.

- Mineral Essence: 2 droppers 3 times daily.

- Goji Berry Tea: 4-10 cups daily .

- ArthroTune: 2-6 capsules 3 times daily.

- Rehemogen: 1-2 droppers n water 2-3 times daily.

- ImmuneTune: 2-3 capsules 3 times daily.

- Exodus: 2-3 capsules 2-3 times daily as needed.

- AlkaLime: 1/2 to 1 level tsp. in water daily.

- EssPro 7: 1/8 tsp. to 1/2 tsp. daily as needed.

Detoxification of the body and strengthening the joint(s) is important, as is eradication of all of the infection. Cleanse the colon and liver (see COLON). Rehemogen cleans and purifies the blood. Toxins block nutrient and oxygen flow into cells (see BLOOD CIRCULATION, BLOOD CLEANING, and DETOXIFICATION).

Apply oils on location followed by massage oil or AromaSilk Satin body lotion. PanAway and Relieve It have cortisone-like action, which give relief of arthritic pain without the cortisone side effects.

Asthma

Researchers have linked most degenerative diseases to lack of nutrients in the body. Minerals and trace minerals account for most of the nutritional deficiencies.

A lot of asthma attacks are triggered by an allergic reaction to pollen, skin particles, dandruff, cat or dogs fur, dust mites, some foods, such as eggs, milk, flavorings, dyes, preservatives, etc. Other causes are infection, particularly respiratory, vigorous exercise, stress, and other psychological factors. However, some attacks start for no apparent reason. Asthma manifests itself in the lungs, chest, eyes, nose, and throat in a manner similar to allergic rhinitis (hay fever) (see ALLERGIES).

Single oils:

- Lavender with Roman chamomile, eucalyptus polybratea, myrtle, peppermint, frankincense, marjoram, or rose.

- Frankincense with ravensara, cypress, fir, spruce, pine, lemon, thyme, rosemary, eucalyptus, helichrysum, birch, or myrtle.

- Rosemary cineol with ravensara, eucalyptus radiata, mountain savory, lemon, or juniper

- Sage with lavender, myrrh, hyssop, or eucalyptus.

Use: Add 1-3 drops to the corresponding single oils above (according to your sensitivity).

Blends:

- Lavender or Roman chamomile (single oils) with Melrose, Di-Tone, Purification, or Thieves.

- Frankincense (single oil) with R.C., Raven, Inspiration Blend, or Sacred Mountain.

- Rosemary (single oil) with R.C., or Raven.

Use: Add 1-3 drops of each single oil to the corresponding blends above (according to your sensitivity).

Supplements: Immune stimulants such as the following: ImmuGel, Radex, Super C, Exodus, Royal Essence, VitaGreen, ImmuneTune, Rehemogen, EssPro 7, Ultra Young, Megazyme, and Royaldophilus.

Athlete's Foot

(See FOOT PROBLEMS.)

Single oils: Melrose and melaleuca.

Use 35% food-grade hydrogen peroxide to clean the area. Apply Melrose and then Rose Ointment. Saturate gauze with oils and wrap infected area.

Attention Deficit Disorder

Single oils: Lavender, sandalwood, cardamon, basil, and frankincense.

Blends: Brain Power and Joy. Diffuse Peace & Calming, Clarity, lavender, chamomile, Joy, and Brain Power.

Supplements: Mineral Essence, Ultra Young, and Power Meal.

Autism

Single oils: Frankincense, sandalwood, melissa, and basil.

Blends: Brain Power and Clarity.

Supplements: Ultra Young and Mineral Essence.

Back Adjustment

(See SPINE.)

Bed Wetting

Blends: Valor and Harmony.

Supplements: K&B

Use K&B tincture once in the afternoon and once before bedtime (2 droppers maximum).

Bell's Palsy

(See NEURITIS.)

Bites

Singles oils: Lavender, citronella, melaleuca, and rosemary.

Blends: Purification, Melrose.

Supplements: Exodus, Super B, and Super C.

Topical application: Purification (reapply until infection is gone). Use lavender for itching.

Bladder Infection, Incontinence

Single oils: Oregano and Melaleuca.

Blends: Inspiration

2-3 drops of Inspiration rubbed over the bladder area may help clear up a bladder infection.

Supplements: K&B

Use K&B tincture (2-3 droppers in distilled water) 3-6 times per day.

Inspiration helps clear up bladder infections. Rub over bladder, on bladder Vita Flex points on feet, and apply in compress over bladder (see COMPRESSES).

Bleeding

Single oils: Cypress, helichrysum, Idaho tansy, and lavender.

Blends: Aroma Life and PanAway.

Supplements: Rehemogen

Blisters

Single oils: Melaleuca, lavender, melissa, clove, and cistus.

Blends: Purification, Inspiration, and Melrose.

Supplements: A. D. & E., Power Meal, and Essential Manna.

Bloating

Single oils: Tarragon, peppermint, anise seed, and fennel.

Blends: Di-Tone

Supplements: Megazyme, Mint Condition, and Royaldophilus.

Blood

Anemia

Single oils: Lemon, lemongrass, and helichrysum.

Blends: Aroma Life

Supplements: Chelex, Rehemogen, Mineral Essence, and Royal Essence.

Lemon stimulates red blood cell formulation and helps anemia. Chelex is great for anemia, helps elevate blood cell count, and brings metals out of the system.

Circulation Problems

Single oils:

- Cypress with basil, rosemary, thyme, lavender, peppermint, helichrysum, ginger, ylang ylang, lemon, geranium, clary sage, sandalwood, black pepper, Idaho tansy, birch, or orange.

Use: Add 1-3 drops to the corresponding single oils (according to your sensitivity).

Blends:

- Cypress (single oil) with Aroma Life, Citrus Fresh, Harmony, Di-Tone, En-R-Gee, Harmony, and PanAway. Cypress strengthens and dilates capillaries and increases circulation, as does lemon. When there is tissue damage, circulation needs to be increased. Myrtle also is a dilator. Marjoram relaxes muscles so that the blood vessels are allowed to return to normal size. Nutmeg is a circulatory stimulant. Helichrysum along with cypress promotes circulation. Cel-Lite Magic is a dilator of capillaries and blood vessels.

Rub Harmony over areas of poor circulation. Add Aroma Life and cypress to the Cel-Lite Magic and do body massage starting at feet, working up towards heart.

Use: Add 1-3 drops of each single oil to the corresponding blends above (according to your sensitivity).

Supplements: Super B, Cel-Lite Magic, HRT, Cardia Care, VitaGreen, Royal Essence, Rehemogen, and JuvaTone.

Vitamin B3 dilates blood vessels, so circulation increases. Super B is a good source of all B-Vitamins. Bay helps increase circulation.

HRT is a very good product for blood system circulation deficiency. Positive results have been produced with 25 drops in 1 ounce of distilled water taken 3 times per day.

Rehemogen may help make or balance platelet production, make more red blood cells, and enhance the blood. JuvaTone taken at the same time enhances the action. Aroma Life also helps; rub on the carotid arteries and pulse points, wherever an artery comes close to the skin. Rub Harmony over areas of poor circulation. Extra cayenne is helpful. Always take with a full glass of water and not at bedtime (see CARDIOVAS-CULAR SYSTEM).

Blood Clot

Single oils: Helichrysum and Idaho tansy.

- Lavender and lemon.

Use: Add 1-3 drops of the single oils (according to your sensitivity).

Supplements: Super Cal, Ultra Young, and Essential Manna.

Take Super Cal internally.

Externally: Massage lemon and lavender with helichrysum on location with or without hot packs (see HOT PACKS).

Helichrysum is good for prevention of clots and helps blood become reabsorbed into tissue. Drink 1-3 drops in water, 2-3 times daily.

Detoxification

Clean, healthy, and detoxified blood assists in beating any disease. Clean blood carries clean nutrients, oxygen, and food to the cells to help one back to good health. Toxins block nutrient and oxygen flow to cells.

Single oils:

- Helichrysum with German chamomile, Roman chamomile, rosemary, geranium, lemon, orange, or cardamom.

Use: Add 1-3 drops to the corresponding single oils above (according to your sensitivity).

Blends:

- Helichrysum (single oil) with Di-Tone, JuvaFlex, Exodus, or EndoFlex.

Use: Add 1-3 drops of each single oil to the corresponding blends above (according to your sensitivity).

Supplements: VitaGreen, Rehemogen, Chelex, Exodus, AlkaLime, and Sulfurzyme.

Do a colon and liver cleanse (see COLON).

Rehemogen is a very powerful assistant for any type of blood disorder, including toxemia, blood toxicity, etc. Chelex helps elevate blood cell count and bring metals out of the blood/system. Use with Cardamom and JuvaTone. MSM (sulfur) found in the Sulfurzyme purifies and cleanses the body and blood, promoting cells to eject toxins and prevent their accumulation.

Dr. J. Hofman, who in 1978, wrote the book, *The Missing Link*, said that the best way to attain perfect health is to have a free-flowing alkaline blood stream (see BODY pH, ACID/ALKALINE BALANCE).

See the following sections: Brain Function, Cardiovascular System, Headaches, and Vascular Cleansing.

Oxygenation

Single oils: Helichrysum, lemongrass, pepper, spruce, and anise.

Blends: Valor, R.C., En-R-Gee, and PanAway.

Supplements: Royal Essence and Super B.

Most oils are oxygenators. Royal Essence increases energy and blood oxygen in as little as 4 seconds. Put under tongue for fastest results. Valor increases oxygen at the cellular level. Spruce dilates and enhances oxygen exchange in the lungs. Through extensive testing, it was found that R.C. increases oxygen.

Hydrogen peroxide (H202), taken orally can show a 9.2% increase in blood oxygen. Essential oils can increase circulation between 22% and 32% (see COLDS - CHEST INFECTIONS).

Blood Pressure

Cholesterol

(See CARDIOVASCULAR SYSTEM.)

Helichrysum and lemon (over the heart and on Vita Flex points), rosemary (massage on heart points and 3 drops under tongue for low blood pressure), HRT, Aroma Life, JuvaTone, and Chelex.

Blood Pressure, High (Hypertension)

Single oils:

- Lavender with ylang ylang, marjoram, cypress, mountain savory, or helichrysum.

- Rosemary with ylang ylang, marjoram, helichrysum, or lavender.

Use: Add 1-3 drops to the corresponding single oils above (according to your sensitivity).

Blends:

- Lavender (single oil) with Aroma Life, Aroma Siez, Peace & Calming, or Citrus Fresh.

- Ylang Ylang (single oil) with Aroma Life, or Joy.

Use: Add 1-3 drops of each single oil to the corresponding blends above (according to your sensitivity).

Supplements: HRT, Garlic, Cel-Lite Magic, ImmuneTune, Super C, Radex, Super B, Mineral Essence,

Super Cal, Stevia, Red Clover Tea (6-10 cups daily), and Desert Breeze Massage Oil.

Do a colon and liver cleanse (see COLON).

To regulate and lower blood pressure, place 1 drop each of Aroma Life and ylang ylang on heart Vita Flex points. Apply heart Vita Flex as for 3 minutes. Also apply a couple of drops of Aroma Life over the heart on the chest during this time. Blood pressure will drop at the 3-minute point and continue to drop for up to 20 minutes. This will continue to be effective for a substantial period of time. It has controlled blood pressure for 5 months before another application was necessary. Monitor the pressure and reapply as required. For increased effect, rub Aroma Life on the carotid arteries at the same time.

Diffuse Aroma Life alternatively with Clarity.

Lowered blood pressure has been reported by taking, 25 drops of HRT in 1 ounce of water, 3 times per day. Stevia lowers high blood pressure.

Extra cayenne pepper is helpful also. Always take with a full glass of water with meals and not at bedtime.

Magnesium acts as a smooth muscle relaxant and supports the cardiovascular system. It will act as a natural calcium channel blocker for the heart, lowering blood pressure and dilating the heart blood vessels (Terry Friedmann, M.D.). Mineral Essence and Super Cal are good sources of magnesium.

Inhalation of jasmine lowers brain activity, while at the same time enhances brain blood supply, thus reducing anxiety and hypertension (see INHALATION THERAPY). Marjoram relaxes muscles, allowing blood vessels to return to normal size and thus helps lower blood pressure.

Also see Cardiovascular and Heart.

Hypotension – Low Blood Pressure

Single oils: Sage, pine, rosemary, and ylang ylang.

Blends: Rosemary with Aroma Life, EndoFlex, or Joy.

Use: Add 1-3 drops of each single oil to the corresponding blends above (according to your sensitivity).

Place 1 drop each of Aroma Life and rosemary on heart Vita Flex points and do heart Vita Flex.

Heart Vita Flex

The foot Vita Flex point is on the sole of the left foot, the ring toe (next to small toe), and behind the knuckle. Vita Flex massaging on this point is as effective as the band and arm together (see

Vita Flex Chapter). The hand point is in the palm of the left hand, one inch below the ring finger joint (at the life line), and the secondary point is on bottom of the left arm in line with the inside of the upturned arm (approximately two inches up the arm from the funny bone), not on the muscle, but up under the muscle. Have another person use thumbs and firmly press these two points alternately for three minutes, in a kind of pumping action. Work all three points when possible; start with the foot first, then go to the hand and arm.

Heart Attack – Myocardial Infarction

Single oils: Helichrysum, lavender, peppermint, lemon, and cypress.

Blends: Aroma Life

- Lavender with Roman Chamomile, rose, or Aroma Life.

Use: Add 1-3 drops of each single oil to the corresponding blends above (according to your sensitivity).

Supplements: CardiaCare, Mineral Essence, Super Cal, and Sulfurzyme Capsules.

Apply heart Vita Flex as above. If not enough time to remove shoes to get at feet, apply pumping action to left hand and arm points. A drop of Aroma Life on each point will increase effectiveness.

Magnesium acts as a smooth muscle relaxant and supports the cardiovascular system. It will act as a natural calcium channel blocker for the heart, lowering blood pressure and dilating the heart blood vessels (Dr. Terry Friedmann). Mineral Essence and Super Cal are good sources of magnesium. MSM (Sulfur), found in Sulfurzyme, normalizes heart functions.

When we are under stress, we are unable to absorb and metabolize magnesium (see STRESS).

Body Frequency (Electrical) Balancing

Single oils: Frankincense , sage, lavender, rose (highest in frequency), sandalwood, and myrtle.

Blends: Valor, Thieves, 3 Wise Men, Harmony, Inner Child, Joy, and Release.

Apply Thieves on the bottom of the feet. Sage is good for balancing frequencies when disease lowers body frequency.

Harmony on the energy centers, (or chakras), helps balance the body, makes the healing process more efficient, and facilitates the release of stored emotions. The energy points corresponding to the endocrine glands:

- The crown (top) of the head (pineal)
- Forehead (pituitary)
- Neck (thyroid)
- Thymus
- Solar plexus (adrenal)
- Navel (pancreas)
- Groin (ovaries/gonads)

Release stimulates harmony and balance by releasing memory trauma from liver cells, which stored emotions of anger, hate, and frustration. Rub neat over liver, apply compress over liver, massage Vita Flex points on feet and hands (see COMPRESSES).

Sandalwood oxygenates the pineal/pituitary gland, thus improving attitude and body balance. Rose has a frequency of 320 Hz., the highest of all oils. Its beautiful fragrance is almost intoxicating and aphrodisiac-like. The frequency of every cell is enhanced, bringing balance and harmony to the body. It is stimulating and elevating to the mind, creating a sense of well being.

The situation where a person has a strong dislike to one or two oils, but enjoys all the other oils, is an indication that the person is not in balance and is fighting, coming into balance. To correct this situation, ask the person which oil or blend is offensive. This traces to a psychological connection. The complementary oil or blend is what is needed to release or change this.

Lavender is very good unless it is the oil that is disliked. Harmony will probably work in most situations. Inner Child is also excellent. One must experiment and find the oil required.

Where the imbalance is due to allergy in sinuses throat, or pituitary insufficiency, apply the complementary oil to the crown of the head, the forehead, and the thymus.

For overall body electrical imbalance, put a couple of drops of the complementary oil in each palm, have the person hold the right palm over the navel and the left palm over the thymus and take three slow, deep breaths. Place the predominate palm/hand over the navel and the other palm/hand over the thymus and rub clockwise three times. This works through the body's electrical circuitry by pulling the frequency in through the umbilicus, the thymus, and the olfactory to the limbic system in the brain to create electrical balance. A lot of the cause of imbalance is in the endocrine glands, which create the electrical balance throughout the physical body.

The person should be in balance. The offending oil should now be pleasing.

Body pH, Acid/Alkaline Balance

Our blood should be alkaline and should not be allowed to become acidic. The naturally occurring yeast/fungi in our bodies thrive in an acid terrain, and secrete a large number of poisons called mycotoxins, which are believed to be among the causes of many diseases and debilitating conditions (see FUNGUS INFECTION).

Research has shown that many diseases can be reversed if the body is kept alkaline (on the inside). This also helps supplements and oils work better. Dairy products and meats produce acidity in the body and thus suppress the immune system. (see DIGESTION).

Single oils: Patchouly with Roman chamomile, lavender, lemon, or lemongrass.

Use: Add 1-3 drops to the corresponding single oils above (according to your sensitivity).

Supplements: AlkaLime, Royaldophilus, Vita-Green, Mineral Essence, Sulfurzyme, Mint Condition, and Rose Ointment.

Do a colon and liver cleanse (see COLON).

The more acidic a person's system blood is, the less effect that the oils have on that person. People who have pronounced reactions to oils, are probably highly acidic. So we must keep our blood on the alkaline side for the oils to work best. This is also our normal and most healthy state.

In chemistry, pH 7.0 is considered neutral. Pure water is pH 7.0. Acidic is lower than pH 7.0. Alkaline is higher than pH 7.0. The ideal pH for the body should average 7.0. Preserving this pH balance is the foundation on which sound health and strong bodies are built and maintained.

Many researchers and doctors believe the best blood plasma pH shaul be 7.0 to 7.5. There are others who believe 6.9 is normal. The Hunza people have a pH average of 7.5. It is impossible to argue with success. Proper blood plasma could range from 6.9 to 7.5 and keeping it as close to 7.0 is the best.

The acids of the body digest essential oils and could create a reaction to the oils if the pH is below 6.9 making the oils less effective. Because the acid of the body digest essential oils, that may be one reason why essential oils do not accumulate in the tissues like vitamins, herb and minerals. There is less chance of a toxic reaction from essential oils than from other natural food products that may tend to build up in the body.

One can test pH with litmus paper strips, available at drug stores. For the most accurate readings, expose the strip to a sample of one's saliva or urine immediately after awakening in the morning and before eating breakfast. Instructions on the kit will give details on how to read the color changes and thus determine the pH.

VitaGreen is a food for alkaline balancing. AlkaLime is a precisely balanced acid neutralizing formula to preserve the body's pH balance.

Squeeze half a Lemon into a glass of water. Drink up to 64 ounces (8 glasses) a day, depending on each person's requirements.

You should be aware of your body's pH balance when using acidic oils and blends. Acidic oils, such as orange, pepper, cinnamon, clove, mandarin, lemon, nutmeg, spruce, etc., should be used with a modifier. The best modifiers to use in these instances are ones that are high in aldehydes, such as lavender, chamomile, and bergamot.

A blend of 2 drops patchouly, 2 drops Roman chamomile, 2 drops lavender, in AromaSilk Satin Body Lotion or Rose Ointment.

Stress, both physical and mental, elevate blood acidity (see STRESS).

Boils

Single oils: Frankincense, lavender, Roman chamomile, patchouly, and myrrh.

Blends: 3 Wise Men, Exodus II, and Thieves.

Supplements: Rehemogen, JuvaTone, A. D. & E., and Essential Manna (Potassium).

Bone Healing, Bruised, Broken, Spurs

Single oils:

- Birch with spruce, fir, pine, cypress, peppermint, tansy, rosemary, basil, or elemi.
- Cypress with spruce, fir, pine, cedarwood, rosemary, peppermint, helichrysum, birch, basil, lemongrass, clove, or ginger.

Use: Add 1-3 drops to the corresponding single oils (according to your sensitivity).

Blends:

- Birch with Aroma Siez, PanAway, or Peace & Calming.
- Cypress with Aroma Life, PanAway, Relieve It, Aroma Siez, Purification, Melrose, Release, or Sacred Mountain.

Use: Add 1-3 drops of each single oil to the corresponding blends above (according to your sensitivity).

Supplements: Ortho Ease, Relaxation, Super Cal, Arthro Plus, Mineral Essence, ArthroTune, and Ortho Sport.

CAUTION: Be gentle on location of new breaks to not disturb the knitting process.

Cypress increases circulation. With damaged tissue, circulation needs to be increased.

Broken Bones

- 10 drops birch
- 3 drops helichrysum
- 2 drops lemongrass
- 3 drops pine
- 4 drops ginger

Mix in teaspoon and apply a few drops to local area neat.

Do a sensitivity test first, or be prepared to apply

V-6 Mixing Oil or Massage Oil Base if burning starts. Oils applied neat are always more effective.

Bone Tissue Regeneration

Recipe #1:
- 8 drops helichrysum
- 4 drops clove
- 2 drops lemongrass
- 12 drops birch
- 6 drops pine

Mix in teaspoon.

Recipe #2:
- 10 drops birch
- 8 drops marjoram
- 4 drops cypress
- 2 drops peppermint
- 1 drop basil

Mix in 1/2 ounce of massage oil or massage oil or V-6 Mixing Oil or Massage Oil Base.

ArthroTune and Super Cal help the repair process.

When selecting oils, particularly for injuries, think through the cause and type of injury and select oils for each segment. For instance, a broken bone could encompass muscle damage, nerve damage, ligament strain or tear, inflammation, infection, bone injury, fever on location, and possibly an emotion. So select an oil or oils for each perceived problem and apply in rotation or prepare a blend to cover all of them. The emotion may be shock, anger, guilt, or the person may have had pain for a long time and need to release or relieve it or need some joy in their lives, etc. Try to work through all factors.

Any time there is tissue damage, there is always inflammation which should be addressed first.

Muscle and Bone Inflammation and Pain Relief

- 12 drops fir
- 10 drops melaleuca
- 8 drops lavender
- 6 drops marjoram
- 3 drops blue chamomile
- 3 drops spearmint
- 2 drops peppermint

Mix in 1 ounce V-6 Mixing Oil or Massage Oil Base.

Shock – to refresh and revitalize

If the injury just happened from an accident or the like, the person may be in shock. Inhaling oils can help to reduce that shock.

Single oils:

- Melaleuca with frankincense, lavender, sandalwood, or rosemary.
- Helichrysum with basil or peppermint.

Use: Add 1-3 drops to the corresponding single oils above (according to your sensitivity).

Blends:

- Melaleuca (single oil) with Clarity, 3 Wise Men, Valor, Harmony, or Present Time.
- Helichrysum (single oil) with Clarity.

Use: Add 1-3 drops of each single oil to the corresponding blends above (according to your sensitivity).

Helichrysum lessens the effects of shock.

Use Clarity, Valor, or 3 Wise Men when a person has passed out from shock due to an accident or from emotional shock.

Bone Spurs

Bone spurs are a calcium deposit/growth that forms generally from the cartilage.

Single oils:

- Cypress with birch, marjoram, or rosemary.
- Cypress with birch and marjoram.
- Cypress with marjoram and rosemary.

Use: Add 1-3 drops to the corresponding single oils above (according to your sensitivity).

Blends: R.C.

Birch helps dissolve calcium deposits.

Apply oils neat on location, then massage using Vita Flex Technique.

Brain Function, Synapse, Neural Cortex

When the nucleus of a neuron cell fires, it sends a signal along the axon to a synapse or synaptic contact point. As the signal reaches the end of the axon, it triggers the release of neurotransmitters across the synapse, which in turn causes the receiving neuron to fire. If these points are blocked by metal or chemicals between them, the neural transmitter has only two options: One is to backfire along the axon, which causes a deterioration of the myelin sheath, which results in multiple sclerosis (MS). The second is to cross to another synaptic point. This results in Parkinson's, Lou Gerhig's, Alzheimer's, and like diseases, depending on where the firing releases.

Dr. Richard Restick, a leading neurologist in Washington, D.C., stated that if we can maintain normal synaptic firing, then we will not have deterioration of the glands or the body. It has also been said that if there were a substance that could go beyond the bloodbrain barrier to heal and regenerate the tissues, perhaps there would be help for diseases like Parkinson's, Lou Gerhig's, MS, and Alzheimer's.

Sesquiterpenes have been documented to cross the bloodbrain barrier. Frankincense, cypress, lavender, and sandalwood are good examples of oils that are high in this constituent.

Essential oils increase synaptic firing, resulting in increased neural transmitter activity in the brain and in the nervous system. Oils also chelate heavy metals and chemicals out of tissues.

People, who get an instant headache from diffusing Clarity have a blockage related to metalics or chemicals in the brain. The main oil in Clarity is cardamom, containing high levels of transphenols, which are very high in oxygen molecules. They can create, almost an instant headache when there are chemicals or metalics in the brain.

Commercial floral perfumes limit the range of brain activity. The use of essential oils increases a wide variation of brain activity and blood/glucose conversion through electro-magnetic fields in the brain. The breathing of oils helps the brain increase blood flow by 15% and brain blood oxygen by 25%, resulting in increased blood glucose conversion and electro-magnetic fields in the brain, thus affecting the immune system. These findings are from the research of Dr. Asawa of Japan and Dr. Richardson of England.

The left brain is logical, rational, judgmental, and conscious and not as responsive as the right side; i.e., students, accountants, and engineers. The right brain is the subconscious and super-conscious part of the limbic system. The limbic system is located on the margin of the cerebral cortex, including the amygdala, hippocampus, and other components, which interact directly with the thalamus and hypothalamus. Acting together, these glands and brain components are the seat of memory, emotions, sexual arousal, and govern aggressive behavior.

When working with oils one becomes much sharper in the right brain than the left brain, actually moving one into balance.

Single oils:

- Helichrysum with frankincense, peppermint, melissa, or nutmeg.

Use: 1-3 drops of single oils (according to your sensitivity).

Blends:

- Brain Power, Helichrysum or Frankincense (single oils) with Aroma Life.

Use: Add 1-3 drops of each single oil to the corresponding blends above (according to your sensitivity).

Supplements: JuvaTone, VitaGreen, Chelex, A. D. & E., and Sulfurzyme.

Seizures: Sugar is the number one cause of brain seizures.

Topical Application: Brain Power and Valor.

Monitor diet for food allergies.

Helichrysum activates the neural cortex (nervous function), increases neural transmitter activity in the axon of nerves, enhances brain synapse and is a chelator. Aroma Life contains helichrysum. Frankincense has been documented to cross the blood-brain barrier. There are indications that other oils do also. Nutmeg is a general cerebral stimulant because it has adrenal cortex-like activity and supports the adrenals.

Put the oils as directly onto the nerve circuitry as is practical. The brain reflex points on the head are as follow: forehead, temple, and mastoids (the bones just behind the ears). Use direct pressure application to the brain stem located on the center of the backbone, on the neck at the skull, and down the spine.

Direct pressure application to the brain stem. What seems to work well is putting the oil on a back brush and rubbing along the spine as vigorously as desired.

NOTE: Use a natural bristle brush, since the oils dissolve some plastics.

To help chelate heavy metals and chemicals, apply oils to the carotid arteries in the neck at pulse points where arteries are closest to the surface, the spine at the base of the skull, mastoids (lumps behind the ears), temples, center of the forehead, and crown (top of the skull). VitaGreen binds with heavy metals in the nervous system to carry them out of the body.

See Blood Circulation, Blood Cleansing - Detoxification. Also see Cardiovascular System and Vascular Cleansing.

(See also NEUROLOGICAL DISEASES.)

Brain Wave Repair

Single oils: Peppermint with basil, frankincense, sandalwood, or rosemary.

Blends: Brain Power and Clarity.

Supplements: Royal Essence

Diffuse, rub on temples and brain stem at back of neck. Take Royal Essence 4 to 5 droppers 2-3 times/day.

Concentration

Single oils: Basil, lemon, and bergamot.

Blends: Brain Power, Clarity, Harmony, and Valor.

Inhale Clarity, rub Harmony on the crown and on throat, and rub Valor on the forehead.

(See also DIFFUSING and INHALATION.)

Memory

Single oils:

- Lemongrass with basil, rosemary, peppermint or rose.

- Rosemary with basil, lemon, peppermint, clove, cardamom, or helichrysum.

Use: Add 1-3 drops to the corresponding single oils above (according to your sensitivity).

Blends: Brain Power

- Lemongrass with Clarity.

- Rosemary with M-Grain.

- Clarity with En-R-Gee (indirectly because of boost in one's energy level).

Use: Add 1-3 drops of each single oil to the corresponding blends above (according to your sensitivity).

Supplements: Royal Essence and VitaGreen.

These oils improve memory by stimulating an opening of emotional blocks.

A drop of peppermint in a glass of water helps some people to wake up brain and memory functions. Rosemary and peppermint is a good combination. Inhaling peppermint has shown a 28% increase in mental accuracy (Dr. Dembar, University of Cincinnati).

Put oils on a cotton ball or tissue, store in a zip lock bag, and inhale during exams or where other mental stimulation is required.

The fragrance of diffused oils as we inhale them helps in increasing memory retention and recall. Lemon has been reported to work here (see Inhalation Therapy).

Improving Memory

- 5 drops basil
- 10 drops rosemary
- 2 drops peppermint
- 4 drops helichrysum

Mix in 1/2 to 1 ounce of massage oil or V-6 Mixing Oil or Massage Oil Base.

Rub on temples, forehead, mastoids (bone behind ears), brain stem (back of neck).

Memory and emotion blend:
- 4 drops lavender
- 3 drops geranium
- 3 drops rosewood
- 3 drops rosemary
- 2 drops tangerine
- 1 drop spearmint
- 2 drops tansy

Blend in 1/2 to 1 ounce V-6 Mixing Oil or Massage Oil Base. Rub on temples, forehead, mastoids (bone behind ears), brain stem (back of neck).

Do a colon and liver cleanse (see COLON).

Vascular cleansing will allow better and unimpeded blood flow, giving improved distribution of oxygen and nutrients (see VASCULAR CLEANSING).

Mental Fatigue

Single oils: Ylang ylang, rosemary, and peppermint.

Blends: Brain Power and Clarity.

Diffuse and wear as a cologne or perfume.

Mental (Mind) Stimulation

Single oils: Cardamom, peppermint, and frankincense.

Blends: Brain Power, Acceptance, and Clarity.

Supplements: Stevia

Ingesting Stevia raises blood sugar levels, increasing energy and mental acuity.

Pineal/Pituitary

Single oils: Sandalwood, lavender, and frankincense.

Blends: Dream Catcher, Forgiveness, Gathering, Harmony, Humility, 3 Wise Men, and ImmuPower.

These blends contain frankincense and sandalwood, which oxygenate the pineal/pituitary gland, thus improving attitude and body frequency balance (see BODY FREQUENCY (ELECTRICAL) BALANCING).

Stroke

Single oils: Helichrysum with cypress, juniper, or peppermint.

Use: Add 1-3 drops of the single oils (according to your sensitivity).

Blends:

- Helichrysum with Aroma Life, Brain Power, or Clarity.

- Lemon with ImmuPower.

Use: Add 1-3 drops of each single oil to the corresponding blends above (according to your sensitivity).

Massage on back of neck, on brain stem, and on the brain Vita Flex points of the feet and hands. Applying ImmuPower over the thymus has helped stroke victims.

Bronchitis

Single oils: Cypress, rosemary, lemon, cinnamon, eucalyptus, frankincense, marjoram, sandalwood, ravensara, thyme, birch, myrrh, dill, fir, spruce, pine, oregano, helichrysum, rose, melaleuca, clove, lavender, spearmint, clary sage, hyssop, and myrtle.

- Mix 1 to 2 drops of cypress with any of the following: rosemary, lemon, cinnamon, eucalyptus, frankincense, marjoram, or sandalwood.

- Mix 2 to 3 drops of frankincense with any of the following: ravensara, cypress, lemon, thyme, rosemary, eucalyptus, birch, myrtle, or hyssop.

- Mix 2 to 3 drops of lavender with any of the following: lemon, lemongrass, ginger, tarragon, peppermint, frankincense, oregano, thyme, spearmint, clary sage, dill, myrrh, or rose.

- Mix 2 to 3 drops of melaleuca or rosemary with any of the following: fir, spruce, pine, oregano, helichrysum, thyme, or cinnamon.

- Mix 1 to 2 drops of thyme with any of the following: ravensara, oregano, melaleuca, frankincense, clove, cinnamon, or lavender.

Add more drops (1 to 5) if desired according to your sensitivity.

Blends: Exodus II, ImmuPower, R.C., Raven, Melrose, Thieves, and Purification.

- Lavender with Melrose or Thieves.

- Cypress or frankincense with Raven, or R.C.

- Melaleuca or rosemary with Melrose, Purification, R.C., or Brain Power.

- Sage with R.C., Thieves, or Raven.

- Thyme with Melrose, Purification, Thieves, or Brain Power.

Use: Mix 1-3 drops of any of the single oils listed first with any of the following blends listed.

Gargle with any combination once every hour.

Rub 1 to 2 drops of Thieves, Exodus, Immu-Power, R.C., or Raven on the bottom of feet and diluted on neck and chest.

Supplements: ImmuGel, Radex, Super C, ImmuneTune, Exodus, Cleansing Trio, and Fresh Essence.

Mouth Wash

- ImmuGel: 1/2 tsp. every 3 to 4 hours. Hold in mouth for 30 seconds for better absorption.

- Radex: 2 to 3 tablets 3 to 4 times daily. Works as a free radical scavenger.

- Super C: 2 to 4 tablets 4 times daily.

- ImmuneTune: 2 to 4 capsules 4 times daily.

- Exodus: 2 to 4 capsules 4 times daily or as desired.

- Cleansing Trio: See Colon and Liver Cleanse.

- Fresh Essence: Gargle whenever desired.

- Diffuse: Raven, Thieves, R.C., ImmuPower, Exodus II, and Purification. Alternate the oils every hour, but diffuse for about 15 minutes or as desired. Alternating Raven and R.C. works very well.

- Alternate Raven and R.C. in an implant and topical application.

- Exodus II: Gargle and massage chest.

Massage the above blends on the bottom of the feet on the Vita Flex points as well as the hands.

Put 2 to 3 drops of any of the oils mentioned in 4 to 6 ounces of water and gargle.

Fresh Essence soothes a sore throat and may be swallowed. Myrrh is very effective for throat problems, and hoarseness. Pine dilates and opens bronchial tubes. Raven strengthens the respiratory system, dilates and opens the pulmonary tract, fights respiratory infections. Rose, sage, and sandalwood help chronic bronchitis. For respiratory conditions combine 1 drop each of, myrtle, mountain savory, and eucalyptus radiata with 4 drops Raven in 1 Tbsp. V-6 Mixing Oil or Massage Oil Base and insert as a rectal implant. An easy way to implant is to buy a small enema syringe, empty out the contents, fill with oil mixture, and insert before going to sleep. Retain throughout the night (*see Rectal Implant*).

Bruising

Some people bruise easily because the capillary walls are weak and break easily, particularly in the skin.

Single oils:

- 1 to 2 drops helichrysum or lavender with cypress, Idaho tansy, lemongrass, geranium, peppermint, rosemary, or Roman chamomile.

- 1 to 2 drops clove with black pepper, peppermint, cypress, marjoram, or geranium.

- 2 to 3 drops cypress in V-6 Mixing Oil or Massage Oil Base

Use: Add 1-3 drops to the corresponding single oils above (according to your sensitivity).

Supplements: Master HIS, Master HERS, Vita-Green, JuvaTone, Rehemogen, and Super C.

Nearly all skin problems are related to liver function. People who bruise easily are usually deficient in vitamin C, which causes poor absorption. Super C is easy to assimilate, is an all-natural product, and contains citrus oils, which are high in flavonoids.

Mix 3 to 4 drops of cypress in 1/2 oz. V-6 Mixing Oil or Massage Oil Base and spread over the area to strengthen capillary walls.

2 to 3 drops of helichrysum works like a natural hemostat and helps to absorb the blood back into the tissue.

- Master Formula HIS/HERS: 2 to 6 tablets 3 times daily (the ingredients of choline bitartrate, inositol, and dl methionine found in Master formula support immune function).

- VitaGreen: 2 to 6 capsules 3 times daily.

- JuvaTone: 2 to 6 tablets 3 times daily. Nearly all skin problems are related to liver function.

- Super C: 2 to 6 tablets 3 times daily or as desired.

Recipe 1:

- 1 drop helichrysum
- 3 drops lavender
- 2 drops lemongrass
- 2 drops geranium
- 1 drop peppermint

Mix in 1/2 oz. V-6 Mixing Oil or Massage Oil Base and apply over area.

Recipe 2:

- 2 drops lavender
- 3 drops rosemary
- 1 drop geranium

Mix together in water and saturate wash cloth or towel and apply as compress over area (see COMPRESSES). Apply 4 to 5 drops neat (undiluted) or mix in V-6 Mixing Oil or Massage Oil Base and rub over affected area.

Deep tissue bruising and pain:
- 8 drops clove
- 8 drops black pepper oil
- 4 drops peppermint
- 5 drops cypress
- 8 drops marjoram
- 5 drops geranium

Mix into 1/2 to 3/4 V-6 Mixing Oil or Massage Oil Base and apply.

Burns

Single oils:

- Lavender with peppermint, Idaho tansy, helichrysum, and rose. Use peppermint sparingly: 1 drop to 5 to 10 drops lavender.

Blends:

- Lavender with Gentle Baby or Sunsation with LavaDerm Cooling Mist.

Use: Add 1-3 drops of each single oil to the corresponding blends above (according to your sensitivity).

Supplements: Colloidal Essence, LavaDerm Cooling Mist, and Rose Ointment.

Colloidal silver (contained in Colloidal Essence) is used externally nationwide in burn units as an antibiotic against microbes on the burnt skin (Dr. Terry Friedmann).

Application: Chill LavaDerm. Keep refrigerated. Apply LavaDerm every 15 minutes the first day. Apply 3 to 5 drops of lavender as needed immediately after misting. On days 2 through 5, mist every 1/2 to 1 hour and follow with lavender. Continue using burn spray 3 to 6 times daily until healed. Apply Rose Ointment to keep tissue soft.

Lavender is very effective on burns and may be applied neat. Add a few drops of AromaSilk Satin Body Lotion to help reduce the pain of burns.

Rose Ointment is soothing and helps keep tissue soft. Add a few drops of lavender to enhance benefit.

Helichrysum is a tissue regenerator and reduces scarring and discoloration.

CAUTION: All burns can be serious, so seek medical attention if necessary.

Peppermint is soothing and cooling to tissue reducing inflammation and fever in damaged tissue. However, it also stings when applied to a fresh burn. Wait 1 to 2 days or mix 1 drop peppermint with 1 drop lavender and dilute in 1/2 oz. V-6 Mixing Oil or Massage Oil Base. After a couple of days, peppermint may be applied to the sealed over burn.

After a burn is healed and is drying and cracking, use Rose Ointment or body lotion with a few drops of lavender added to keep skin soft and promote faster healing.

Shock

If the burn is large or if it is from an accident, the individual may be in shock. Inhaling oils may help reduce the shock. Use 1 to 2 drops of Trauma Life on temples, back of neck, and under nose. Put 1 to 2 drops in hands and then cup over nose and breathe deeply.

Single oils:

- Melaleuca with frankincense, lavender, sandalwood, or rosemary.

- Helichrysum with basil or peppermint.

Use: Add 1-3 drops to the corresponding single oils (according to your sensitivity).

Blends:

- Apply 1 to 2 drops Clarity, 3 Wise Men, Brain Power, Trauma Life, Valor, Harmony, or Present Time.

- Apply 1 to 2 drops of helichrysum with Clarity.

Helichrysum lessens the effects of shock.

If a person has passed out from shock, apply 1 to 2 drops of Clarity, Trauma Life, or peppermint under the nose, on the thymus, on temples, back of neck, and the thymus. Clarity should restore consciousness. Valor and 3 Wise Men are also excellent for emotional shock.

Bursitis

Single oils: Marjoram, basil, lavender, pepper, spruce, fir, pine, birch, Idaho tansy, and elemi

- Birch with oregano.

Blends: Relieve It and PanAway.

Use: Add 1-3 drops to the corresponding oils above (according to your sensitivity).

Supplements: Arthro Plus, ArthroTune, AlkaLime, Super Cal, Essential Manna, and Sulfurzyme

Bursitis may signal the beginning of arthritis.

Cancer

Researchers have linked most degenerative diseases to lack of nutrients in the body. Minerals and trace minerals are a large part of our nutritional deficiencies.

With this type of degenerative situation in the body, it is important to have strong cleansing and nutritional building programs, regardless of the type of problem. The following is a suggested program that you may tailor to fit your particular needs. Other suggestions would be in addition to these programs.

Cleansing: Cleansing Trio with JuvaTone

Megazyme program:

Phase 1: Start with 3 tablets 3 times daily. Increase amount by 1 tablet every day until vomiting starts. At this point, stop Megazyme for 24-36 hours.

Phase 2: Start again with 4 tablets 3 times daily. Increase daily amount until vomiting starts again. Stop and rest for 24-36 hours.

Phase 3: Start with 5 tablets 3 times daily. Increase amount by one tablet every day until vomiting starts. Rest for 24-36 hours.

Phase 4: Go back to the amount taken before vomiting occurred the third time. Continue this amount for 6 weeks.

Phase 5: Start enzyme (Megazyme) saturation again.

Anyone with cancer should skip phase 3 and rest at least 1 day per week.

When starting this program, it is best to be monitored by a health care professional:

Supplements: Master Formula HIS/HERS, VitaGreen, Super C, Radex, ImmuneTune, Ultra Young, Seagal Power Meal, Thyromin, Exodus, Sulfurzyme, AlkaLime, Rehemogen, Mineral Essence, and Royaldophilus.

- Master HIS/HERS: 6 to 8 tablets per day.

- VitaGreen: 8 to 18 capsules per day.

- Super C: 8 to 18 tablets per day.

- Radex: 8 to 12 tablets per day.

- ImmuneTune : 6 to 12 capsules per day.

- Ultra Young: 3 squirts 3 times daily.

- Seagal Power Meal or Body Balance: 2 to 3 scoops 3 times daily.

- Megazyme: 2 to 6 tablets 3 times daily according to blood type.

- Thyromin: Start 1 before bedtime and increase as needed.

- Exodus: 6 to 8 capsules daily

- Sulfurzyme: Begin with 1 tsp. 3 times daily and work up to 1-3 Tbsp. daily.

- AlkaLime: 1 Tbsp. in water daily.

Drink AlkaLime 1 hour before meals or 1 hour after meals. Do not drink with food and do not mix with any juice or milk. **Drink only with water**. Degenerative disease flourishes in an acid environment but will not grow in an alkaline environment. (See BODY pH - ACID/ALKALINE BALANCE.)

- Rehemogen: 3 droppers 3 times daily. Detoxifies blood.

- Mineral Essence: 3 to 4 droppers 3 times daily.

- Royaldophilus: 2 to 3 capsules 3 times daily. Ensures good digestion and assimilation.

With cancer there is always a deficiency in vitamin B5 and pantothenic acid. Super B is a good source of all B vitamins. Exodus is a good source of pantothenic acid complex. An adequate supply of all vitamins and minerals is important so that the body has the required nutrients to fight any disease.

Blood Types

0 blood types need higher amounts of supplements and will find that they generally can take as many supplements as desired and not over do.

Single oils:

- Frankincense with helichrysum, clove, lavender, inula, Idaho tansy, or clary sage.

Blends:

- ImmuPower and Grounding (for emotions related to the disease).

Use: Add 1-3 drops of oil to the corresponding oils above (according to your sensitivity).

General application of oils: Neat, direct on skin cancers, cancerous nodes, or on Vita Flex points for internal cancers. Apply on the spine up to 3 times daily.

Supplements: ImmuneTune, Super C, Radex, Master Formula HIS/HERS, and VitaGreen.

Terry S. Friedman, M.D., conducted an experimental cancer program. All ten people that were on the program are now healthy. One little girl had a massive tumor on her forehead, spinal problems, and was on morphine. Three days into this program she was off of the morphine; 2 weeks later off Tylenol; 1 month later her tumor was gone; she had gained 7 pounds and her spine was 75% regenerated. Dr. Friedmann's program is as follows:

- ImmuneTune: 1 capsule

- Super C: 6 tablets

- Radex: 3 tablets

- Master Formula HIS/HERS: 1 tablet

- Vitagreen: 2 capsules

Use: Take 6 to 7 times daily:

Apply frankincense on tumorous growths and ImmuPower on spine and bottom of feet 2 times daily. Mix 6 to 10 drops each of frankincense and clove and massage on location.

Cancer cells cannot live or grow in the presence of pure essential oils.

They will only grow in an oxygen starved environment. Hormone imbalance is also a factor in serious disease. Natural progesterone helps restore proper cellar oxygen. EssPro 7 helps restore balance as well as providing a good source of natural progesterone.

Clean, healthy blood, assists in overcoming any disease. Rehemogen cleans blood, carries nutrients and oxygen to the cells to help bring back good health. (See BLOOD.)

Mix:

- 12 drops frankincense
- 5 drops lavender
- 6 drops bergamot
- 6 drops helichrysum

Use neat for serious conditions or in 1 oz. V-6 Mixing Oil or Massage Oil Base for maintenance and long-term use.

Wolfberry detoxifies and cleanses. The Chinese who eat Wolfberry are not recorded as developing cancer.

When people have terminal illness, their minds are fractured, and they have difficulty focusing and bringing their thoughts together. Gathering helps you gather your thoughts and feelings for greater focus and clarity.

Damage and burns from radiation (see RADIATION DAMAGE).

Brain Tumors

Single oils:

- Frankincense with clove.

Use: Add 1-3 drops (according to your sensitivity).

Take supplements as suggested above under Cancer.

Cleanse: Cleansing Trio and JuvaTone.

Brain: Inhale frankincense until nauseated and massage frankincense on brain stem and carotid arteries. Apply frankincense orally on the roof of the mouth and the boucle cavity with your finger.

Start Megazyme program:

- Take 20 Radex, 15 to 20 Immune Tune, 15 Exodus, and 20 Super C per day.
- Maintain a concentrated carrot juice diet. Potassium is critical. Drink plenty of Dandelion Tea (diuretic) and Yellow Dock Tea (iron).

Blood flow to the brain is extremely important. This can be obtained in vertical positions.

Application:

- Mix 4 drops frankincense and 5 drops ImmuPower and massage on the neck.

- Mix 15 drops frankincense and 6 drops clove in 1/2 oz. V-6 Mixing Oil or Massage Oil Base and rub several times per day on the brain stem (spine at base of skull), temples, mastoids (behind the ears), forehead, and crown (top of head).
- Put 10 drops frankincense and 1 drop clove in diffuser. Sit in front of the diffuser and breathe vapors for 1/2 hour, 3 times a day. If you get a headache or feel nauseous, reduce to what is tolerable, but do not quit.
- AlkaLime: 1 Tbsp. in water 1 hour before or after meals to help restore pH balance.

Bone Tumors

Single oils: Frankincense and clove.

Mix 15 drops frankincense and 6 drops clove in 1/2 oz. V-6 Mixing Oil or Massage Oil Base and massage on location daily.

Blends: ImmuPower

Apply 2 to 3 drops each of frankincense and ImmuPower on the spine, 3 times per day.

Supplements: Cleansing Trio

Cleanse: Cleansing Trio

Breast Lumps (Benign and Malignant)

Single oils: Frankincense, lavender, clove.

Blends: Present Time and Brain Power.

Supplements: As suggested, including Femi-Gen, EssPro 7, Femalin, Seagal Power Meal, Body Balance, Mineral Essence, and Super Cal.

Rub frankincense on breast Vita Flex points on feet, which is on top of the foot at the base of the three middle toes. Massage Vita Flex areas after applying the oils. (See VITA FLEX.)

Prevention: Keep lymphatics open with deep breathing exercise and aerobics. Have a body massage with Cel-lite Magic once per month to work the lymph nodes in the abdomen and the thoracic region.

Oil Application: Massage oils for 4 days and then rest for 4 days. Layer 15 drops frankincense, 10 drops lavender, and 3 drops clove. Apply 3 drops of Present Time in a clockwise rotation on the sternum. Put 30 to 60 drops of frankincense in a capsule and swallow daily. Diffuse frankincense and Brain Power.

Do Colon and Liver Cleanse (see COLON).

Cancer cells will only grow in an oxygen-starved environment. Natural progesterone helps restore proper cell oxygen levels. EssPro 7 is a good source of natural progesterone.

The soy in the Body Balance helps protect the hormone (estrogen) receptors and therefore assist hormone regulation. Mix 2 to 3 Tbsp. Body Balance with water or juice and drink 1 to 2 times daily.

Discontinue use of antiperspirants and monitor calcium levels.

Do not take colloidal minerals as they block energy in the body's meridians, which may cause nodules to develop in the lymphatic system.

Colon

Single oils: Clove, frankincense, and lavender.

Day 1: Put 23 drops of frankincense in a capsule and swallow 3 to 4 times daily

Day 2: Mix 18 drops frankincense and 5 drops clove and put in capsule. Swallow 3 to 4 times daily.

Day 3: Frankincense and Lavender (equal parts) capsule 3 to 4 times per day

Day 4: Frankincense capsules 3 to 4 times per day.

Rest for 4 days and continue.

Supplements: Cleansing Trio

Begin with Megazyme to digest toxic waste.

ComforTone: Begin 2 capsules 3 times daily. Increase by one everyday until the bowels move. Afterwards begin reducing. If diarrhea occurs, reduce amount and increase I.C.P. Drink plenty of purified or distilled water.

I.C.P. Fiber cleanse: Begin with 1 Tbsp. in water 3 times daily. Increase to 2 Tbsp. 3 times daily or as desired until bowels are moving regularly.

Leukemia

Single oils: Frankincense

Use: Apply in a full body massage.

Blends: Thieves

Use: Apply on bottom of the feet.

Supplements: Rehemogen, Radex, Super C, ImmuneTune, VitaGreen, and Royal Essence.

Take the following, daily throughout the day:

- Rehemogen: 3 droppers 3 times daily in water.
- Radex: 10 tablets daily.
- Super C: 12 tablets daily.
- ImmuneTune: 15 capsules daily.
- Vitagreen: 9 capsules daily.
- Royal Essence: 9 droppers daily in water.
- Fresh Carrot Juice: 1/2 gallon.

Do not eat white flour, sugar, salt, or red meat.

Liver

Single oils: Frankincense, lavender, clove.

- 30 drops frankincense, 20 drops lavender, and 10 drops clove in a castor oil compress 5 nights per week.

Blends: JuvaFlex

- Rub JuvaFlex over the liver, with or without compresses or hot packs, alternating with rubbing on liver Vita Flex points on the feet (see COMPRESS).

Supplements: JuvaTone and Ultra Young (with supplement program as stated).

Vita Life Juice Drink (see CLEANSING).

Cleansing is extremely important since an optimal functioning liver is necessary to rid the body of toxins. The emotions of anger and hate are stored in the liver and cause extreme toxicity and eventually disease.

Lung Cancer

Single oils:

- Frankincense with sage, myrrh, clove, raven, or hyssop.

Use: Add 1-3 drops to the corresponding single oils (according to your sensitivity).

Blends:

- Frankincense with ImmuPower.

Use: Add 1-3 drops (according to your sensitivity).

Diffuse R.C. and frankincense.

Day 1 rectal implant: R.C. (20 drops) and frankincense (20 drops).

Day 2 rectal implant: Raven and frankincense equal parts.

Day 3 rectal implant: Frankincense and lavender equal parts.

Day 4 rectal implant: Frankincense.

Day 5 rectal implant: R.C. and frankincense.

Rest 2 days and continue. If a noticeable improvement is not detected, do not rest.

Alternate:

Eucalyptus globulus: 10 drops

Frankincense: 10 drops (expectorant)

Peppermint and frankincense: 10 drops each (to break up mucus)

Tangerine: 40 drops

Cypress: 10 drops

Peppermint: 5 drops for edema in the cavity due to tumor on outside of lung.

Diffuse oil combinations used in rectal implants consistently.

Take internally, in a capsule, clove (10 drops) and frankincense (5 drops).

Do full body massages:
- Clove: 10 drops
- Frankincense: 5 drops

1 tsp. V-6 Mixing Oil or Massage Oil Base. Alternate with clove and lavender every day for a minimum of 7 days.

Mix in sequence for a rectal implant:
- 2 drops sage
- 4 drops myrrh
- 5 drops clove
- 6 drops Raven
- 5 drops frankincense

Mix in 1/2 oz. (1 Tbsp.) V-6 Mixing Oil or Massage Oil Base. Use enema syringe to implant and retain through the night (see RECTAL IMPLANT).

Rub ImmuPower up the spine, daily. Compress on back and chest twice daily.

Supplements: Super C, K & B, Goji Berry Tea, Super Cal, and Essential Manna.

Take daily Super C, 30 to 40 capsules, Dandelion Tea, raw lemon juice, red clover tea, K & B, and Goji Berry Tea.

Edema: Super Cal, Essential Manna, pomegranate juice, or organic bananas

Lymphoma - cancer of lymph glands

Both Hodgkin's disease and non-Hodgkin's disease are characterized by swollen lymph gland nodes, generally first appearing on the neck, armpit or groin. Other possible symptoms for non-Hodgkin's are feeling generally ill, loss of appetite, loss of weight, fever and night sweats. Other possible symptoms for Hodgkin's, which often occur in early adulthood are fever, sweating, fatigue, weakness, itching.

A major cause of lymphoma is pollution from petrochemicals in the air and water. The lymphatic system tries to clear out the pollution but often becomes clogged.

Single oils:

- Frankincense with myrrh and sage.

Use: Add 1-3 drops (according to your sensitivity).

Mix:
- 10 drops frankincense
- 5 drops myrrh
- 3 drops sage
- 1/2 to 1 oz. V-6 Mixing Oil or Massage Oil Base.

Apply on swollen nodes daily. Every second day apply 1 or 2 drops of frankincense. For faster results apply in a rectal implant.

Rub along spine twice daily. Every other day rub frankincense, neat, along spine. Rub Immu-Power 3 times per day on spine.

A program for lymphoma stage 4 (very fatty bone marrow):

Body massage:
- 15 drops frankincense
- 6 drops clove
- 1 oz. (2 Tbsp.) V-6 Mixing Oil or Massage Oil Base.

Supplements: ImmuneTune, Super C, Vita-Green, Cleansing Trio, and Radex.

Take 4 ImmuneTune 3 times per day, 6 Super C 3 times per day, 6 VitaGreen 3 times per day, and 3 Radex 4 times per day.

Follow this program for 1 month, then gradually reduce. If lymphoma goes into remission, continue program for 1 month, then gradually reduce. It is best to be on a total vegetarian diet. For 0 blood types that may need more protein, eat fresh stream trout or arctic salmon.

Do a colon and liver cleanse (see COLON). JuvaTone is particularly important, since the liver is the detoxifying organ of the body.

(See LYMPHATIC SYSTEM.)

Melanoma - Skin Cancer

Single oils:

- Frankincense with inula, lavender, Idaho tansy, melaleuca, lemongrass, or tarragon.

Use: Add 1-3 drops to the corresponding single oils above (according to your sensitivity).

Blends:

- Frankincense with Release, JuvaFlex, EndoFlex, Purification, or Gentle Baby.

Use: Add 1-3 drops of each single oil to the corresponding blends above (according to your sensitivity).

Apply frankincense neat, on location, 2 or 3 times daily. For prevention, apply frankincense to any odd lumps, rough moles, or red rough lesions that develop on the skin. Idaho tansy has been reported to help reduce odd lumps and growths as well.

Mix:
- 3 drops lavender
- 4 drops frankincense

Mix in 3/4 oz. V-6 Mixing Oil or Massage Oil Base. Apply 3 times daily.

Rawhide or Pharaoh Aftershave help to reduce the incidence of melanoma. Add 2 to 3 drops of frankincense to each.

Ovarian Cancer

Single oils:

- Frankincense with myrrh and geranium.

Use: Add 1-3 drops to the corresponding single oils above (according to your sensitivity).

Blends:

- Frankincense with ImmuPower.

Use: Add *1-3 drops of each single oil to the corresponding blends above (according to your sensitivity).*

Supplements: FemiGen, Femalin, Body Balance, EssPro 7, Protec, and ArthroTune.

Supplements as suggested.

- Drink 3 to 4 cups Goji Berry Tea daily.

- Mix 1 to 2 scoops of Body Balance in water or juice and drink 3 times daily. Soy helps protect the hormone (estrogen) receptors assisting in hormone regulation.

Mix:
- 15 drops frankincense
- 5 drops myrrh
- 6 drops geranium
- 1/2 oz. V-6 Mixing Oil or Massage Oil Base

Alternate vaginal retention implant 1 night and rectal implant the next night. (See VAGINAL and RECTAL IMPLANTS.)

Rub 3 to 4 drops ImmuPower up the spine, on the feet, and on the throat, daily.

Protec: Use as douche. Start with 1/2 tsp. at night and work up to 1 to 2 Tbsp. Retain throughout the night. Protec is already diluted. If irritation occurs, discontinue for 3 days and start again with a smaller amount. To make stronger, extra oils may be added and used for alternating applications. Add 3 to 4 drops of frankincense. The next night add 3 to 4 drops of clove. The next night add 3 to 4 drops of myrrh, etc.

Rub topically over the abdomen, over the ovaries, and also over the reproductive Vita Flex areas on hands and feet. These Vita Flex areas are inside of wrists and around the front of the ankles in line with the ankle bone, and particularly inside and outside of the foot just above the ankle bone and up along the achilles tendon.

Prostrate Cancer

Single oils:

• Frankincense with myrrh, sage, or anise seed oil.

Use: Add 1-3 drops to the corresponding single oils above (according to your sensitivity).

Blends: Mister

Supplements: Super B, ProGen, EssPro 7, Protec, Cleansing Trio, and JuvaTone.

Supplements as suggested.

Mix:
• 10 drops frankincense
• 5 drops myrrh
• 3 drops sage

Mix in 1 Tbsp. (15 ml.) V-6 Mixing Oil or Massage Oil Base for rectal implant (see RECTAL IMPLANT).

Protec is very beneficial as a rectal implant. Start with 1 Tbsp. the first night and work up to 1 to 2 Tbsp. and continue for 7 consecutive nights. If irritation occurs, discontinue for 3 days before restarting Protec. If irritation occurs, discontinue for 3 days and start again with smaller amount. To make stronger, extra oils may be added and used for alternating applications. Add 3 to 4 drops of frankincense. The next night add 3 to 4 drops clove. The next night add 3 to 4 drops myrrh, etc.

This application has taken PSA (prostate specific antigen) counts from 23.5 down to 5.5, which is considered high end to normal in 2 months.

Rub topically on the area between the rectum and scrotum and also on the reproductive Vita Flex areas on hands and feet. These areas are inside of the wrists and around the front of the ankles in line with the ankle bone and particularly inside and outside of the foot just above the ankle bone and up along the achilles tendon. This has helped reduce the pain and has been credited for moving into remission.

Do a colon and liver cleanse (see COLON).

Uterine Cancer

Environmental pollutants become lodged in fatty tissue, such as the breasts, thyroid, ovaries, and uterus. Many chemicals mimic or imitate our natural hormones and can fit the hormone receptors, thus tricking and over-stimulating these organs. This can become a major source of cancer of the breast, uterus, and lymph nodes.

(Same program as OVARIAN CANCER.)

Candida

Single oils: Melaleuca, rosemary, thyme, and hyssop.

Blends: Melrose and Mister.

Supplements: ImmuGel, Thyromin, Protec, Megazyme, and Mineral Essence.

(See VAGINAL YEAST INFECTION, SKIN CANDIDA, FUNGUS)

Canker Sores

These tend to occur because of stress, illness, weakened immune system, injury caused by such things as hot food, rough brushing of teeth, or dentures. Herpes Simplex, a virus, that causes blisters, may develop into an ulcer.

Single oils:

• Sage with clove or lavender.

Use: Add 1-3 drops to the corresponding single oils above (according to your sensitivity).

Blends:

• Sage with Thieves.

Use: Add 1-3 drops (according to your sensitivity).

Cardiovascular System

Plaque Removal

High Cholesterol

Single oils:

- Rosemary with helichrysum.

- Helichrysum with German chamomile, Roman chamomile, clary sage, geranium, or fennel.

Use: 1-3 drops to the corresponding single oils above (according to your sensitivity).

Blends:

- Rosemary with Clarity, Aroma Life, or JuvaFlex.

- Helichrysum with Di-Tone, JuvaFlex, or EndoFlex.

Use: Add 1-3 drops of each single oil to the corresponding blends above (according to your sensitivity).

Apply neat on arteries at pulse points where the arteries are close to the surface, or mix with V-6 Mixing Oil or Massage Oil Base for body massage.

Aroma Life is a help and benefit to regulate and lower blood pressure. Aroma Life contains helichrysum. Rosemary breaks down plaque. Helichrysum is a chelator; it lowers and regulates cholesterol and is an anticoagulant. (For application, see Heart Vita Flex under Blood Pressure.)

Supplements: JuvaTone, Cleansing Trio, Vita-Green, Radex, Super C, Super Cal, ImmuGel, Royal Essence, Mineral Essence, Chelex, and Goji Berry Tea.

Do a colon and liver cleanse using the Cleansing Trio, JuvaTone, and JuvaFlex (see COLON). JuvaTone is particularly useful for high cholesterol. I.C.P. helps break down plaque.

Mix 25 drops of HRT in 6 ounces of distilled water, 3 times daily. Supports blood system and circulation deficiency.

Sheep milk lowers cholesterol. Goji Berry Tea helps reduce cholesterol and burn fat.

Magnesium acts as a smooth muscle relaxant and supports the cardiovascular system. It acts as a natural calcium channel blocker for the heart, lowering blood pressure and dilating the heart blood vessels (*Dr. Terry Friedmann*). Mineral Essence and Super Cal are good sources of magnesium.

Aneurysm

Single oils:

- Frankincense with helichrysum and cypress.

Use: 1-3 drops (according to your sensitivity).

Apply oils by gently massaging along blood vessel towards the heart.

Cypress strengthens capillary and vascular walls. Helichrysum helps absorb blood back into tissues.

Diffuse and inhale: (see DIFFUSING and INHALATION).

Mix:
- 5 drops frankincense
- 1 drop helichrysum
- 1 drop cypress

Blends: JuvaFlex

Supplements: Cleansing Trio and JuvaTone.

Arrhythmia

Single oils: Lavender and cypress.

Blends: Aroma Life, JuvaFlex, and Melrose.

Rub oils over affected areas.

Supplements: Cleansing Trio, JuvaTone, and Cel-Lite Magic Massage Oil.

Drink chamomile tea. Body massage with Cel-Lite Magic Massage Oil.

Hardening of the Arteries

Singles: Helichrysum and cypress.

Blends: Aroma Life

Phlebitis (Inflammation of Veins)

Single oils:

- Helichrysum with lavender, German chamomile, Roman chamomile, or geranium.

Use: Add 1-3 drops to the corresponding single oils above (according to your sensitivity).

Blends:

• Helichrysum or lavender with Aroma Life.

Use: Add 1-3 drops of each single oil (according to your sensitivity).

Helichrysum with lavender is excellent. Helichrysum prevents phlebitis. Use the oil on location with cold packs (see COLD PACKS).

Carpal Tunnel Syndrome

(See NERVOUS SYSTEM.)

Cataracts/Glaucoma

(See EYES.)

Cel-Lite

(See FATS.)

Chemical Sensitivity Reaction

Environmental poisoning and chemical sensitivity is fast becoming a major cause of discomfort and disease. Strong chemical compounds, such as insecticides, herbicides, formaldehydes found in paints, glues, cosmetics, and finger nail polish easily enter the body. Symptoms include indigestion, upper and lower gas, poor assimilation, poor electrolyte balance, rashes, hypoglycemia, allergic reaction to foods and other substances, along with emotional mood swings, fatigue, irritability, lack of motivation, lack of discipline and creativity.

Single oils: Frankincense and sandalwood.

Blends: Purification, Clarity, Brain Power, and JuvaFlex.

Supplements: Radex, ImmuneTune, Exodus, Rehemogen, Chelex, JuvaTone, and Cleansing Trio.

People who get an instant headache from diffusing oils, usually have a blockage relating to metallics or chemicals in the brain. High levels of transphenols are very high in oxygen molecules, which will create an instant headache as the brain oxygen increases.

For headache relief:

• 6 Radex

• 4 ImmuneTune or ArthroTune

Drink 2 to 3 large glasses of water.

(See VASCULAR CLEANSING.)

Absorption of Chemicals

Handling refuse or any type of contaminate without protective gloves may cause discoloration of hands.

Single oils: Lavender and lemon.

Blends: Purification

Use good rubber gloves and change them often or at least wash them out with strong soap, rinse well, and dry well. If hands become discolored through chemical absorption, soak them in a solution of hydrogen peroxide 3%, available at drug stores. This helps remove chemicals from the skin. Rub lavender, lemon, or purification neat on hands and cover with clean cotton gloves or wrap lightly with cotton bandages all night.

Chicken Pox

Single oils: Lavender

Add lavender to calamine lotion and dab on spots.

Cholera

Single oils: Clove, ravensara, and rosemary.

Cholesterol

Single oils: Rosemary, Roman chamomile, and helichrysum italicum.

Supplements: I.C.P. (work up to 2 Tbsp. twice daily) and JuvaTone.

Rub along spine twice daily. Every other day rub frankincense, neat, along spine. Rub ImmuPower 3 times per day on spine.

Mix:
- 10 to 15 drops rosemary
- 5 drops Roman chamomile
- 3 drops helichrysum italicum

Put in capsules and take 3 times daily

Chronic Fatigue

Single oils: Rosemary, melaleuca, thyme, nutmeg, and blue tansy.

Blends: EndoFlex, Exodus II, Thieves, Di-Tone, and ImmuPower.

Supplements: Cleansing Trio, Thyromin, Exodus, ImmuGel, Master HIS/HERS, Vita-Green, Ultra Young, Seagal Power Meal, and Mineral Essence.

Cold Sores - Blisters from Herpes Simplex Virus Type 1

Single oils:

- Lavender with peppermint, melaleuca, Idaho tansy, melissa, ravensara, bergamot, lemon, helichrysum italicum, oregano, thyme, or mountain savory.

Dilute with V-6 Mixing Oil or Massage Oil Base.

Use: Add 1-3 drops to the corresponding single oils (according to your sensitivity).

Blends: Melissa, Hope, and Purification.

- Lavender with Melrose.

Use: 1-3 drops (according to your sensitivity).

As soon as a cold sore is noticed or suspected, apply neat, 1 drop lavender and 1 drop melaleuca or melrose.

Oils can sting on an open sore. Wait until the sore is sealed over before applying or dilute in V-6 Mixing Oil or Massage Oil Base. Mix 10 drops lavender with 1 drop peppermint. If drying is uncomfortable, mix 10% essential oil in V-6 Mixing Oil or Massage Oil Base.

Supplements: Super C, ImmuGel, Radex, Royal Essence, VitaGreen, ImmuneTune, Stevia, Cleansing Trio, and JuvaTone.

Apply Stevia directly on lip sores. Helps healing without scarring.

Colds - Sore Throat, Tonsillitis, Laryngitis, Influenza

Single oils:

- Lavender with lemon, lemongrass, Roman and German chamomile, marjoram, ginger, tarragon, peppermint, oregano, frankincense, thyme, fennel, jasmine, or laurus nobilis.

- Frankincense with cypress, oregano, thyme, lemon, rosewood, eucalyptus, myrrh, hyssop, or mountain savory.

- Melaleuca with thyme, Idaho tansy, myrrh, eucalyptus, ravensara, or rosemary.

- Rosemary with ravensara, eucalyptus, lemon, or juniper.

- Sage with mountain savory, fir, spruce, oregano, clary sage, helichrysum, thyme, cinnamon, cedarwood, or spearmint.

Use: Add 1-3 drops to the corresponding single oils above (according to your sensitivity).

Blends:

- Lavender with Melrose, Di-Tone, Immu-Power or Thieves.

- Frankincense with Peace & Calming, R.C., Raven, Sacred Mountain, Inspiration Blend, or Exodus II.

- Melaleuca with Raven, R.C., Thieves, or ImmuPower.

- Rosemary with R.C. or Raven.

- Sage with Melrose, Purification, R.C., Christmas Spirit, Di-Tone, or Sacred Mountain.

Use: Add 1-3 drops of each single oil to the corresponding blends above (according to your sensitivity).

Application of oils:

Massage oils on the Vita Flex points on the feet and hands. Apply 4 drops oregano and 4 drops thyme to Raindrop Therapy. Other oils and blends may be substituted for oregano and thyme (see RAINDROP THERAPY).

Diffuse Purification, Raven, R.C., or your favorite blend to kill airborne germs and bacteria.

Sacred Mountain and Inspiration blends are powerful antiseptics for the respiratory tract (see DIFFUSING).

Mix R.C., frankincense, and lemon for congestion.

Peppermint removes mucous, reduces fever and throat infection.

Myrrh is very effective on throat troubles and phlegm.

Jasmine helps coughs, hoarseness, and laryngitis.

Myrtle is good for chronic coughs.

Hyssop for colds and cedarwood for congestion and coughs.

Laryngitis:1 drop Melrose or lemon on tongue.

For relief of general cold symptoms:

Mix:
- 2 drops rosemary
- 2 drops melaleuca
- 1 drop eucalyptus
- 3 drops lemon.

Put in a steam vaporizer or add to hot bath (add to bath gel).

Mix:
- 1 drop lemon
- 2 drops eucalyptus
- 3 drops rosemary
- 2 drops peppermint

Inhale or put on a tissue, store in a zip lock bag, and inhale when desired.

Mix 1 tsp. (5 ml) V-6 Mixing Oil or Massage Oil Base, massage around sinuses, forehead, nose, cheek bones, chest, and upper back.

Rub 6 drops R.C. and 2 drops Raven on chest, neck, and throat. Works well with cypress, birch, lemon, peppermint, and eucalyptus.

Mix:
- 10 drops rosemary
- 8 drops Raven
- 8 drops frankincense
- 2 drops oregano
- 2 drops peppermint

Gargle 2-4 times daily.

Mix:
- 2 drops raven
- 1 drop thyme
- 3 drops frankincense
- 3 drops lemon
- 3 drops rosemary

Mix in 3/4 tsp. honey. The first week gargle 4 times daily, 2nd week 2 times daily, 3rd week 3 times daily, and 4th week 1 time daily. Stop for 1 month and repeat if necessary.

To prevent relapse, apply chamomile on thoracic vertebrae T4 and T5 (neck to shoulder intersection).

The phenols in lavender and chamomile help reduce over-production of mucous. Apply to bottom of feet to slow down the parasympathetic system reducing the over-production of mucous.

(See Whooping Cough and Strep Throat under INFECTION and MUCUS).

Supplements: ImmuGel, Radex, Super C, Royal Essence, VitaGreen, ImmuneTune, Royaldophilus, Rehemogen, Colloidal Essence, Stevia, and Exodus.

ImmuGel helps the body recover and may serve as an antibiotic (do not mix with citrus juices). Take 2 capsules of Royaldophilus 3 times daily. This helps to restores healthy bacteria in intestinal tract and bowels. Do a colon and liver cleanse, including JuvaTone (see COLON). Clean, healthy, and detoxified blood assists in the recovery from any disease. Take 3 droppers of Rehemogen 3 times daily. Rehemogen cleanses the blood, which carries nutrients and oxygen to the cells to help the healing process. Toxins block nutrient and oxygen flow into cells. Colloidal Essence is a powerful bacteria, fungus, and virus fighter. It may be taken internally or applied externally as required. Take 2 to 6 Exodus capsules 3 times daily. Exodus is a powerful immune builder, which speeds the body's healing process. Exodus II is a the companion product to Exodus.

Colitis

Single oils: Peppermint, spearmint, tarragon, anise seed oil, and fennel.

Blends: Di-Tone 20 drops in a capsule 2 times daily.

Supplements: Royaldophilus, Kefir, AlkaLime, Mint Condition, and ImmuGel.

Take oils orally in water or topically.

Colitis, Viral

Single oils:

- Thyme with melaleuca, lemon, basil, lemongrass, rosemary, lavender, eucalyptus, geranium, bergamot, patchouly, clove, or cinnamon.

- Helichrysum with myrrh, German chamomile, Roman chamomile, lavender, or tarragon.

Use: Add 1-3 drops to the corresponding single oils above (according to your sensitivity).

Blends:

- Thyme with Di-Tone, Melrose, Purification, Thieves, or 3 Wise Men.

- Helichrysum with Di-Tone.

Use: Add 1-3 drops of each single oil to the corresponding blends above (according to your sensitivity).

Use helichrysum with tarragon or helichrysum with Di-Tone, in a compress application, which is very good for viral colitis.

Supplements: Mint Condition, Colloidal Essence, ImmuGel, VitaGreen, Master HERS and Master HIS.

Colon and Liver Cleanse: Cleansing Trio, JuvaTone, and JuvaFlex (see COLON). Take Mint Condition, along with ComforTone. Wait about 2 weeks or more before adding I.C.P. Start with a small amount of the I.C.P. and increase slowly. If any discomfort is experienced, reduce to a level of comfort and take it slower. Listen to your body.

Colloidal Essence is a powerful bacteria, fungus, and virus fighter. It may be taken internally or applied externally as required.

Colon

Colon and Liver Cleanse (Digestive System Cleanse)

The first step to good health is detoxification. For degenerative diseases, allergies, Alzheimer's, arteriosclerosis, arthritis, asthma, bursitis, diabetes, cancer, hypertension, insomnia, multiple scleroses (MS), and rheumatism, and of course infections, colds, and influenza, and often just sluggishness and general poor health, the first thing to do is a digestive system cleanse. This allows the body to work towards fighting off the disease and not be encumbered or overloaded with the accumulation of toxins, mucous, and parasites that have built up over the years.

Poor health many times can be traced to an unhealthy digestive tract and colon. It is important to cleanse the bowels because from here, toxins are released into the blood and travel to all parts of the body. Loss of energy is the first indication of toxic overload.

A colon and liver cleanse help prepare the cells of the small intestine for proper assimilation and elimination of parasites. Parasites can infest all areas of the body and affect many people. This cleansing program, particularly ComforTone, Di-Tone, and ParaFree, are very effective against bowel parasites (see PARASITES). They are able to regenerate and build the immune system if the body is not polluted and bogged down by toxins.

Our modern day food chain contains more than 37,000 chemicals, many of which are carcinogenic, including radioactive isotopes known as metallics. With many of these chemicals, the level at which ingestion or breathing becomes harmful has not yet been determined.

DDT is still produced in the U.S.A. Although banned for use in the U.S.A and Canada, DDT is exported to third world countries and used in agriculture and is found in the produce imported into our country. High levels of DDT have even been found in the fat of seals in Antarctica, where there is no agriculture.

Our bodies have the amazing ability to ward off unwanted pathogens, but the body must be in top condition. Staying healthy today is a full-time and life-time job. If you have a problem, you can never go back to the lifestyle and habits that created the problem.

The best way to protect ourselves is to have proper digestive and endocrine functions. The body must be able to assimilate substances that provide oxygen and nutrients compatible with good health for which the body must have a clean digestive tract, colon, liver, and pancreas, a clean properly flowing blood stream, a lymphatic system clear of accumulated toxins and mucous, and a good functioning neurological system. These systems give the body the tools that it needs to carry out its work.

Our bodies are designed to be active. They must have exercise. Since the lymphatic system is not a powered system, it gets its activation by muscle movement and activity. A sedentary lifestyle may cause the system to become clogged.

Single oils:

* Sage with helichrysum, carrot seed oil, or patchouly.

Use: Add 1-3 drops to the corresponding oils (according to your sensitivity).

Blends:

* Helichrysum or sage with JuvaFlex, Endo-Flex, Di-Tone, or Purification.

* For mood swings: Frankincense with Valor, Sacred Mountain, or Peace & Calming.

Use: Add 1-3 drops of each single oil to the corresponding blends above (according to your sensitivity).

Supplements: ComforTone, I.C.P., Megazyme, JuvaTone, ParaFree, Royaldophilus, VitaGreen, Master HIS, Master HERS, Radex, Super B, Super C, Super Cal, Thyromin, Mint Condition, Royal Essence, Mineral Essence, and Exodus.

Cleansing Program:

ComforTone cleans the colon and the small intestines, and is particularly effective in enhancing peristalsis, which controls bowel movement.

ComforTone: Start with one capsule first thing in the morning and last thing before going to bed. Increase up to 5 capsules, morning and evening, as time progresses adding only one capsule per day.

Drink plenty of distilled or purified water, at least 6 ounces 6 to 8 times daily. This is in addition to any other fluids, such as juice.

Thin or hard stools indicate insufficient water. The stool should pass easily and should be about 1 inch in diameter, 10 to 12 inches long. When bowel movements occur 3 to 4 times per day, ComforTone has done its job. If you retain this regularity, after stopping ComforTone, you have taken enough. An ideal bowel movement is 1 movement for each meal consumed per day; i.e.: 3 meals per day equal 3 bowel movements per day. When the movement slows to 1 or 2 per day or you begin to feel sluggish, begin again with ComforTone.

It is best not to rush the cleansing process. As the mucous, toxins, and plaque in the lining of the colon are removed, one may experience flu-like discomforts that come and go. Some aches continue longer than others and seem to be more severe if large dosages of the ComforTone are maintained. If this happens, reduce the dosage but do not stop completely. The discomfort will soon go away.

CAUTION: Anyone, including pregnant women, should stop ComforTone if diarrhea occurs for 1 to 2 days Restart again with a smaller amount. Other than this, it is safe to take the supplement through the entire pregnancy.

I.C.P. Fiber Cleanse:

After being on ComforTone for 2 to 3 days, add I.C.P. Start with 1 small tsp. in juice, water, or rice/soy milk at bedtime. Carrot juice is very tasty and produces excellent cleansing. Apple juice and water, half and half also aid in cleansing. Citrus juices will produce and increase acidity, which may not be desired. Over several days work up to 1 heaping tsp. and as much as 2 Tbsp. Take with ComforTone in the morning if your system seems to need it.

I.C.P. helps the cleansing process by providing bulk to help move the stool. This also has ingredients that loosen deposits on intestine walls, polish and lubricate those walls, and root out parasites. It is more specific for the small intestine because it contains enzymes and digestive stimulants that work as a mild laxative, helping to restore proper bowel function, facilitating good assimilation of nutrients.

Mint Condition soothes related symptoms of colitis, diverticulitis, or ulcers. Take this with ComforTone. Mint Condition is soothing, helps digestion, and relieves upset stomach.

Wait for about 2 weeks before adding I.C.P. to the program. Start with a small amount and increase slowly to avoid irritation. With any irritation simply reduce to a level of comfort and go slower.

Royal Essence and Mineral Essence help keep electrolytes balanced. Some people who have taken Royal Essence have reported a colon release simular to ComforTone. This indicates an improper electrolyte balance in the colon.

Beta carotene, as found in carrot juice and beet juice, also helps elimination.

Carrot seed oil detoxifies the liver, expels kidney stones, cleanses the bowel, and relieves flatulence.

To maintain a healthy colon, it is best to stay away from dairy products, cheeses, white sugar, and yeasts.

If ComforTone or I.C.P. produces heartburn, this indicates that the gut is not working properly. If the cleansing process reduces the intestinal flora, add the following the program:

- Royaldophilus: 2 to 3 times daily.

- Megazyme: 1-3 per meal and up to 6 with heavy meat meals late in the day or at night.

- Yogurt: Take 1/2 hour before meals on an empty stomach.

These supplements provide the stomach with the friendly bacteria and enzymes necessary for good digestion, conversion, and assimilation. Master Formula HERS/HIS and CHILDREN'S, Royal Essence, and Mineral Essence provide trace minerals that the body requires to make enzymes.

Heartburn could also be an indication of candida (See VAGINAL YEAST INFECTION and FUNGUS).

ComforTone and Megazyme are very synergistic. When used together, one may be able to reduce the amount of ComforTone being taken.

Dr. Terry Friedman reports that Exodus shows phenomenal results in cleansing the digestive system when used with the colon cleansing program (reported Aug. 1997). Take 2 capsules 2 to 3 times daily.

Di-Tone aids digestion and elimination, and reduces cramping, gas, and nausea. Put 2 to 15 drops in the palm, rub over stomach around navel, over the area of the small intestine, on the mastoids behind the ears, and on Vita Flex areas on bottom of the feet. In severe cases, apply hot compresses over the stomach (see COMPRESSES). Di-Tone is also excellent for parasite removal. (See PARASITES.)

Add JuvaTone to the cleansing process after being on ComforTone and I.C.P. for 2 to 3 days. JuvaTone acts as a liver detoxifier. It increases urine flow, which helps to rid the body of excess water. Start with 1 capsule at mid-morning and mid-afternoon (at least 2 hours after a meal or 1 hour before the next meal). Work up to 3 tablets 2 times daily. In order to overcome addictions from smoking, alcohol, sugar, chocolate, and drugs, it may be necessary to take up to 9 tablets per day.

Take JuvaTone and ComforTone at least 1 hour apart. Do no take at the same time. The cleansing may be too much as some people have reported uncomfortable reactions, such as bloating, gas, diaphragm and chest pains. If this happens, massage Di-Tone or JuvaFlex around the navel and on the spine. Mint Condition will help alleviate this discomfort. The reaction should subside in 10 or 15 minutes.

CAUTION: It is best not to use JuvaTone for cleansing after 6 months into a pregnancy.

If you feel that you still need to cleanse, then massage JuvaFlex over the liver and on the liver Vita Flex points on the bottom of the feet, and around the navel to assist in liver detoxification. JuvaFlex is a good companion to JuvaTone.

With the pollution of our environment today, it is not unusual to find parasites in the body. They can cause all kinds of illness and disease and may go undetected for years. This cleansing program, particularly ComforTone, Di-Tone, I.C.P., ParaFree, and Colloidal Essence, are very effective against bowel parasites.

Sage, carrot seed oil, and helichrysum also assist in liver detoxification. Helichrysum is a great stimulant to the detoxifying organs of the body; i.e., pancreas, spleen, kidneys, liver, lymphatic system, and blood system. When doing a colon and liver cleanse, diffuse or rub Purification (may add sage or helichrysum) on the bottom of feet. Patchouly also digests toxic wastes and may be used as a massage oil during the cleanse. Mix 10 drops patchouly with 3 Tbsp. V-6 Mixing Oil or Massage Oil Base.

When you are cleansing, body energy must be maintained, or the cleansing process will stop. EndoFlex will help boost body metabolism and the circulatory system, which is necessary for detoxification.

The following supplements will help maintain body energy:

- Master HIS/HERS: 2-4 tablets 3 times daily.

- VitaGreen: 2-6 capsules 2-3 times daily.

- Super B: 1 tablet daily with food.

- Super C: 2-4 tablets 1-2 times daily.

- Radex: 2-4 tablets 2-3. times daily

- Super Cal: 2-4 capsules 1-2 times daily.

- Thyromin: 1-2 capsules before betimes: (See THYROID).

Liver problems are often indicated by brown spots on the skin (called liver spots or sometimes age spots), by cracking around fingernails, and rough, dry skin. As the liver is cleaned, the skin turns soft and silky, particularly on the upper arms. This how you can tell that you have taken enough JuvaTone. Many people have reported that liver spots have disappeared and faded.

JuvaTone and VitaGreen both work to cleanse the vascular system and to chelate heavy metals, metallics, and plaque out of the body.

These high-quality cleansing products have up to a 6 year shelf life due to the addition of essential oils and the proper formulating process necessary to hold oils in the herb powder. The oils help restore bowel movement (peristalsis). The longer one has been taking these supplements, the less one needs. Amounts should be reduced over time.

Marjoram increases peristalsis. You need only to add marjoram in very special cases when extra help is necessary.

Occasionally there will be an emotional reaction to cleansing. This is because of high levels of heavy metals, such as lead, mercury, etc., being expel through the blood stream. This may upset the hormonal balance and result in mood swings. Apply Valor, Sacred Mountain, and Peace & Calming to help balance these mood swings. Reduce amount of JuvaTone but do not quit. Quitting allows the toxins to remain and a greater effect will be felt. Massage Valor on the bottom of the feet and inhale or diffuse other blends, such as Joy, Peace & Calming, Harmony, White Angelica, and Brain Power. Again, begin to slowly increase the amount of JuvaTone until a comfortable level is found.

The first digestive system cleanse will probably require about 90 days on the program before a significant change is detectable. Thereafter, a colon and liver cleanse should be done 3 to 4 times per year for about 30 days each time. When the system is clean and working well, the following program may work well:

- ComforTone and I.C.P., 5 to 10 days per month.

- JuvaTone 45 days, 2 times per year.

Maintenance:

- 1-3 ComforTone daily. This is a balanced product so one will not become addicted nor immune to it.

- 1 Tbsp. I.C.P. 5 times per week.

- Megazyme: After 30 years of age, 2 to 3 tablets 3 times daily or as desired

- Royaldophilus throughout the week.

As the system becomes clean and balanced, cravings for sweets, chocolate, nicotine, and even red meats, will diminish allowing you to pursue a more healthy diet regime.

It may take 2 to 2 1/2 years of very diligent work to establish proper digestive functions. You should be prepared to listen to the body and modify the program as your body indicates.

Colonics

Mix:
- 5 drops rosemary
- 5 drops basil
- 4 drops juniper

Add to colonic water and mix well.

Diverticulosis

Single oils: Peppermint

Blends:

- Frankincense with Di-Tone or Melrose.

Use: Add 1-3 drops of each single oil to the corresponding blends above (according to your sensitivity).

Supplements: ComforTone, Mint Condition, ImmuGel, and Royaldophilus

Mix:
- 15 drops Di-Tone
- 5 drops melrose

Mix in 1 Tbsp. of V-6 Mixing Oil or Massage Oil Base.

Mix:
- 10 drops Di-Tone
- 15 drops frankincense

Mix in 1 Tbsp. of V-6 Mixing Oil or Massage Oil Base.

Rub on feet, use as a hot compress on stomach, and as a rectal implant.

Mix: 1 drop peppermint in 1 tsp. of honey and sip.

Irritable Bowel Syndrome

Supplements: Royaldolphilus and Mint Condition.

Spastic Colon

Single oils:

- Oregano with thyme, Roman chamomile, clove, cinnamon, or peppermint.

Blends:

- Oregano with Purification or Di-Tone

Use: Add 1-3 drops of each single oil to the corresponding blends or single oil above (according to your sensitivity).

Massage on Vita Flex point on feet, Raindrop Therapy on the spine:

Mix:
- 2 drops oregano
- 2 drops thyme
- 3 drops Purification
- 2 drops Roman chamomile
- 2 drops clove or cinnamon
- 2 drops Di-Tone

Mix with 1 oz. V-6 Mixing Oil or Massage Oil Base and use in a rectal implant.

Coma

Single oils: Frankincense, sandalwood, cypress, pepper, and peppermint.

Blends: Trauma Life, Hope, and Surrender.

Supplements: Mineral Essence and Ultra Young.

Concentration/Confusion

Single oils: Peppermint, rosemary, basil, and cardamom.

Blends: Clarity, Brain Power, M-Grain, and Gathering.

Supplements: Mineral Essence, Super B, and Ultra Young.

Congestion

Single oils: Sandalwood, coriander, cypress, eucalyptus radiata, fennel, and rosemary.

Blends: Di-Tone, R.C., Raven, and Exodus II.

Supplements: Cleansing Trio and Cel-Lite Magic Massage Oil.

Connective Tissue - Weak, Repair, Sprains, Tendonitis, Tensonovitis

Tendonitis, often called Tennis Elbow and Golfer's Elbow, is a torn or inflamed tendon, probably from strain or injury. Tenosynovitis, sometimes called "Trigger Finger," is a tendon being restricted by its sheath (particularly thumbs and fingers) by being swollen and inflamed. Repetitive use or infection may be the cause.

Connective tissue is an essential part of every structure in the body.

Single oils:

- Basil with lemongrass, lavender, marjoram, helichrysum, birch, or Idaho tansy.

- Lemongrass with helichrysum, cypress, lavender, or ginger.

- Helichrysum with lemongrass, cypress, or rose.

- Rosemary with eucalyptus or peppermint.

Use: Add 1-3 drops to the corresponding single oils above (according to your sensitivity).

Blends:

- Basil with PanAway.

- Lemongrass with Aroma Life, PanAway, R.C., or Citrus Fresh.

- Helichrysum with Relieve It or Release.

Use: Add 1-3 drops of each single oil to the corresponding blends above (according to your sensitivity).

Supplements: Master HIS/HERS, ArthroTune, Super Cal, Super B, Super C, VitaGreen, Royal Essence, Mineral Essence, Sulfurzyme, Cel-Lite Magic, Ortho Ease, and Ortho Sport Massage Oils.

ArthroTune and Super Cal help the repair process. Sulfurzyme, formulated with MSM (methyl sulfonyl methane), equalizes water pressure inside the cells so that the cell protein envelope will allow water transfer in and out freely. When water pressure is higher inside the cells than outside, it creates pain.

PanAway and lemongrass make a potent combination. PanAway keeps the pain down and lemongrass promotes the repair of connective tissue.

Helichrysum and lemongrass also make a powerful combination for repairing torn ligaments. Lavender and lemongrass, and marjoram and lemongrass work well together for inflamed tendons. Ortho Sport and Ortho Ease Massage Oils also help with the healing.

Rub 4 to 5 drops of oils over the area and then cover with massage oil.

Tendonitis

Mix:
- 10 drops basil
- 8 drops birch
- 6 drops cypress
- 3 drops peppermint

Rub neat on location. Mix with V-6 Mixing Oil or Massage Oil Base to massage larger areas. For general aching, do Raindrop Therapy.

Tennis Elbow (Tendonitis)

Pain Relief:
- 10 drops rosemary
- 10 drops eucalyptus
- 10 drops peppermint

Mix with 2 Tbsp. V-6 Mixing Oil or Massage Oil Base and use with ice packs.

Sprain - Torn Ligament Blend

Pain Relief:
- 1 drop lemongrass,
- 2 to 3 drops Aroma Siez.

Mix with V-6 Mixing Oil or Massage Oil Base and apply.

CAUTION: For sprains, use cold packs. For any serious sprain or constant pain, always consult a health care professional.

When selecting oils, particularly for injuries, think through the cause and type of injury and select oils for each segment. For instance, tendonitis could encompass muscle damage, nerve damage, ligament strain or tear, inflammation, infection, fever on location, and possibly an emotion. Therefore, select an oil or oils for each perceived problem and apply in rotation or prepare a blend to cover all problems. The emotional distress may be anger or guilt, or the person may have had pain for a long time and needs to release.

Any time that there is tissue damage, there is always inflammation, which needs to be reduced first.

Constipation

Single oils: Ginger and anise seed oil.

Blends: Di-Tone

Supplements: Cleansing Trio, AlkaLime, Royaldophilus, Goji Berry Tea, Body Balance, Royal Essence, and Seagal Power Meal.

- Megazyme: 3 to 6 capsules, 3 times daily.

- AlkaLime: 1 Tbsp. in water, 2 times daily before or after meals.

- ComforTone: Start with 1 capsule and increase next day to 1 more capsule. Continue to increase 1 capsule each day until bowels start moving.

- I.C.P.: 1 week following beginning ComforTone, start with 1 Tbsp. 2 times daily and then increase to 3 times daily up to 2 Tbsp. 3 times daily.

- Drink aloe vera juice, water, prune juice, and raw fruit and vegetable juices.

Convulsions

Monitor diet. Discontinue sugar and dairy products.

Blends: Brain Power and Valor.

Apply these oils at base of skull, across the neck, C1 to C6 receptors, and bottom of feet (for relief only).

Supplements: Master Formula CHILDREN'S, Vita Life Juice, and Ultra Young.

Corns

(See FOOT PROBLEMS.)

Coughs

(See COLDS.)

Cramps, Charley Horses, Night Leg Cramps

(See MUSCLES.)

Crohne's Disease

Chronic inflammation of the digestive tract, most commonly the last section of the small intestine. Usual symptoms include periodic attacks of cramping, lower right abdominal pain, diarrhea, and a general sense of feeling ill. **Attacks may occur once or twice a day** for the rest of your life. If the disease continues for years, it can cause deterioration of bowel function, leaking bowel, poor absorption of nutrients, loss of appetite and weight, intestinal obstruction, severe bleeding, and increased susceptibility to intestinal cancer.

Single oils: Peppermint

Blends: Di-Tone

Supplements: Mint Condition, Royaldophilus, ImmuGel, AlkaLime, Body Balance, VitaGreen, Goji Berry Tea, Cleansing Trio, Seagal Power Meal, and Mineral Essence.

- Mint Condition: 2 to 4 capsules 3 times daily.

- Royaldophilus: 2 to 4 capsules 3 times daily. Empty capsules and add to water or yogurt if desired twice daily.

- ImmuGel: 1/2 tsp. 5 times daily.

Each phase is for 1 week and is to be added to the previous phases.

Phase I: Do not use ComforTone, Megazyme, or I.C.P.

Take Mint Condition in Yogurt or kefir, liquid acidophilus, and charcoal tablets.

Phase II: Add AlkaLime if no diarrhea. Body Balance for 2 to 3 weeks.

Raw juices (5 oz. celery and 2 oz carrot).

Phase III: VitaGreen, Goji Berry Tea.

Phase IV: (1 week after blood spots stops).

- ComforTone (1 capsule morning and night) until stools loosen.

- I.C.P.: Start with 1 level tsp. 2 times daily and gradually increase.

- Megazyme: Start 1 tablet 3 times daily.

If irritation occurs, rest from Cleansing Trio for a few days and start again. Switch from Body Balance to Seagal Power Meal.

- Mineral Essence: Start the second week: 1 dropper 2 times daily.

Raindrop Therapy on the spine with ImmuPower.

Chronic Fatigue Syndrome

(See HYPOGLYCEMIA.)

Symptoms can include indigestion, upper and lower gas, poor assimilation, poor electrolyte balance, allergic reaction to food and other substances, mood swings, fatigue, irritability and lack of motivation, discipline, and creativity. Hypoglycemia is a precursor and even causes chronic fatigue syndrome. Overcome hypoglycemia, and the symptoms of chronic fatigue syndrome will probably disappear.

Cuts

(See WOUNDS.)

Cystitis

Single oils:

- Thyme with German chamomile, frankincense, Roman chamomile, melaleuca, lemongrass, geranium, helichrysum, fennel, lavender, peppermint, patchouly, spearmint, and tangerine.

Mix:
- 3 drops thyme
- 4 drops blue chamomile
- 8 drops frankincense
- 6 drops Roman chamomile
- 9 drops melaleuca
- 13 drops lemongrass
- 10 drops geranium
- 4 drops helichrysum
- 10 drops fennel
- 8 drops lavender
- 6 drops peppermint
- 6 drops patchouly
- 11 drops spearmint
- 10 drops tangerine

Mix in 2 oz. V-6 Mixing Oil or Massage Oil Base.

Mix:
- 3 droppers of K & B Tincture
- 1 drop mountain savory

Mix in water and drink every 2 hours.

Use cistus, ImmuPower, Inspiration in Raindrop Therapy application or massage along lower back and pubic area.

Take 1 tsp. of AlkaLime daily, in water only, 1 hour before or after meal.

Dandruff

(See SKIN CARE.)

Dandruff may be caused from allergies, parasites, and chemicals.

Single oils: Cedarwood, lavender, rosemary, and sage.

Blends: Citrus Fresh

Supplements: Lavender Shampoo and Lemon Sage Shampoo.

Decongestants

(See MUCUS.)

Dental

Infection

Single oils: Clove, cinnamon, and peppermint.

Blends: Thieves

- Helichrysum with PanAway.

Use: Add 1-3 drops of each single oil with corresponding blends above (according to your sensitivity).

Before going to the dentist, rub helichrysum with PanAway on gums and jaw.

Brush with Thieves and Dentarome. If infection is due to leukemia, saturate gauze with ImmuGel and Thieves. Lay over gums and change morning and night. Massage abscessed area with Thieves. Irrigate mouth with Fresh Essence.

Pulling Teeth

Single oils: Birch, helichrysum, melaleuca, eucalyptus, clove, thyme, and oregano. May be diluted if necessary.

Blends:

- Helichrysum with Thieves and R.C.

Use: 1-3 drops of each single oil with corresponding blends above (according to your sensitivity).

Before having teeth pulled, rub helichrysum with Thieves and R.C. around gums.

Rub R.C. on gums to bring back feeling from numbness of Novacaine.

Deodorant

Excessive body odor indicates putrefaction in the system and possibly poor digestion from the lack of enzymes in the digestive tract. A colon and liver cleanse may be needed (see COLON).

Single oils: Lavender, geranium, bergamot, cypress, eucalyptus, and myrtle

Blends: Aroma Siez, Acceptance, Dragon Time, EndoFlex, Harmony, Joy, Mister, R.C., Release, White Angelica, and Peace & Calming.

Supplements and Skin Care: Dragon Time and Relaxation Massage Oils, Aroma Silk Satin Body Lotion, Sandalwood Moisture Cream, Sunsation Suntan Oil, Dragon Time Bath and Shower Gel, and Evening Peace .

These products contain the single oils of lavender, geranium, and bergamot, which inhibit proliferation of odor-causing bacteria on the skin. To enhance the fragrant influence or get the synergistic effect of a favorite blend or product, add one or more of the single oils.

You can also use oils under your armpits or on the skin, neat or in the V-6 Mixing Oil or Massage Oil Base. You can also put a couple of drops on a face cloth when washing.

Deodorant Mix:

- 4 ounces of unscented talcum powder
- 2 ounces of baking soda
- 3 drops lavender (or your favorite oil or blend)

Mix well. Use under arms, on the feet (or in shoes), or any other place on the body.

Dermatitis - Eczema

Eczema and dermatitis are both inflammations of the skin and are most often due to allergies. Dermatitis is more a result of external factors, such as poison ivy, contact with some metals (wrist watch, ear rings, jewelry, etc.), or sunburn, etc. Eczema is more from internal factors, such as irritant chemicals, soaps and shampoos, allergy to wheat (gluten), etc. In both dermatitis and eczema, skin becomes red, flaky and itchy, small blisters may form and if broken by scratching, can become infected.

Single oils: Lavender and cistus.

- Lavender with Roman or German chamomile, helichrysum, geranium, rosewood, patchouly, sage, or thyme.

Use: Add 1-3 drops to the corresponding single oils above (according to your sensitivity).

Blends: JuvaFlex

- Lavender with Purification, Melrose, Sensation, or Gentle Baby.

Use: Add 1-3 drops of each single oil to the corresponding blends above (according to your sensitivity).

Oils for treating dermatitis and eczema are probably best if applied when diluted in V-6 Mixing Oil or Massage Oil Base.

Supplements: Cleansing Trio, JuvaTone, Rehemogen, and Rose Ointment.

Most skin problems are a result of a toxic liver. It is therefore, extremely important to cleanse the liver and blood and make that the elimination system is working properly.

Diabetes - Blood Sugar Imbalance

The pancreas produces insulin, which enables the body to use glucose. If there is no insulin, or not enough insulin is produced, the body cannot regulate the sugar levels in the body. This disorder is called diabetes mellitus, which causes low energy and abnormally high blood glucose (sugar).

Single oils:

- Coriander with cinnamon, fennel, dill, cypress, rosemary, or ylang ylang.

Use: Add 1-3 drops to the corresponding single oils above (according to your sensitivity).

Blends:

- Cypress with Thieves or EndoFlex.
- Lavender with Thieves, JuvaFlex, or Di-Tone.
- Helichrysum with Thieves.

Use: Add 1-3 drops of each single oil with corresponding blends above (according to your sensitivity).

Supplements: Vita Green, Stevia, Master HIS/ HERS, Megazyme, Super B, Body Balance, Seagal Power Meal, Royal Essence, Mineral Essence, EssPro 7, Sulfurzyme, Goji Berry Tea, and Wolfberry Power Bars.

- Body Balance and Seagal Power Meal.
- VitaGreen: 8 to 16 capsules daily.

- Sulfurzyme: 1 to 4 Tbsp. daily.
- Massage on pancreas Vita Flex points on bottom of feet: Thieves, coriander, fennel, and dill to lower glucose levels. Apply as compress over pancreas area.
- Cleansing Trio, JuvaTone, and JuvaFlex (see COLON).

CAUTION: Do not use fennel longer than 10 days at a time, since it excessively increases flow through the urinary tract.

VitaGreen is high in plant protein, which helps balance blood glucose (sugar). The MSM/sulfur found in the Sulfurzyme is significant for insulin production.

Megazyme supports enzyme production, which helps keep the pancreas from premature wasting and enlargement, a condition linked to diabetes and premature aging.

Super B is a good source of B vitamins to support pancreas function.

The Stevia leaf (whole or ground) is one of the most health-restoring plants on earth. It is a natural sweetener, has no calories, and does not have the harmful side effects of processed sugar or sugar substitutes. Stevia increases glucose tolerance, inhibits glucose absorption, and helps normalize blood sugar fluctuations. The FDA has approved it for use as a dietary supplement.

Goji Berry Tea helps prevent diabetes. Wolfberry balances the pancreas and is a detoxifier and cleanser. Diabetes is not common in China, where wolfberry is consumed regularly.

Digestion Problems - Diarrhea, Constipation, Flatulence (intestinal gas), Intestinal Infections

Any of the following indicate that the stomach is not digesting properly:

- Burping, belching, flatulence, and bloating.
- Rumbling or gurgling sounds in the abdomen.
- Heartburn (may be a possible indication of candida).
- Constipation and diarrhea.

- Constant hunger or fatigue after eating.

- Food intolerance or food allergies.

- Intestinal parasites.

  Poor bowel function is linked to enzyme deficiency, low fiber, insufficient liquid, bad diet, and stress.

Single oils:

- Basil with tarragon, peppermint, fennel, juniper, ginger, geranium, black cumin, or pepper.

- Lavender with patchouly, peppermint, Idaho tansy, tarragon, sandalwood, lemon, bergamot, eucalyptus, myrrh, oregano, thyme, spearmint, mandarin, melaleuca, nutmeg, orange, tangerine, laurus nobilis, or rose.

- Lemongrass with tarragon, ginger, peppermint, patchouly, cinnamon, spearmint, grapefruit, mandarin, or spikenard.

- Rosemary with clary sage, sage, marjoram, lavender, Roman chamomile, German chamomile, caraway seed, or neroli.

Use: Add 1-3 drops to the corresponding single oils above (according to your sensitivity).

Blends:

- Basil with Di-Tone.

- Lavender with Di-Tone or JuvaFlex.

- Lemongrass with Di-Tone or JuvaFlex.

- Sage with Di-Tone.

Use: Add 1-3 drops of each single oil to the corresponding blends above (according to your sensitivity).

Supplements: Megazyme, Royaldophilus, Royal Essence, Mineral Essence, Master HIS/HERS, Mint Condition, Body Balance, Vita-Green, Colloidal Essence, AlkaLime, Stevia, and Sulfurzyme.

A colon and liver cleanse should be done and repeated until digestion deficiency is cleared up (see COLON). Repeat program 2 to 4 times per year in order to maintain proper digestion.

Between 1:00 and 3:00 PM the body stops producing the protein digestion substances pepsin and hydrochloric acid (HC1). So protein digestion shuts down at about 2:00 PM. After 2:00 PM, heavy protein will be difficult to digest. Meat protein does not digest at all after 2:00 PM and will wait and ferment in the gut, making gas and upsetting the digestive system until the body again produces pepsin and HC1 at about 6:00 AM the next morning. This produces nightmares, restless sleep, and waking up fatigued in the morning.

Excess gas and poor digestion indicate a deficiency of enzymes. One should have about 3500 enzymes; most of us have only 500-600 enzymes. This indicates a need to balance the body and increase enzyme activity. Inadequate digestive enzyme activity has also been linked to chronic inflammations elsewhere in the body: fibromyalgia, herpes, inability to gain or lose weight, bad breath, body odor, skin rashes, and migraines.

The stomach requires high acidity to start digestion. The small intestine requires an alkaline environment to fully digest and assimilate fats, carbohydrates, and proteins. Without enough alkalinity, the body can only extract simple sugars from food, leaving the rest to ferment unused in the intestinal tract. These putrefying proteins and fats feed yeasts and fungi, which then run rampant in the intestines. The result is that the body gets calories but few vitamins, minerals, and proteins from the food.

AlkaLime helps reduce acidity in our internal environment, providing the alkalinity necessary for proper digestion, destroying damaging yeast, fungi, and negative bacteria.

Megazyme helps provide necessary enzymes. Most people require this supplement daily.

Dr. Radwan Farag of Cairo University found in his studies that microwaving food for 2 seconds destroys all enzymes and alters the food's frequency. Thus, microwaved food increases our enzyme deficiency.

Red meat takes 24 hours to move into the intestines and up to 72 hours to go through the system if the body is working properly. At 98° F the meat putrefies and ferments, creating a lot of gas. It takes 1 quart of blood to digest a meat meal, thus reducing the oxygen level in the blood which reduces blood and oxygen to the brain making one tired and sleepy.

A or AB blood types have low metabolism and do not digest meat well. These people have a low protein requirement and can get most of their protein requirements from grains. They also tend to have low thyroid and require more thyroid support than people with type O blood. People with type A and AB blood put on weight easily.

People with type B blood can eat meat at times.

People with type 0 blood have a higher metabolism, digest meat easily, and generally need meat in their diet. 0 blood types generally do not make the best total vegetarians and would probably require protein from perhaps organic fish or chicken. These people require more food intake and need to eat more often. They do not tend to put on weight but have a shorter life expectancy.

The body produces CO gas and other toxins from every-day metabolism. Enzymes are needed to digest this toxic residue. If we are too enzyme deficient, we absorb the toxins created from daily activity. Poor digestion also builds mucous and putrefactive material along the intestinal walls.

The gas we produce has to go somewhere. Some is expelled as flatulence and some goes into the blood and lymphatics and removes oxygen (CO gas is oxygen starved, so it steals any oxygen it can find). Since the liver cleans the blood, it also absorbs gas and toxins. When cells become oxygen-deficient, their frequency drops, and they start to mutate.

The result of gas and toxins in the liver will produce insomnia, frequent recurring migraine headaches, skin eruptions, discoloration, change in pigmentation, acne, and bumpy skin (like turkey skin).

In order to provide the stomach with the friendly bacteria and enzymes necessary for food digestion, conversion, and assimilation, these dietary supplements are very beneficial.

1/2 an hour before breakfast and heavy meals:

- Royaldophilus: 1-3 capsules.

- Megazyme: 2 to 6 tablets depending on blood type.

Most of us have depleted our enzyme supply and therefore need supplementation every day. Master HIS/HERS and CHILDREN'S, and Mineral Essence will provide the trace minerals that the body requires to make enzymes. Royal Essence, along with Mineral Essence, is particularly supportive of digestion and should be taken before meals.

Yogurt taken before lighter meals also helps provide friendly bacteria. The need for yogurt is sometimes indicated by an intolerance of dairy products.

A clean, healthy, detoxified system, provided with sufficient enzymes and trace minerals can process any food.

Mint Condition taken before eating helps with digestion and upset stomach. When heaviness is felt in the stomach, Mint Condition is a beneficial synergistic companion to Di-Tone.

Stevia improves digestion and gastrointestinal function and soothes upset stomach.

Di-Tone stimulates enzyme production and aids digestion and elimination. It is also carminative (reducing gas, belching, bloating, indigestion, and digests toxic material). Place up to 15 drops in the palm and rub over stomach and around navel. In severe cases apply hot compress over stomach. Massage 3 drops on stomach Vita Flex points on bottom of each foot.

Lemon neutralizes acids and helps heartburn. Place several drops in water and sip slowly.

1 drop of peppermint on the end of your tongue aids digestion and expels gas. Put 1 to 2 drops of peppermint in a glass of water, stir, and sip slowly.

Infants cannot go through the colon and liver cleanse. Use 3 drops of Di-Tone in a tsp. of V-6 Mixing Oil or Massage Oil Base, rub around the navel, and place warm "hot packs" over the stomach. Apply the same mix on the bottom of the feet.

For stomach cramps, diarrhea, nausea, and heartburn, rub Di-Tone or peppermint over the stomach around the navel and on the colon Vita Flex points on the bottom of feet.

For heartburn:
- 2 drops basil
- 2 drops Idaho tansy
- 8 drops sage
- 3 drops sandalwood

Blend in 1/2 to 1 oz. V-6 Mixing Oil or Massage Oil Base. Rub over your navel and on the colon Vita Flex area on bottom of feet.

Single essential oils to aid digestion:

- Rosemary or ginger for stomach cramps.

- Carrot seed oil helps relieve flatulence.

- Idaho tansy rubbed on the bottom of the feet has been reported to ease vomiting and diarrhea.

- Grapefruit seed oil helps digestive complaints and dyspepsia (indigestion).

- Sage, marjoram, and tangerine are digestive stimulants.

- Thyme and mandarin are stomach/digestive tonics.

- Patchouly digests toxic waste.

- Nutmeg aids digestion of starchy foods and fats, is an intestinal antiseptic, and helps flatulence, nausea, chronic diarrhea, indigestion, and sluggish digestion.

- Orange helps ease constipation, dyspepsia (indigestion), and chronic diarrhea.

- Tarragon prevents fermentation, is a digestive stimulant, reduces anorexia, dyspepsia (indigestion), flatulence, hiccups, intestinal spasms, and nervous digestion.

- Idaho tansy soothes the bowels and helps dyspepsia (indigestion), stomach sickness, and diarrhea.

- Lemongrass helps eliminate lactic acid (from fermentation of lactose in milk).

One will get the maximum benefit from supplements if taken before meals and spread throughout the day. For example, take the ComforTone as soon as you get up, then the other supplements after you shower, shave, comb your hair, etc. The supplements are dissolved and assimilated within 1/2 an hour.

Guidelines for the healthiest diet:

Breakfast is the most important meal of the day. Some people get up and work for an hour or two until they have a good appetite and the digestive system is awake. Then they have breakfast.

Eat breakfast between 6 and 7 a.m. Do not eat any fruit. The exception to this is strawberries with cereal or occasionally bananas. Yogurt is good since it supplies friendly bacteria. Cereals may be oatmeal, millet, wheat, barley, triticale, or a mixture of these, with coconut milk, rice milk, soy milk, whey powder, or goat milk. Since we do not have enough enzymes to handle multiple foods, it is best to not mix over 3 grains or different foods at a time. Bread should always be toasted; this changes it from a wet food to a dry food, making it more digestible.

Breakfast is the best meal of the day for eating proteins, such as beans and rice, or if you eat meat, then meats, eggs, fish, etc. Avoid meat after the noon meal; meat is best for breakfast. This will provide more energy and stamina in the afternoon because in the morning the enzymes are in place for meat digestion.

Our bodies cannot absorb vitamins and minerals without the presence of protein (protein powders suffice). This is particularly true for those who have had their gall bladder removed. Seagal Power Meal, Sulfurzyme, and Megazyme magnify the nutritional effects of vitamins vital to the production of amino acids that are responsible for protein synthesis.

Lunch should consist of carbohydrates and complex carbohydrates in the form of pasta, fruit, vegetable broth (not solid vegetables), or juices.

Dinner should be eaten as close to 3 p.m. as possible. It is better not to eat late at night. Both fruit and solid vegetables are fine for the evening meal.

If one gets trapped into a heavy large meal late in the day or evening, an extra portion of Megazyme is most beneficial. This will assist with digestion and assimilation of the heavy food, allowing restful sleep and a reduction of gas production.

Be patient. It may take 2 to 2 1/2 years of very diligent work to establish good digestive function. Listen to your body and modify the program with body changes.

We are programmed from years of eating meat to think our bodies require meat. In actuality, we can get the proteins we need from a variety of foods, such as grains, occasional cheeses, and eggs. The older a person, the more difficult the conversion to vegetarianism. The desire for meat has been programmed into our RNA and DNA. The best way to change over is to fast.

Hiatal Hernia

Single oils:

• Peppermint with lavender, lemongrass, or helichrysum.

Use: Add 1-3 drops to the corresponding single oils above (according to your sensitivity).

Supplements: Megazyme, Mint Condition, and Cleansing Trio.

(See COLON.)

Intestine Detoxification

Single oils:

• Helichrysum with tangerine, ginger, peppermint, or tarragon.

Use: Add 1-3 drops to the corresponding single oils above (according to your sensitivity).

Blends:

• Di-Tone with EndoFlex, JuvaFlex, or helichrysum.

Use: Add 1-3 drops of each single oil to the corresponding blends above (according to your sensitivity).

Traveler's Diarrhea

Single oils: Peppermint, ginger, lemon, mountain savory, and oregano.

Blends: Di-Tone

Supplements: ComforTone, I.C.P., Megazyme, and JuvaTone.

A maintenance dosage of ComforTone has protected travelers going to other countries from diarrhea, and other digestive discomforts.

One drop of peppermint on the end of the tongue or a couple of drops in water sipped slowly helps to settle the stomach.

Travel Sickness

Single oils:

• Peppermint with ginger.

Use: Mix 4 drops peppermint and 4 drops ginger in 1 ounce V-6 Mixing Oil or Massage Oil Base. Rub on chest and stomach before traveling.

Diverticulitis

Singles: Patchouly, anise seed oil, tarragon, rosemary, fennel, peppermint, and mountain savory.

Blends: Di-Tone

Supplements: Cleansing Trio and Mineral Essence.

Disinfectant

(See WOUNDS or ANTISEPTIC.)

Dizziness

Single oils: Cypress, tangerine, peppermint, basil, and cardamom.

Blends: Aroma Life, Clarity, Brain Power, and Thieves.

Apply Thieves to pancreas point on bottom of foot.

Supplements: Cel-Lite Magic Massage Oil, VitaGreen, and Essential Manna.

Blood circulation can be a factor (see CIRCULATION).

Dysentery

Singles: Lemon, mountain savory, oregano, and peppermint.

Blends: Thieves and Di-Tone.

Mix Thieves with 5 drops of peppermint and take orally.

Supplements: Mint Condition, Royaldophilus, Megazyme, I.C.P., and Mineral Essence.

Ears

Single oils:

- Helichrysum with juniper, peppermint, or geranium.

- Lavender with basil.

Use: Add 1-3 drops to the corresponding single oils above (according to your sensitivity).

Blends:

- Helichrysum with Purification, ImmuPower, and Melrose.

Use: Add 1-3 drops of each single oil to the corresponding blends above (according to your sensitivity).

Use ImmuPower on a cotton ball and place in the ear.

Lavender and basil, layered on temples and forehead, has helped ringing (tintinitus).

Hearing Vita Flex

Vita Flex Ear Points:

- Make sure that your fingernails are short. Place 1-2 drops of helichrysum, on each index finger.

- Standing behind the person, gently insert index fingers into the person's ears. Have the person hold head firmly against your chest.

- Rotate your hands (with the index fingers still inserted in ears) until the palms face upward. Lift fingers alternately (in a rocking motion) 10 times in each ear to a count of 20.

- Rotate hands 90 degrees until the palms face backwards. Pull back alternately 5 times in each ear to a count of 10.

- Rotate hands 90 degrees until the palms face downward. Press down alternately 5 times in each ear to a count of 10.

- Rotate hands 90 degrees until the palms face backward. Put thumbs behind the fingers. Push forward alternately 5 times in each ear to a count of 10.

- Rotate hands 90 degrees back to starting position (palms facing upward). Lift both fingers up once and let down slowly.

- Rotate fingers 90 degrees back and remove slowly.

- Grasp ear lobes, pull down and release.

For the average hearing loss problem, massage Purification on ear lobe, behind the ears, and down the jaw line (along the Eustachian tube). With ringing in the ears (tintinitus), which is often caused from plaque in the Eustachian tubes, massage helichrysum with juniper. Additionally, apply juniper with peppermint and geranium on tips of toes and fingers, also on the brain stem so that the oils get into the nerve pathways. It generally takes 12 to15 minutes to notice a change in hearing. Apply 1 drop of helichrysum in each ear.

Ear Infection

Single oils:

- Lavender with melaleuca, rosemary, helichrysum, Roman chamomile, hyssop, peppermint, or eucalyptus (radiata).

- Helichrysum with ravensara.

Use: Add 1-3 drops to the corresponding single oils above (according to your sensitivity).

Blends: Lavender with Melrose, Purification, PanAway, Thieves (diluted), or ImmuPower.

Use: Add 1-3 drops of each single oil to the corresponding blends above (according to your sensitivity).

Application of oils: Mix 1 to 2 drops of selected oils in 1 tsp. (5 ml) of warm olive oil. Apply in the ear with finger or cotton swab and around the ear and down the Eustachian tubes (externally) and on ear Vita Flex points on the feet. You can also put 2 or 3 drops of selected oil on a cotton ball and insert carefully into ear as a plug. Then lay a warm hot pack over the ear area to ease the pain.

CAUTION: Do not drop oil directly on the eardrum. First place oil on a cotton swab or put on finger and then place into ear.

Ear pain can be very serious. Always seek medical attention if pain persists.

Supplements: Super C, ImmuGel, Radex, Royal Essence, VitaGreen, ImmuneTune, Rehemogen, Cleansing Trio, and JuvaTone.

Ear Mites

Blends: Purification

1 Drop Purification oil on piece of cotton and put in ear.

Ebola Virus

Single oils:

• Rosemary with Geranium and Lemon.

Use: Add 1-3 drops to the corresponding single oils above (according to your sensitivity).

Mix:
• 10 drops rosemary
• 10 drops geranium
• 10 drops lemon
• 1/2 raw lemon
• 1 tablespoon honey

Mix in 8 oz. warm water. Drink every 2 hours. Every hour take 2 JuvaTone. Do a rectal implant of 2 tablespoons of Protec. Drink a mixture of 1/2 cup sauerkraut juice, 1/2 cup tomato juice, and 2 Tbsp. olive oil.

Eczema

(See SKIN DISORDERS.)

Edema

(See KIDNEY DISORDERS.)

Emotional Trauma - Heavy

Supporting a Person to move forward in Life.

Single oils:

• Frankincense with lavender, orange, tangerine, lemon, German chamomile, patchouly, sandalwood, myrrh, juniper, or geranium.

Blends:

• Frankincense with Present Time, Valor, Peace & Calming, Citrus Fresh, Christmas Spirit, White Angelica, 3 Wise Men, Sacred Mountain, or Trauma Life.

Supplements: Royaldophilus

Apply oils by anointing the crown of the head and the forehead and also by diffusing (see EMOTIONAL CLEARING). It is best if done in a quiet and dark room or at least in a low lit room.

Place 1-3 drops of Present Time over the thymus and rub clockwise 3 times and up to 3 times per day as desired. This is important to help people move out of the past and out of their negative thinking.

The synergistic combination of frankincense with Valor applied at night for a couple of days helps one to wake up in the morning ready to face the world and get on with life.

The effect of heavy emotional trauma can disrupt the stomach and digestive system. You may need 2 capsules of Royaldophilus, 2 or 3 times per day during the period of trauma and for 10 to 15 days thereafter (see DIGESTION).

Emphysema

Abnormal presence of air or gas in body tissue; wasting of lung substance.

Endocrine Balancing

Place EndoFlex on the tongue, roof of the mouth, thyroid, kidneys, liver, all of the glands, and the Vita Flex points for these glands on the feet and hands.

Use helichrysum on the Vita Flex points on the bottom of the feet and hands to stimulate the pineal and pituitary glands, which are considered the most important of the endocrine system.

Essential oils enable oxygen to transport and increase oxygen levels in the brain, which enables the pituitary and other glands to secrete neural transmitters and endorphins that support the endocrine and immune systems.

The thyroid is an important gland for balancing all the body systems (see THYROID).

Endocrine System

The endocrine system encompasses the hormone-producing glands of the body. These glands cluster around blood vessels and release their hormones directly into the bloodstream. The pituitary gland exerts wide range of control over the hormonal (endocrine) system and is often called the master gland. Other glands include the pancreas, adrenals, thyroid and parathyroid, ovaries (in women), and testes (in men). The limbic system lies along the margin of the cerebral cortex (brain) and is the hormone-producing system of the brain. It includes the amygdala, hippocampus, pineal, pituitary, thalamus, and hypothalamus.

Single oils:

- Helichrysum with nutmeg, clove, rosemary, bergamot, spearmint, or pepper.

Use: Add 1-3 drops to the corresponding single oils above (according to your sensitivity).

Blends:

- Helichrysum with EndoFlex, En-R-Gee, or Humility.

Use: Add 1-3 drops of each single oil to the corresponding blends above (according to your sensitivity).

Supplements: Thyromin and EssPro 7.

Energy, Lack of

Single oils:

- Lemongrass or juniper with basil, lemon, peppermint, rosemary, nutmeg, pepper, geranium, rosemary, Roman chamomile, melissa, ylang ylang, cypress, patchouly, or thyme.

Use: Add 1-3 drops to the corresponding single oils above (according to your sensitivity).

Blends:

- Lemongrass or juniper with En-R-Gee, Clarity, Hope, or Citrus Fresh.

- Ylang Ylang with Joy, Motivation, or Awaken.

Use: Add 1-3 drops of each single oil to the corresponding blends above (according to your sensitivity).

These oils stimulate brain function.

Supplements: Royal Essence, VitaGreen, Master HIS/HERS, Thyromin, Super B, and Stevia.

Place Royal Essence under the tongue for quick energy boost by increasing blood oxygen. Nutmeg has adrenal cortex-like activity and thus supports the adrenals for increased energy.

Environmental Toxic Poisoning

(See CHEMICAL SENSITIVITY.)

Epilepsy

Blends: Valor, Brain Power

Apply on brain stem (back of the neck at base of skull) and on brain Vita Flex points on the bottom of the feet.

Supplements: Cleansing Trio

(See COLON.)

Epstein-Barr Syndrome or Virus

(See HYPOGLYCEMIA.)

Symptoms include indigestion, upper and lower gas, poor assimilation, poor electrolyte balance, allergic reaction to foods and other substances, emotional mood swings, fatigue, irritability, and lack of motivation, discipline and creativity.

Hypoglycemia is a precursor and can render the body susceptible to the Epstein-Barr virus. Treat the hypoglycemia, and the symptoms of the Epstein-Barr virus will probably disappear.

Blends: ImmuPower

Supplements: Radex, ImmuGel, Super C, ImmuneTune, Cleansing Trio, and JuvaTone.

Do Raindrop Therapy on the spine with a mixture of ImmuneTune.

Exhaustion (Physical) - Fatigue

Single oils:

- Lemongrass with lavender, peppermint, mountain savory, sage, thyme, rosemary, or clove.

Use: Add 1-3 drops to the corresponding single oils above (according to your sensitivity).

Mountain savory is a tonic and stimulant for the body.

Blends:

- Lemongrass with En-R-Gee

Use: Add 1-3 drops of each single oil to the corresponding blends above (according to your sensitivity).

En-R-Gee helps with alertness.

Supplements: Vitagreen, Seagal Power Meal, Master HIS/HERS, Mineral Essence, Royal Essence, Super B, Thyromin, and EssPro 7.

Vitagreen is a plant-derived high-protein energy formula that athletes use to boost endurance. Royal Essence increases energy and endurance.

Digestion and colon problems may cause fatigue. A colon and liver cleanse unburdens the gut and therefore increases energy

Eyes

Supplements: Mineral Essence, Royal Essence, A. D. & E., Chelex, and VitaGreen.

Selenium supports the eyes. Mineral Essence and Royal Essence are good sources of all minerals, including selenium. A. D. & E. is beneficial for all eye problems.

Dr. Terry Friedman no longer needs his glasses after using sandalwood and juniper around the eyes (eyelids). He also used the supplements of Chelex, VitaGreen, the Cleansing Trio, and JuvaTone for a complete colon and liver cleanse (see COLON).

Blocked Tear Ducts

Single oils: Lavender

1 drop lavender oil rubbed over the bridge of the nose has been reported to work in seconds.

Cataracts and Glaucoma

Single oils:

- Lemongrass or lemon with cypress and eucalyptus.

Use: Add 1-3 drops to the corresponding single oils above (according to your sensitivity).

Eyes:
- 10 drops lemongrass
- 5 drops cypress
- 3 drops eucalyptus radiata

Mix in 1 oz. V-6 Mixing Oil or Massage Oil Base and apply around the eyes, temples, and Vita Flex points on the hands and feet, (the undersides of your two largest toes, index and middle fingers). This will also help with puffiness.

Mix:
- 10 drops lemon
- 5 drops cypress
- 3 drops eucalyptus

Mix in 1 oz. V-6 Mixing Oil or Massage Oil Base. Apply daily as above.

Eyewash formula:
- 2 parts pure honey
- 1 part pure apple cider vinegar
- 5 parts distilled water

Use as an eye wash, 3 or 4 times a day, while using the above oils.

Apply as desired for maintenance.

CAUTION: Do not get into eyes. If this happens, dilute with V-6, milk, butter, or any other oil based substance. NEVER rinse with water.

Drooping Eyelids

Single oils: Lavender and helichrysum.

Blends:

- Lavender or helichrysum with Aroma Life.

Use: Add 1-3 drops to the corresponding single oils above (according to your sensitivity).

Recipe:
- 5 drops lavender
- 1 drop helichrysum
- 2 drops Aroma Life

Mix in 1/2 oz. V-6 Mixing Oil or Massage Oil Base.

Supplements: VitaGreen

Inflamed Eyes

Single oils: Idaho tansy, lavender, and lemon (dilute in V-6 Mixing Oil or Massage Oil Base).

Apply to eyelids only and massage around the eyes.

Recipe:
- 10 drops lemongrass
- 5 drops cypress
- 3 drops eucalyptus radiata
- 1/2-oz. V-6 Mixing Oil or Massage Oil Base

Massage neat into fingertips and end of toes.

Supplements: A. D. & E., Ultra Young, and Sulfurzyme.

Bleeding

Single oils: Tansy, helichrysum, lavender, and peppermint.

Blends: Aroma Life or PanAway.

Supplements: Master Formula HERS/HIS, VitaGreen, and Sulfurzyme.

Blurred Vision

Single oils: Tansy, helichrysum, lavender, and peppermint.

Blends: Aroma Life or PanAway.

Supplements: Master Formula HERS/HIS, VitaGreen, Sulfurzyme, Super B, Super Cal, and Power Meal.

Fainting

Shock

Single Oils: Peppermint, spearmint.

Blends: Clarity, Brain Power, and Trauma Life.

Fasting

The best way to convert to vegetarianism is by fasting. To be healthy, have energy, be free of sickness and disease, you must learn to discipline yourself and listen to the needs of your body, not the desires of your body.

Our bodies do not need meat to maintain good health. We have programmed our RNA and DNA through years of meat consumption to have the desire to eat meat. Our bodies can get the protein required from a diet containing a wide variety of non-meat foods: beans, lentils, vegetables, whole grains, seeds, some cheeses, dairy products (preferably unpasteurized and natural colored), and occasionally eggs. However, you must be sure to eat enough protein to maintain a balanced, healthy body.

To change a lifestyle or habit, we must re-program our DNA and RNA. The DNA (deoxyribonucleic acid) contains the instructions for reproducing cells of the same kind. The RNA (ribonucleic acid) controls the chemical processes in cells, such as the production of proteins from amino acids. Fasting will help to change both the DNA and RNA.

Anyone young, old, or even lactating mothers, can fast. Wastes are eliminated through urine and stools. Mammary glands act as are filters, helping the baby to get proper nutrients from a lactating mother.

People with blood type A and AB are natural vegetarians and have the easiest time converting to a vegetarian diet. However, these people also have a tendency for thyroid problems and tend to be overweight. For them, exercise that increases heartrate is necessary to have weight reduction.

People with type B blood are probably the most balanced in nutritional needs and can go either way.

People with type 0 blood need additional protein, possibly through meat consumption. They have a more difficult time converting to vegetarianism. These people can get the protein they need if they consume the correct portions of seeds, nuts and grains. VitaGreen should be a mainstay for this group. These people often have digestive deficiencies. They eat more but assimilate less, have excess gas, get full quickly but are hungry sooner, and tend to weigh less.

Start with the master cleanse drink as follows:

- 8 ounces of water (preferably distilled).

- Juice from 1/2 of a fresh lemon.

- 1 or 2 tablespoons of grade C maple syrup.

- A shake or two of red cayenne pepper (work up to 1/4 teaspoon of the pepper per 8 ounces water, to taste). Cayenne dilates capillaries for better cleansing.

Drink at least ten 8 ounce glasses of this mixture per day, or better yet sip all day, but consume at least 80 ounces per day, plus all the plain water one can drink. During a fast, one cannot drink too much water. Be sure to drink distilled or purified water. Do not drink chlorinated tap water.

Grade C maple syrup is the best sweetener and the most balanced sugar, since it contains a balance of positive and negative ions. It is processed in open kettles without formaldehyde. Other grades are processed in pressurized containers with formaldehyde added.

Cayenne pepper provides vitamin A and is also a blood vessel dilator and thermal warmer.

People who have type 0 blood tend to have poor circulation and as a result tend to be cold when fasting. Cayenne pepper improves this situation. Put some cayenne in one's shoes and socks to warm the feet. Cayenne becomes damp from foot perspiration creating warmth to the feet.

Exercise makes fasting work better, particularly if one is trying to lose weight.

To change body chemistry, one will have to stay on the master cleanse as described above for at least 30 days. This gives the fastest and deepest cleanse and gets the quickest results.

To aid the transition to vegetarianism and help re-program the system, drink Power Meal 3 or 4 times per week. Also, for 2 weeks take VitaGreen, then follow the master cleanse for a further 30 days.

During the fast, 0 blood types may require more protein. During the first 2 weeks these people should take Power Meal twice a day and VitaGreen 3 times a day. These supplements will provide the necessary proteins. The body will convert its minimal protein requirements as needed. Individuals can go 60 days on a water-only fast before there is tissue breakdown.

Anyone fasting for more than 24 days should do so under supervision.

Never begin a shut-down fast unless you have been fasting regularly for at least two years. This type of a fast should always be done under supervision.

A regular fast is nothing but water. The above fast is really a cleanser, just as effective, but easier to do. By eating Power Meal and VitaGreen, you could stay on the master cleanse program as long as you desire.

As you progress on this program, your body chemistry will change. You should begin to feel an increase in energy. However, during the program you may also experience headaches, upset stomach, and low energy. These will be short lived and will pass.

Contrary to popular belief, lemon is not acidic in the body. It turns alkaline in the mouth. If an acid-like reaction is observed when putting lemon into water, it is because of the minerals in the water. Distilled water will not react.

Diabetics and those who react adversely to sugar (get hyper, cannot sleep, etc.) will have to substitute black strap molasses or stevia for the maple syrup. Start with 1 teaspoon molasses. In this way they will still be able to fast.

(See DIGESTIVE PROBLEMS.)

Fatigue

Single oils: Pepper, peppermint, and nutmeg.

Blends: En-R-Gee and Motivation.

Supplements: Thryomin, Power Meal, Vita-Green, Master Formula, Mineral Essence, and Royal Essence.

Fats (hard in the system) - Cellulite

Cellulite is one of the harder types of fats to dissolve in the body. Cellulite is an accumulation of old fat cell clusters that are solidifying and getting hard, while the surrounding tissue is losing its elasticity.

Overweight, excess fat is undesirable for two reasons:

1. The extra weight puts an extra load on all body systems, particularly the heart and cardiovascular system, but also on the joints (knees, hips, spine, etc.).

2. The body is unable to expel toxins and chemicals (pesticides, herbicides, metalics, etc.), that are stored in fatty tissue.

Single oils:

- Rosemary with grapefruit, lemon, cypress, fennel, juniper, spearmint, tangerine, lemongrass, or cedarwood.

Use: Add 1-3 drops to the corresponding single oils above (according to your sensitivity).

Blends:

- Rosemary with Citrus Fresh or EndoFlex.

Use: Add 1-3 drops of each single oil to the corresponding blends above (according to your sensitivity).

Supplements: Thyromin, EssPro 7, Power Meal, Cel-Lite Magic Massage Oil, and Goji Berry Tea.

Mix:
- 5 drops rosemary
- 10 drops grapefruit
- 2 drops cypress

Massage over area of concern at least once daily. Before exercising, massage the oils into the skin. Cellulite is slow to dissolve. Work on those areas for a month or more in conjunction with other methods of weight loss.

Recipe:
Mix:
- 9 drops lemon
- 9 drops cypress
- 2 ounces of jojoba oil

Recipe:
Mix:
- 10 drops grapefruit
- 5 drops lavender
- 3 drops helichrysum
- 3 drops patchouly
- 4 drops cypress
- 1/2 to 1 oz. V-6 Mixing Oil or Massage Oil Base.

Tangerine and grapefruit dissolve and digest fat cells and cellulite.

Spearmint increases metabolism to burn fat and toxins.

Lemongrass helps burn fat.

Goji Berry Tea helps to burn fat.

Cel-Lite Magic Massage Oil helps dissolve cellulite.

Add 3 to 5 drops of grapefruit to increase action in areas of fat rolls, puckers, dimples, etc.

The combination of grapefruit and cypress break up and digest the molecules of chemicals stored in the fat cells and stimulate the lymphatic system and blood to remove these chemicals.

Apply 1-3 times daily, depending on extent of problem and the person's age. Old fat and cellulite take longer to dissolve, so be patient. You should begin to see results in 6 to 8 weeks. Of course, a weigh-loss regime is recommended at the same time.

Bath:
- 5 drops juniper
- 3 drops orange
- 3 drops cypress
- 3 drops lemon
- 2 tbs. honey

Dissolve in warm bath water. Massage with Cel-Lite Magic afterwards.

Thyromin helps to balance or increase metabolism.

EssPro 7 helps balance hormones. Both assist the body in burning unwanted fat.

Fertility

Single oils:

- Clary sage with sage, fennel, yarrow, geranium, or bergamot.

Use: Add 1-3 drops with the corresponding single oils above (according to your sensitivity).

Blends: Dragon Time, Mister, and Sensation.

Application: Rub on the reproductive Vita Flex areas on the hands and feet. These areas are inside of wrists, around the front of the ankles in line with the anklebone, particularly inside and outside of the foot on either side of the anklebone, and along the achilles tendon.

In addition, women may rub on the lower back and area of lower bowels near the pubic bone or use as a vaginal retention implant.

Women: FemiGen 3-6 capsules daily to nourish reproductive system.

Use VitaGreen 3-8 capsules, 2-3 times a day and Essential Manna.

Men: Progen 2-4 capsules daily to nourish reproductive system.

Use VitaGreen and Essential Manna.

In addition for men, rub on the lower bowel near the pubic bone and in the area between the scrotum and rectum or use as a rectal implant.

Fever - Fever Blisters

Single oils:

- Lavender with peppermint, clove, or sandalwood.

Use: Add 1-3 drops to the corresponding single oils above (according to your sensitivity).

Blends:

- Lavender with Melrose.

Use: Add 1-3 drops of each single oil to the corresponding blends above (according to your sensitivity).

Supplements: AlkaLime, Super C, ImmuGel, Radex, Royal Essence, and Cinnamint Lip Balm.

Mix 5 drops each of lemon and peppermint. Diffuse or inhale.

Drink 1-2 drops of lemon or peppermint in an 8 oz. glass of water and sip slowly.

(See COLON.)

Fibroids

Single oils: Frankincense, inula, labdanom, lavender, and helichrysum.

Blends: Valor, EndoFlex, Cel-Lite Magic, and Protec.

Supplements: EssPro 7, Ultra Young, Thyromin, VitaGreen, AlkaLime, Power Meal, and Megazyme.

Fibromyalgia

Symptoms include general body pain, in some parts worse than others, brought on by only short periods of exercise. The pain is ubiquitous and continuous. It interrupts sleep patterns so that the fourth stage of sleep is never attained, and thus the body cannot rejuvenate and heal. Fibromyalgia is an acid condition in which the liver is toxic (see LIVER DETOXIFICATION).

Researchers have linked most degenerative diseases to lack of nutrients in the body. Insufficient minerals and trace minerals account for most of the nutritional deficiencies.

Blends:

- Birch or spruce with PanAway, Relieve It, or ImmuPower.

Use: Add 1-3 drops of each single oil to the corresponding blends above (according to your sensitivity).

Supplements: Ultra Young, Essential Manna, Power Meal, Super B, Super C, VitaGreen, Megazyme, ImmuneTune, Super Cal, Royal Essence, Mineral Essence, Rehemogen, EssPro 7, Royaldophilus, Vitamin E, Ortho Ease, and Ortho Sport Massage Oils.

Cleanse: (See COLON).

Eat less acidic foods and more alkaline foods, such as wheat sprouts or barley sprouts. VitaGreen is a food for alkaline balancing. This may be taken up to 4 times daily (see BODY pH ACID/ALKALINE BALANCE).

- Super C: 4-6 tablets daily.

- ImmuneTune: 2-6 times daily.

- Mineral Essence: 2-3 droppers 2 times daily in water or cold apple juice will supply the trace minerals needed without increasing the acid condition.

- Super Cal: 2-4 daily or as needed.

Rehemogen was formulated to cleanse and purify the blood. Clean blood more easily carries nutrients and oxygen to the cells to promote the healing process. Toxins block nutrient and oxygen flow into cells as well the absorption. (See BLOOD CIRCULATION, and DETOXIFICATION.)

- ImmuPower: Apply 4-6 drops along the spine and back with the Raindrop Therapy (see RAINDROP THERAPY).

- PanAway: Mix 20 drops in 2 Tbs. V-6 Mixing Oil or Massage Oil Base. Massage wherever there is pain until dry. Follow with the Ortho Ease or Ortho Sport Massage Oils. Add 3-4 drops of birch or spruce to make it stronger if needed.

Massage small areas with PanAway, neat (undiluted).

Mix:
- 10 drops PanAway
- 8 drops birch
- 8 drops marjoram
- 6 drops spruce

Mix in 1/2 oz. (4 Tbs.) of V-6 Massage Oil or Massage Oil Base and massage the entire body.

EssPro 7 has been reported to help cases of fibromyalgia, particularly in older people who may have a hormone imbalance.

Flatulence

Single oils: Peppermint, tarragon, anise seed, and fennel.

Blends: Di-Tone

Supplements: Megazyme, AlkaLime, and Royaldolphilus.

Flu

Single oils: Idaho tansy, lemon, mountain savory, oregano, and peppermint.

Blends: Di-Tone, Thieves, ParaFree, Megazyme, and Mint Condition.

Tansy rubbed should be applied topically on stomach and bottom of feet.

Food Poisoning

Single oils: Tarragon, patchouly, and rosemary cineol.

Blends: Di-Tone, Exodus II, and Thieves.

Supplements: Megazyme and Exodus.

Foot Problems

Athlete's Foot

- Mix 2-4 drops of melaleuca with any of the single oils listed: lemon, lemongrass, thyme, basil, rosemary, lavender, eucalyptus, geranium, or bergamot.

- Mix 2-4 drops of lavender with any of the single oils listed: melaleuca, frankincense, rosemary, thyme, geranium, bergamot, patchouly, tarragon, or myrrh.

- Mix 2-4 drops of the single oil of melaleuca with Thieves.

- Mix 2-4 drops of the lavender with any of the following: Melrose, Purification, Mister, Di-Tone, or Thieves.

Mix
- 2 drops melaleuca
- 2 drops melaleuca
- 1 drop lavender.
  Apply to infected areas, between toes and around toenails.

Mix:
- 11 drops geranium
- 6 drops myrrh
- 13 drops melaleuca
- 6 drops patchouly

Mix in 1/2 oz. V-6 Mixing Oil or Massage Oil Base or blend in a mixture of cocoa butter, glycerol, and lecithin. Use in place of the first blend.

Supplements: ImmuGel, Exodus, and Rose Ointment.

Blisters on Feet

Single oils:

- Mix 1 drop lavender with 1 drop Roman chamomile. Mix 1 drop lavender with 1 drop melaleuca. Gently pat on thoroughly, but carefully.

Bunions

Single oils:

Mix:
- 6 drops eucalyptus
- 3 drops lemon
- 4 drops raven
- 1 drop birch

Apply over area. Dilute if desired with 1 oz. V-6 Mixing Oil or Massage Oil Base if concerned about skin sensitivity.

Corns

Single oils: Lemon, tangerine, grapefruit, and myrrh.

Blends: Citrus Fresh

Apply 1 drop of oil, neat, directly on the corn.

Frigidity

(See SEXUAL PROBLEMS.)

Fungus Infection - Ringworm - Thrush - Skin Candida

Fungi and yeast are responsible for decomposing dead tissues. They exist everywhere: inside our stomachs, on our skin, and out on the lawn. When kept under control, the yeast and fungi populating our bodies are harmless and digest what our bodies cannot or do not use.

Fungus grows from the fermentation of yeast and sugar, but not the sugar or the yeast as individual substances. When we feed the naturally occurring fungi in our bodies too many acidic foods, such as sugar, animal proteins, and dairy products, the fungi population grows out of control. They secrete large numbers of poisons called mycotoxins, which are believed to be one of the causes of many diseases and debilitating conditions.

Ringworm is a fungus called Tinea that infects the skin, causing scaly round itchy patches. It is infectious and can be caught from an animal or any one else with the condition. If it is in the hair, sterilize or throw away the combs, brushes, hats, and clothes that contact the patches.

Skin candida is a fungus infection that can erupt almost anywhere on the skin. It shows up in various places, such as behind the knees, inside the elbows, behind the ears, on temple area, and between the breasts.

Thrush (candida albicans) is a fungus infection of the mouth and can go into the throat as well.

Warts are another form of skin candida.

Researchers have linked most degenerative diseases to lack of nutrients in the body. Insufficient minerals and trace minerals account for many nutritional deficiencies.

Research has found that most diseases are linked to acid-based yeast and fungus dominance, which include the following symptoms:

- Fatigue/low energy
- Unexplained aches and pains
- Overweight
- Low resistance to Illness
- Allergies
- Unbalanced blood sugar
- Headaches
- Irritability
- Mood swings
- Indigestion
- Colitis and ulcers
- Diarrhea/constipation
- Urinary tract infections
- Rectal itch
- Vaginal itch

Single oils:

- Lavender with melaleuca, frankincense, Roman chamomile, German chamomile, rosemary, thyme, geranium, bergamot, black cumin, patchouly, Idaho tansy, mountain savory, tarragon, palmarosa, helichrysum, mandarin, marjoram, or rose.

- Melaleuca with rosemary, tarragon, lavender, spruce, thyme, eucalyptus, clove, lemon, lemongrass, basil, geranium, bergamot, cinnamon, or spikenard.

- Thyme with oregano, rosemary, tarragon, lavender, spruce, eucalyptus, hyssop, clove, or cinnamon.

- Rosemary with clary sage, sage, mountain savory, fennel, bergamot, sandalwood, ylang ylang, jasmine, rosewood, geranium, yarrow, myrrh, neroli, peppermint, spearmint, or cistus.

Use: Add 1-3 drops to the corresponding single oils above (according to your sensitivity).

Blends:

- Lavender with Melrose, Purification, Mister, ImmuPower, Inspiration, Di-Tone, Thieves, Abundance, Acceptance, or Exodus II.

- Melaleuca with Melrose, Purification, Thieves, R..C, Di-Tone, or Raven.

- Rosemary with Melrose, Purification, R.C., Di-Tone, Raven, Christmas Spirit, or Clarity.

- Thyme with Melrose, Purification, Thieves, Sensation, or 3 Wise Men.

Use: Add 1-3 drops of each single oil to the corresponding blends above (according to your sensitivity).

Supplements: Rose Ointment, Master Formula HIS/HERS, Femigen, Royaldophilus, Megazyme, ImmuGel, ImmuneTune, VitaGreen, Arthro-Tune, Thyromin, Super C, Radex, Mineral Essence, Rehemogen, Colloidal Essence, Alka-Lime, Exodus, corn starch, and baking soda.

Heartburn is a possible indication of fungus infections. Fermentation of sugars is what feeds candida. A healthy, fully functioning digestive system will not allow this fermentation, and thus fungus will not develop or progress. Royaldophilus will help to provide the friendly, intestinal flora to aid digestion. You should take 1 dose before each meal (3 per day).

Cleanse: (see COLON).

Candida/fungus overgrowth in stomach: 5-10 drops Di-Tone over stomach and 3 drops on the feet.

Mineral Essence: 3 droppers 3 times daily. Fungi will not grow in the presence of sufficient trace minerals (electrolytes) and enzymes.

Megazyme: 3 tablets 3 times daily with meals provides necessary enzymes for good absorption through mouth and throat tissue.

Thyromin: Strengthens endocrine glands. The thyroid secretes antibodies that regulate fungus overgrowth (see THYROID).

Super C: Provides necessary bioflavinoids.

Radex: Necessary for antioxidant and free radical scavenging.

Colloidal Essence: Powerful antibacterial, antifungal, and antiviral. May be taken internally or applied externally as required.

ImmuPower: 3 drops in 4 oz. of water, 3 times daily after meals. Boosts the immune system and fights fungus. Also apply to bottom of feet.

Rosewood: Helps rid skin of candida (fungus).

Melrose: Beneficial for treating fungus.

Myrrh: Fights against athlete's foot, ringworm, eczema, cracked and chapped skin, wrinkles, etc.

Oregano: Antifungal and antiparasitic.

Ring worm fungus:
- 3 drops melaleuca
- 3 drops spearmint
- 1 drop peppermint

Mix in 1/2 ounce V-6 Mixing Oil or Massage Oil Base.

Fungus itching:
- 2 drops tansy
- 10 drops melaleuca
- 1 drop oregano
- 2 drops patchouly

Neat or mix in 1/2 oz. V-6 Mixing Oil or Massage Oil Base. Apply oils neat on location, to spinal Vita Flex points on the feet, and hands and around the heel up to the anklebone.

Fungi tend to reside in the spinal fluid. Microorganisms have a tendency to hibernate along the spinal chord. The body has the ability to hold viruses in a suspended state for long periods of time. When the immune system becomes compromised from stress, fatigue or other factors, the virus can be released and manifest illness and disease.

Oregano, thyme, or hyssop along the spine in Raindrop Therapy application may help to drive the dormant fungi out of the spinal fluid.

Thieves: 1-2 drops in V-6 Mixing Oil or Massage Oil Base massaged on the thymus, stimulates the immune system.

ImmuPower: Apply to the bottom of the feet, on the throat, and chest.

Diffuse: Alternate Thieves with ImmuPower for protection from airborne bacteria and viruses. Diffuse 15 to 30 minutes every 2 to 3 hours. With heavy saturation, the cinnamon in Thieves may irritate the nasal passages.

Rose Ointment: Maintains soft and supple skin.

Overuse of antibiotics increases the resistance of pathogenic microorganisms, kills the beneficial bacteria in our bodies generating yeast and fungi overgrowth.

Fungus infections may clear up, only to erupt again in a few weeks. The fungus lies dormant in the lymphatic system or spinal fluid. Lymphatic pump therapy will assist in cleaning a sluggish lymphatic system and help remove dormant fungi.

The lymphatic system pump is performed as follows:

- Have the person lie on his/her back or sit in a comfortable chair. With one hand, support one foot by lifting it just above the heel. Grasp the toes of that foot by clamping your other hand over them, covering both sides of the toes. Bend the toes up as far as comfortable and hold the toes in that position; pull the foot down as far as is comfortable. Bend the toes down as far as comfortable. Holding the toes in this position, push the foot up as far as is comfortable. Bend the toes up as far as comfortable and repeat. Pump like this 2 to 6 times. Less for the first time and more as the lymph system clears. Change to the other foot and repeat. (See LYMPHATIC PUMP under CLEANSING.)

Gall Bladder

Single oils:

- Lavender with geranium, juniper, Roman chamomile, German chamomile, rosemary, or eucalyptus.

Use: Add 1-3 drops to the corresponding single oils above (according to your sensitivity).

Blends:

- Lavender with JuvaFlex, PanAway, or Release.

Use: Add 1-3 drops of each single oil to the corresponding blends above (according to your sensitivity).

Apply oils on Vita Flex points on feet and hands, on location, and around navel.

JuvaFlex stimulates the gall bladder.

Supplements: Sulfurzyme

Our bodies cannot absorb vitamins and minerals without the presence of protein (protein powders suffice), particularly those who have had their gall bladders surgically removed. The MSM (sulfurr) found in Sulfurzyme is vital to the amino acids responsible for protein synthesis. MSM (sulfur) magnifies the nutritional effects of vitamins and aids bile secretion.

Gall Stones

Single oils:

- Lavender with rosemary, geranium, juniper or nutmeg.

Use: Add 1-3 drops to the corresponding single oils above (according to your sensitivity).

Blends: JuvaFlex stimulates the gall bladder. Rosemary or nutmeg is supportive.

Recipe:
- 10 drops lavender
- 10 drops rosemary
- 10 drops geranium
- 10 drops juniper

Mix in juice and drink.

Rub oils over gall bladder or apply a hot compress over area, massage Vita Flex points on bottom of feet.

Gangrene

Single oils: Oregano, mountain savory, thyme, ravensara, and cistus.

Blends: Exodus II, Thieves, ImmuPower, and Melrose.

Supplements: Exodus, Radex, ImmuGel, Immu-Tune, and Super C.

Gastritis

Single oils: Tarragon, peppermint, and fennel.

Blends: Di-Tone

Supplements:

- Megazyme: 3-4 capsules 3 times daily.

- Mint Condition: 3-4 capsules 3 times daily.

- Royaldophilus: 2-4 capsules 3 times daily.

- Mineral Essence: 2-3 droppers 3 times daily.

- ComforTone and I.C.P.: Begin after 2 weeks.

Gingivitis, Phyorrhea

(See GUMS.)

Glaucoma

(See EYES.)

Gout

Single oils:

- Mix 1-3 drops with any of the following: Geranium, juniper, rosemary, Roman chamomile, lemon, melaleuca, nutmeg, or Idaho tansy.

Blends: PanAway and JuvaFlex.

Supplements: Thyromin, Essential Manna, Mineral Essence, Super C, Super Cal, Arthro-Tune, VitaGreen, Sulfurzyme, Cleansing Trio, JuvaTone, Ortho Ease Massage Oil, and Ortho Sport Massage Oil.

With gout, the kidneys, adrenal, and immune functions are not fully functional, and there is an excess of uric acid in the body. Detoxify by cleansing and drinking plenty of fluids, water, juices, and herbal teas.

Uric acid:

- 10 drops geranium
- 8 drops juniper
- 5 drops rosemary
- 3 drops Roman chamomile
- 4 drops lemon
- 8 drops melaleuca

Put 6 drops in water and drink 3 times daily.

Mix in 1 teaspoon of V-6 Mixing Oil or Massage Oil Base for massage on affected areas. May be applied neat 1-3 drops.

Supplements:

- Mineral Essence - 3 droppers, 3 times daily.

- ArthroTune - 3 capsules, 3 times daily.

- JuvaTone - up to 18 per day, cutting back after 2 weeks.

- Super Cal: 2-4 capsules 1-2 times daily.

- Super C: 2-4 tablets 2-3 times daily.

- VitaGreen: 2-6 capsules 2-3 times daily.

Mix:
- 10 drops birch
- 6 drops fennel
- 2 drops tansy
- 3 drops patchouly
- 10 drops tangerine

Mix in 1/2 to 1 teaspoon. V-6 Mixing Oil or Massage Oil Base. This is helpful for liver, kidneys, and water retention.

Grand Mall Seizures

Blends: Brain Power, Clarity, Valor, Peace & Calming, Joy, Sacred Mountain, and Aroma Siez.

- Valor: Massage on bottom of feet.

- Diffuse: Brain Power, Peace & Calming.

- Joy: Rub over heart.

- Sacred Mountain: 2-3 drops on back of neck and on crown.

- Aroma Siez: Raindrop Therapy on Spine. (See RAINDROP THERAPY.)

Supplements: Master HIS/HERS, VitaGreen, Super B, Mineral Essence, Royal Essence, Power Meal, Sulfurzyme, Body Balance, and Ultra Young.

Growing Pains, Children

Single oils:

- Pine and elemi.

- Birch with cypress or peppermint.

Use: Add 1-3 drops to the corresponding single oils above (according to your sensitivity).

Blends: PanAway and Relieve It.

Supplements: Mineral Essence, Super Cal, and ArthroTune.

Super Cal provides calcium for growing bones.

ArthroTune: 2-4 capsules daily.

Massage birch, cypress, and peppermint, wait five minutes, and then cover with Ortho Ease Massage Oil.

Gums

Bleeding

Single oils: Mountain savory, clove, and cistus.

Supplements: Dentarome, Dentarome Plus, and Fresh Essence Mouth Wash.

For infection use mountain savory, clove and cistus.

Gingivitis

Single oils: Helichrysum, mountain savory, cistus, and clove.

Blends: Exodus II and Thieves.

Supplements: Super C, Dentarome, Dentarome Plus, and Fresh Essence Mouth Wash.

Super C: 14 tablets spread throughout the day.

For infection use mountain savory and cistus.

Pyorrhea

Single oils: Helichrysum, mountain savory, cistus, and clove.

Blends: Exodus II and Thieves.

Supplements: Dentarome, Dentarome Plus, and Fresh Essence Mouth Wash.

For infection use mountain savory and cistus.

Hair Care - Dandruff

Single oils:

- Rosemary or lavender with clary sage, sage, fennel, cedarwood, juniper, ylang ylang, sandalwood, lemon, Roman chamomile, German chamomile, cypress, rose, rosewood, geranium, or patchouly.

Use: Add 1-3 drops to the corresponding single oils above (according to your sensitivity).

Supplements: ParaFree, Thyromin, Super B, Master HIS/HERS, Royal Essence, EssPro 7, Morning Start Bath Gel, Shampoo: Lavender

Massage: 4-8 drops of the single oils listed above into the scalp or add to any AromaSilk Hair and Scalp. Sandalwood helps restore hair color by helping the body utilize nutrients. Sage supports the hair follicle and helps deliver nutrients to the hair shaft.

Premature graying is thought to be from a deficiency of biotin. Super B and Super C are a good source of all B vitamins.

NOTE: Shampoos containing essential oils do not lather up because they do not contain harmful foaming chemicals.

Lemongrass has been reported to clear acne and balance oily skin and scalp conditions. Lavender shampoo helps to balance skin pH, decongest the lymphatics, and stimulate circulation.

Sandalwood oil rinse retards graying. Rosewood will lighten hair color.

A rinse to help restore the acid mantle of the hair:

- 1 drop rosemary, 1 tsp. pure apple cider vinegar, and 8 oz. water. Use as a final rinse on hair. Rosemary adds body and conditions the hair. Rub 1 or 2 drops on as hairdressing or on hairbrush to prevent static electricity.

Dandruff:
- 5 drops lemon
- 1 drop rosemary or sage
- 1 drop lavender
- 1 quart/litre of water

Use as a rinse

Dry Hair:
- 2 drops ylang ylang
- 8 drops rosewood
- 4 drops geranium

Oily Hair:

- 6 drops patchouly
- 2 to 5 oz. of lavender shampoo
- 6 drops lemon

Split Ends
- 1 drop rosemary
- 3 drops sandalwood
- 1 drop ylang ylang

To keep hair dark:
- 1 drop geranium
- 3 drops sandalwood
- 1 quart/liter of water

Use as a rinse. May add 2 drops sandalwood.

To keep hair light:
- 2 drops Roman chamomile
- 1 drop lemon
- 2 drops rosemary
- 1 quart/liter of water

Use as a rinse.

Hair Loss

Single oils:

- Lavender or rosemary with any of the following: ylang ylang, sage, cedarwood, sandalwood, sage, or clary sage.

Use: Add 1-3 drops to the corresponding single oils above (according to your sensitivity).

Oils cleanse, nourish, and strengthen the hair follicle and shaft.

Rosemary encourages hair growth and cleanses.

Supplements: Super B, Thyromin, EssPro 7, Sulfurzyme.

Lavender shampoo may decrease hair loss.

Mix 1 drop of any 3 or more of the above oils and massage into the scalp nightly.

Premature Balding:
- 3 drops rosemary
- 5 drops lavender
- 4 drops cypress
- 2 drops clary sage
- 2 drops juniper

At night add a drop of the above blend to 1 tsp. of water and massage into scalp where balding; then rub gently into rest of scalp.

To stop hair from falling out:
- 10 drops cedarwood
- 8 drops rosemary
- 10 drops sandalwood
- 10 drops lavender

Mix in shampoo base or massage individually into scalp one oil per day.

Body massage:
- 10 drops frankincense
- 8 drops Roman chamomile
- 5 drops lemon

Mix with V-6 Mixing Oil or Massage Oil Base:.

Hair growth:
- 3-4 drops rosemary
- 4 drops ylang ylang
- 6 drops cedarwood
- 6 drops clary sage

Mix in V-6 Mixing Oil or Massage Oil Base and rub into scalp at night.

Hair growth:
- 10 drops rosemary
- 3 drops cedarwood
- 3 drops birch
- 2 drops ylang ylang

Mix in V-6 Mixing Oil or Massage Oil Base. Rub into scalp at night.

Halitosis - Bad Breath

Single oils: Nutmeg, peppermint, and tarragon.

If one has persistent bad breath or gum disease, it may be a sign of poor digestion, or other health problems.

Infection

Mix:

- 2 to 5 drops of clove
- 2 drops of thyme
- Thieves
- Exodus

Rub on gums. Melrose can also be used on gums.

Place ImmuGel on a piece of gauze. Roll like a piece of rope and place along the gum. This works particularly well for leukemia patients because their gums tend to inflame, swell, and become infected.

Brush with Dentarome and Dentarome Plus toothpaste.

Gargle with Fresh Essence Mouth Wash.

Single oils:

- Mix 1-2 drops of birch with sage or myrrh.

Blends:

- Birch or sage with Melrose or Thieves.

Use: Add 1-3 drops of each single oil to the corresponding blends above (according to your sensitivity).

Mouth Ulcers

Single oils: 1 drop of Myrrh with Oregano.

Blends: 1 drop of Thieves with Exodus II.

Brush with Dentarome or Dentarome Plus Toothpaste.

Gargle with Fresh Essence Mouth Wash. Add 1-2 drops of Thieves, clove, and Exodus II to make stronger.

Head Lice

Single oils:

- Eucalyptus with lavender, peppermint, or geranium.

Use: Add 1-3 drops to the corresponding single oils above (according to your sensitivity).

Mix:

- 2 drops eucalyptus
- 1 drop lavender
- 1 drop geranium

Mix into 1 tsp. of V-6 Mixing Oil or Massage Oil Base. Massage into scalp. Leave for 1/2 hour. Shampoo and rinse well.

Antiseptic rinse:

- 2 drops eucalyptus
- 2 drops lavender
- 2 drops geranium
- 1/2 ounce vinegar
- 8 oz. water

Pour over hair making sure every hair is rinsed. Dry naturally. Repeat daily until lice and eggs are gone.

Pulling Hair:

Blends: EndoFlex, Harmony, Joy, Valor, and Peace & Calming.

Supplements: Master Formula HIS/HERS, and CHILDREN'S, VitaGreen, Megazyme, and Thyromin.

Headaches

Headaches are due to a shortage of oxygen, stress, and sugar imbalance (hypoglycemia). Oils boost the oxygen-carrying capacity of the blood and oxygen infusion into the cell. When a person's frequency drops, a headache begins.

Single Oils: Tansy, Roman chamomile, peppermint, lavender, basil, spearmint, bergamot, lemon, and rosemary.

Blends: M-Grain, Brain Power, Clarity, and Thieves.

Diffuse, rub on back of neck, temples, or put under nose.

Headaches:

- 4 drops Idaho tansy
- 5 drops Roman chamomile
- 2 drops peppermint
- 2 drops lavender
- 1 drop basil
- 3 drops rosemary

To relieve headaches:

- 2 drops Idaho tansy
- 1 drops Roman chamomile
- 3 drops spearmint
- 7 drops lavender
- 9 drops basil

Mix in 1/2 oz. V-6 Mixing Oil or Massage Oil Base.

Calming and soothing a headache:
- 12 drops bergamot
- 2 drops lavender
- 3 drops geranium
- 2 drops rosemary
- 5 drops lemon

Blend in V-6 Mixing Oil or Massage Oil Base.

- Thieves: 1 drop on tongue and push against roof of mouth.
- Clarity: 1-2 drops on back of neck, under nose, and on temples. Put 1-2 drops in palm of hands, rub hands together, cup over nose, and breathe deeply.

Supplements: VitaGreen, Power Meal, Body Balance, and Brain Power.

Stress

Single oils:

- Lavender with patchouly, birch, spruce, lemongrass, rosemary, or basil.

Use: Add 1-3 drops to the corresponding single oils above (according to your sensitivity).

Blends:

- Lavender with Valor or Aroma Siez.
- Lemongrass with Valor or Aroma Siez.

Use: Add 1-3 drops of each single oil to the corresponding blends above (according to your sensitivity).

Children's Migraine

Single oils: German chamomile, grapefruit, peppermint, and rosemary.

Mix:
- 1 drops German chamomile
- 10 drops grapefruit
- 5 drops peppermint
- 3 drops rosemary

Mix in 1 teaspoon of V-6 Mixing Oil or Massage Oil Base. Rub on temples, forehead, and brain stem. Also massage on thumbs and big toes.

Headache from Diffusing - Clarity, Brain Power, and other oils

People who get an instant headache from diffusing usually have a blockage related to metalics or chemicals in the brain. The main oil in Clarity is cardamom, which contains high levels of trans-phenols, which are very high in oxygen molecules.

Single oils:

- Helichrysum with rosemary.

Use: Add 1-3 drops to the corresponding single oils above (according to your sensitivity).

Blends: Aroma Life, M-Grain, and Clarity.

Helichrysum is a chelator. Rosemary breaks down plaque. Aroma Life and M-Grain both contain helichrysum. Apply these oils to the arteries in the neck on the pulse points where arteries are closest to the surface.

Continue to diffuse Clarity or the offending oil, but in small amounts until the body clears itself and the diffused oil does not cause the headache any more. Clarity will also help the chelation process.

Hormonal Imbalance

Single oils:

- Lavender with clary sage, sage, fennel, bergamot, or geranium.

Use: Add 1-3 drops to the corresponding single oils above (according to your sensitivity).

Blends:

- Lavender or basil with Mister, Dragon Time, EndoFlex, or M-Grain.

Use: Add 1-3 drops of each single oil to the corresponding blends above (according to your sensitivity).

Supplements: Femalin, Thyromin, Super B, VitaGreen, Royal Essence, EssPro 7, Dragon Time Massage Oil, and Dragon Time Bath and Shower Gel.

Oils may be rubbed on the reproductive Vita Flex areas on hands and feet. These areas are inside of wrists and around the front of the ankles in line with the anklebone and particularly inside and outside of the foot just above the anklebone and up along the Achilles tendon. They may also be rubbed on the lower back and groin (see MENOPAUSE and HORMONAL IMBALANCE).

Hypoglycemic Migraine

Single oils:

- Lavender, lemongrass, clove, caraway, thyme, or geranium.

Use: Add 1-3 drops to the corresponding single oils above (according to your sensitivity).

Blends: Clarity

- Lavender with Thieves, M-Grain, JuvaFlex, or Di-Tone.

Use: Add 1-3 drops of each single oil to the corresponding blends above (according to your sensitivity).

Supplements: Power Meal, Body Balance, VitaGreen, Royal Essence, and EssPro 7

From low blood sugar or sugar imbalance:

- Thieves: 1 drop on tongue and push against roof of mouth.

- Clarity: 1-2 drops on back of neck, under nose, and on temples. Put 1-2 drops in palm of hands, rub hands together, cup over nose and breathe deeply.

Application of oils: Apply neat on pancreas Vita Flex points on feet. Thieves will boost blood sugar levels, as will VitaGreen and Body Balance. Apply M-Grain on thumbs.

Migraine

Single oils:

- Rosemary with basil, peppermint, melissa, lavender, ylang ylang, German chamomile, eucalyptus, or marjoram.

- Helichrysum with sandalwood.

Use: Add 1-3 drops to the corresponding single oils above (according to your sensitivity).

Blends:

- Rosemary or peppermint with M-Grain or Clarity.

Use: Add 1-3 drops of each single oil to the corresponding blends above (according to your sensitivity).

Supplements: A. D. & E. and Megazyme.

The vast majority of migraine headaches are from colon congestion. Poor digestion can also be a factor. The Cleansing Trio is most important for cleansing the colon.

M-Grain is specially formulated for migraine headaches. Put a couple of drops in your palm (can also add a drop of peppermint). Rub hands together clockwise; then cup hands over your nose and breathe deeply. Put on temples, forehead, and brain stem (back of neck at skull). Massage on thumbs and big toes. Lavender and basil, layered on temples and forehead, has relieved migraine headaches

Apply 1 drop helichrysum and 1 drop sandalwood to the inside of nasal passages, also on temples and brain stem.

A. D. & E. vitamin supplement is important for vision. Eye strain and decreased vision can accompany migraine headaches.

Muscle-Related Headache

Single oils:

- Lavender with marjoram, rosemary, peppermint, lemongrass, basil, valerian, marjoram, or cardamom.

Use: Add 1-3 drops to the corresponding single oils above (according to your sensitivity).

Blends:

- Lavender or lemongrass with M-Grain or Aroma Siez.

Use: Add 1-3 drops of each single oil to the corresponding blends above (according to your sensitivity).

Supplements: Relaxation, Ortho Ease and Ortho Sport Massage Oils.

Use peppermint around the hairline, on the back of the neck, and across the forehead.

Sinus-Related Headache

Single oils:

- Rosemary with bergamot, melaleuca ericifolia with eucalyptus, lavender, lemon, or geranium.

Use: Add 1-3 drops to the corresponding single oils above (according to your sensitivity).

Mix:
- 5 drops melaleuca ericifolia
- 9 drops rosemary
- 2 drops bergamot
- 7 drops lavender
- 3 drops lemon
- 4 drops geranium

Mix in 1 oz. V-6 Mixing Oil or Massage Oil Base.

Structural - Bone-Related Headache

Single oils:

- Lavender with birch, basil, marjoram, lemongrass, or rosemary.

Use: Add 1-3 drops to the corresponding single oils above (according to your sensitivity).

Blends:

- Lavender or lemongrass with M-Grain and Aroma Siez or PanAway.

Use: Add 1-3 drops of each single oil to the corresponding blends above (according to your sensitivity).

Supplements: Ortho Ease, Relaxation and, Sensation Massage Oils, Evening Peace Bath and Shower Gel.

Hearing

(See EARS.)

Heart

Heart Vita Flex

The foot Vita Flex point related to the heart is on the sole of the left foot, on the ring toe (2nd toe) and behind the knuckle. Massaging this point is as effective as massaging the hand and arm together. The hand Vita Flex point related to the heart is in the palm of the left hand, 1 inch below the ring finger joint (at the lifeline). The secondary point is on the bottom of the left arm in line with the inside of the up-turned arm (approximately 2 inches up the arm from the funny bone), not on the muscle but up under the muscle. Have another person use thumbs and firmly press these two points alternately for 3 minutes, in a kind of pumping action. Work all 3 points when possible. Start with the foot first; then go to the hand and arm.

Heart Attack - Myocardial Infarction

Interruption of blood supply to an area.

Single oils:

- Lavender with Roman chamomile, helichrysum, or rose.

Use: Add 1-3 drops to the corresponding single oils above (according to your sensitivity).

Blends:

- Lavender or marjoram with Aroma Life, Valor, Peace & Calming, Harmony, PanAway, or Relieve It.

Supplements: Cardia Care, HRT Tincture, Mineral Essence, Super Cal, Power Meal, and, Sulfurzyme.

Apply to heart Vita Flex points on feet, hand, and arm as described above. If there is not enough time to remove shoes to get at the feet, apply pumping action to left hand and arm points. Using 1 drop of Aroma Life on each point will increase effectiveness and may even revive an individual having a heat attack while waiting for medical attention.

Applying Valor on bottom of feet improves effectiveness of other oils. Apply Harmony to the energy or chakra points (crown of head, forehead, throat (thyroid), thymus, navel, stomach, groin) to balance body frequencies. Inhale Peace & Calming to relax the individual.

Magnesium, the most important mineral for the heart, acts as a smooth muscle relaxant and supports the cardiovascular system. Magnesium will act as a natural calcium channel blocker for the heart, lowering blood pressure and dilating the heart blood vessels (*Dr. Terry Friedmann*). Mineral Essence along with Super Cal are good sources of magnesium.

MSM (sulfur), found in Sulfurzyme, normalizes heart function.

Angina

Single oils: Ginger

False Angina

Single oils: Orange

Arrhythmia (Heart Rhythm Disorders)

Single oils:

- Ylang ylang with marjoram or Idaho tansy.

Use: Add 1-3 drops to the corresponding single oils above (according to your sensitivity).

Blends:

- Ylang ylang or marjoram with Aroma Life or Joy.

Use: Add 1-3 drops of each single oil to the corresponding blends above (according to your sensitivity).

Place 1 drop of each oil on heart Vita Flex points and do heart Vita Flex application. Marjoram and Aroma Life stimulate regeneration of smooth muscle tissue, particularly in the heart. Rub Joy over the heart and diffuse in the room.

Supplements: CardiaCare, Mineral Essence, Super Cal, Sulfurzyme, and HRT.

Arterial Fibrillation

This is when the upper heart chambers contract at a rate of over 300 pulsation's per minute. The lower chambers cannot keep this pace, so efficiency is reduced, and not enough blood is pumped. Palpitations, a feeling that the heart is beating irregularly, more strongly, or more rapidly than normal, is the most common symptom.

Single oils:

- Ylang Ylang with marjoram, helichrysum, or orange.

Use: Add 1-3 drops to the corresponding single oils above (according to your sensitivity).

Blends: Aroma Life

Supplements: HRT, CardiaCare, Mineral Essence, Super Cal, and Sulfurzyme.

Place 1 drop of each oil on heart Vita Flex points and do Vita Flex (see HEART).

Cardiac Spasm

Single oils: Marjoram, basil, and valerian

Nervousness

Single oils:

- Lavender with marjoram, ylang ylang, peppermint, Roman chamomile, valerian or basil.

Use: Add 1-3 drops to the corresponding single oils above (according to your sensitivity).

Blends:

- Lavender with Aroma Life, Peace & Calming, Valor, Joy, or Harmony.

Use: Add 1-3 drops of each single oil to the corresponding blends above (according to your sensitivity).

Supplements: HRT

Rub Joy over heart every day as needed (see BLOOD PRESSURE, CARDIOVASCULAR SYSTEM).

Shortness of Breath

(Due to enlarged heart valve)

Blends: Aroma Siez and R.C.

Supplements: HRT, CardiaCare

Strengthen Heart

Blends:

- Marjoram with Aroma Life.

Use: Add 1-3 drops of each single oil to the corresponding blends above (according to your sensitivity).

Supplements: HRT, CardiaCare

Tachycardia

Heart rate that suddenly increases to 160 per minute or faster for no reason.

Single oils: Lavender, ylang ylang, and Idaho tansy.

Blends:

- Ylang ylang with Aroma Life or Joy.

Use: Add 1-3 drops of each single oil to the corresponding blends above (according to your sensitivity).

Supplements: CardiaCare, HRT, and Sulfurzyme.

Place 1 drop of each oil on heart Vita Flex points and do heart Vita Flex.

Rub Joy over the heart and diffuse in the room

Tonic - Stimulant

Single oils: Anise, mandarin, rosemary, peppermint, and thyme.

Anise is a tonic and stimulant to the heart.

Heart Burn

Single oils: Peppermint, spearmint

Blends: Di-Tone

Supplements: AlkaLime and Mint Condition.

Heat Stroke

Single oils: Helichrysum, cypress, sandalwood, and peppermint.

- Rub 1 drop lavender with 1 drop peppermint on back of neck and on forehead.

Use: Add 1-3 drops to the corresponding single oils above (according to your sensitivity).

Supplements: CardiaCare and HRT.

Heavy Metals

(See CHEMICAL POISONING.)

Hematoma

A tumor-like mass of coagulated blood, caused by a break in the blood vessel or capillary wall.

Single oils:

- Helichrysum with German chamomile, rose, cypress, Roman chamomile, or geranium.

Use: Add 1-3 drops to the corresponding single oils above (according to your sensitivity).

Blends:

- Helichrysum with Aroma Life.

Use: Add 1-3 drops of each single oil to the corresponding blends above (according to your sensitivity).

Supplements: Super C, A. D. & E., and Mineral Essence.

Apply oils neat on location, with or without cold compresses (See COMPRESSES).

Cypress strengthens capillary walls. Helichrysum helps blood absorb back into the tissue.

People who bruise easily are usually low in vitamin C, which may be caused by insufficient intake or poor absorption.

Hemorrhaging

Single oils: Helichrysum and cypress.

Hemorrhoids

Single oils:

- Cypress with helichrysum, birch, patchouly, myrrh, myrtle, or clary sage.
- Basil with cypress, basil, or peppermint.

Use: Add 1-3 drops to the corresponding single oils above (according to your sensitivity).

Blends:

- Basil with Aroma Siez, Citrus Fresh, Aroma Life, or PanAway.
- Cypress with PanAway.

Use: Add 1-3 drops of each single oil to the corresponding blends above (according to your sensitivity).

Supplements: Cel-Lite Magic, Acidophilus, Megazyme, Mint Condition, VitaGreen, Super B, and Royal Essence.

Mix with V-6 Mixing Oil or Massage Oil Base before application.

Cleanse using the Cleansing Trio (see COLON AND LIVER CLEANSE).

Mix:
- 3 or 4 drops of basil
- 1 drop of birch
- 1 drop of cypress
- 1 drop of helichrysum

Mix with V-6 Mixing Oil or Massage Oil Base and place on location. This may sting, but one application works on hemorrhoids.

Mix:
- 3 drops cypress
- 2 drops helichrysum
- 10 drops myrtle

Mixed in V-6 Mixing Oil or Massage Oil Base.

Hepatitis

(See VIRAL HEPATITIS under LIVER.)

Herpes

(See SEXUAL DISEASES.)

Hiccups (Hiccoughs)

This is usually caused by irritated nerves of the diaphragm, possibly caused from a full stomach or indigestion (dyspepsia). (See DIGESTIVE PROBLEMS).

Single oils: Tarragon

Using 2-4 drops of Tarragon may relax intestinal spasms, nervous digestion and hiccups.

Hives

Single oils: Patchouly

Supplements: Super Cal

Patchouly may help itching.

Hodgkin's Disease

Single oils: Clove, lavender, frankincense, and labdamon.

Hormone Imbalance - In Women

(See MENOPAUSE.)

Hyper Activity

Single oils: Lavender, Roman chamomile, peppermint, and valerian.

Hypoglycemia

Low blood glucose (sugar). Hypoglycemia is the opposite of diabetes. The signs of hypoglycemia can include:

- Fatigue, drowsiness, and sleepiness after meals.
- Headache or dizziness if periods between meals are too long.
- Craving for sweets. When a coke or a chocolate bar supplies us with a short-lived spurt of energy, we have a problem.
- Allergic reaction to foods and other substances.
- Palpitations, tremors, sweats, rapid heart beat.
- Inattentiveness, mood swings, irritability, anxiety, nervousness, inability to cope with stress, feeling of emotional depression, and confusion.
- Lack of motivation, discipline, and creativity.
- Feeling a loss of energy in early afternoon.
- Indigestion, upper and lower gas, poor assimilation, poor electrolyte balance, protein deficiency.
- Recognizing that if one does not have protein intake, one cannot remain active.
- Hunger that cannot be satisfied.

Often people with even some of the above symptoms are labeled as fatigued or even neurotic. Instead, they may be hypoglycemic.

The interesting part of this is that animal protein will actually increase the hypoglycemic symptoms. This is because hypoglycemics do not digest protein well. Protein intake gives a boost because of an adrenaline rush, which is relatively short lived. Then the protein starts to putrefy, giving off a glucose gas that feeds the sugar in the body and causes candida overgrowth. Hypoglycemia is a precursor to candida, Epstein Barr virus, allergies, Chronic Fatigue Syndrome, depression, chemical sensitivity, and universal reactors. All of these have essentially the same signs as hypoglycemia.

If the hypoglycemia is treated first, the other symptoms will probably disappear. If you do not have hypoglycemia, you will not be susceptible to the related diseases listed above.

One of the problems of hypoglycemia is low thyroid function. Correct thyroid function is necessary. (See THYROID) Another hypoglycemia-related problem is an inability to assimilate protein and to balance blood glucose levels. Thus, digestion is also a factor. A colon and liver cleanse (See Colon) is most important to rid the body of toxic gases and putrefied materials. The first step to overcome hypoglycemia is to bring the digestive tract back in order.

Excessive consumption of sugar or honey will also cause hypoglycemia.

Single oils:

- Lavender with cinnamon, cumin, clove, caraway, thyme, lemongrass, geranium, coriander or dill.

Use: Add 1-3 drops to the corresponding single oils above (according to your sensitivity).

Blends:

- Lavender with Thieves, JuvaFlex, or Di-Tone.
- Ylang Ylang with Thieves, JuvaFlex, Di-Tone, or Exodus II.

Use: Add 1-3 drops of each single oil to the corresponding blends above (according to your sensitivity).

Apply neat on pancreas Vita Flex points on feet. Thieves will boost blood sugar levels.

Supplements: Power Meal, Body Balance, VitaGreen, Stevia, Exodus, EssPro 7, Mineral Essence, and Essential Manna.

These supplements are all sources of protein and will help the body assimilate protein for balancing blood glucose (sugar) levels.

Stevia has been known to raise blood sugar levels, thus rapidly increasing energy and mental acuity.

Exodus is an immune support with its companion being Exodus II.

Raw carrot sticks, celery sticks, broccoli, and cauliflower make good snacks to boost blood glucose. Green foods give body nitrogen, which converts to protein.

Hysterectomy

(See MENOPAUSE.)

Immune System

The immune system is probably the most important body system or function. It must be strong and responsive in order to produce the antibodies and antitoxins to fight germs and virus antigens and toxins and the other toxins that we produce or encounter. Some 40% of immune system function is found in the intestinal tract and is called *pirus patchet*. Another 40% is accounted for by the thymus gland, which produces immune-stimulating cells (Terry Friedmann, M.D.).

Single oils:

- Frankincense with ravensara, thyme, helichrysum, oregano, rosemary, chamomile, Idaho tansy, mountain savory, melissa, lavender, grapefruit, lemon, cinnamon, clove, black cumin, cistus, melaleuca, myrrh, myrtle, rose, vetiver, or lemongrass.

Use: Add 1-3 drops to the corresponding single oils above (according to your sensitivity).

Blends:

- Frankincense with Thieves, ImmuPower, Exodus II, Abundance, Acceptance, Humility, Raven, or 3 Wise Men.

Use: Add 1-3 drops of each single oil to the corresponding blends above (according to your sensitivity).

Supplements:

ImmuGel, Radex, Super C, Super B, Royal Essence, Mineral Essence, VitaGreen, Power Meal, Thyromin, ImmuneTune, ArthroTune, Colloidal Essence, Goji Berry Tea, Rehemogen, AlkaLime, Ultra Young, Exodus, Cleansing Trio, JuvaTone, and Wolfberry Power Bar.

It is important to first cleanse the colon and liver (see COLON).

When we are caught up in fear, nervousness, anxiety, and depression, we compromise our immune function.

Improper and incorrect eating habits also compromise immune function and status (see DIGESTION PROBLEMS). Fatigue is also a factor (see EXHAUSTION).

Contaminated water compromises immune function (see WATER).

ImmuneTune can build and support the immune system. Exodus can also be a powerful immune support. Exodus II is a companion to both supplements.

Roman chamomile, cinnamon, oregano, thyme, clove, and melissa are used in Europe to strengthen the immune system.

Grapefruit, lemon, lemongrass, and Raven promote leukocyte (white blood cell) formation.

Essential oils increase the oxygen levels in the brain, which enables the pituitary and other endocrine glands to secrete neural transmitters, endorphins, and antibodies, which support the endocrine and immune systems.

Stress is a major factor in immune dysfunction. Continual daily use of essential oils is optimal to overcome stress (see STRESS).

Viruses and bacteria have a tendency to hibernate along the spine. The body may hold a virus in a suspended state for long periods of time. When the immune system is compromised, these viruses may be released and then manifest into illness. Raindrop Therapy along the spine may help bring out these microorganisms and rid them from the body.

Oregano and thyme are generally used first for the Raindrop application. However, other oils may also be used and may be more desirable for some people. ImmuPower, Raven, and Purification all work well in the Raindrop application method. Other oils and blends may be used depending on perceived requirements.

Parasites compromise immune function by overloading the system (see PARASITES).

Inhalation of essential oils and massage application increase immune function by as much as 32%, but only when pure unadulterated oils are used (see INHALATION THERAPY).

Commercial floral perfumes limit the range of brain activity because the oils in the perfumes have been chemically altered through extraction methods. However, the use of pure unadulterated essential oils increases a wide variation of brain activity and increases blood/glucose conversion through electromagnetic fields in the brain. Inhalation of pure oils increases blood flow to the brain by 15% and brain blood oxygen levels by 25%. The result is increased blood glucose conversion and electromagnetic fields in the brain, stimulating the immune system. These findings are from the research of Dr. Asawa of Japan and Dr. Richardson of England.

Thieves applied to bottom of feet with ImmuPower on the throat and chest helps the immune system. Also, 1 or 2 drops of Thieves in massage oil or V-6 Mixing Oil or Massage Oil Base massaged on the thymus stimulates the immune system.

Mountain savory and Abundance are both powerful immune stimulants.

Exodus II can also be taken internally. Use 3 drops four to six times daily for seven days. Repeat the cycle again, if needed, after four days.

For prevention of and protection from airborne viruses, alternate diffusing ImmuPower and Thieves periodically.

CAUTION: Do not diffuse Thieves more than 15 to 30 minutes at a time as the cinnamon may irritate the nasal passages. Also be sure that the room is well ventilated.

It is important to diffuse oils in the home or office in order to reduce airborne pathogens that overload the immune system.

Research from the Universities of Cairo, Geneva, and Paris indicate that essential oils are one of the highest known sources of antioxidants.

Chlorine inhibits thyroid function and therefore slows down metabolism, circulation, and immune function. Chlorine shuts down thyroid function by stopping it from taking in iodine and the amino acid tyrosine. Drinking chlorinated water is damaging to one's health. Add 1 drop of lemon, peppermint, or spearmint to reduce chlorine levels. Chlorine-free water for showering and bathing is more difficult to achieve.

However, there are carbon filters that remove chlorides from water, which may be attached to faucets. When showering, use a showerhead into which you can put essential oils and bath salts.

Today, there is a lot of radiation and radioactive materials in the atmosphere that severely challenges the immune system.

Thyromin strengthens the thyroid, which is very important for the endocrine system (see ENDOCRINE SYSTEM and THYROID).

VitaGreen encourages healthy blood and boosts immune function.

Radex provides immune support and detoxifies the body. Radex is necessary for its antioxidant and free radical scavenging.

Super C contains bioflavonoids, which are a strong immune support.

For maintenance, a standard dosage of these formulas is generally adequate. If you know you have been exposed to radiation, feeling fatigued from it, or if you are flying with commercial airlines (because of the greater exposure to radiation high in the atmosphere), or similar experiences, an increased daily amount of these supplements would be beneficial. When flying, increase intake 10 days before the trip and continue this higher dosage for 10 days after the trip.

One of the ways you can tell if you have been affected by radiation is to take Radex by itself for a couple of days. Most people who do this will find an energy increase.

People who have disease are deficient in vitamin B5. Super B is a good source of all B vitamins.

Body acid/alkaline balance is also a factor in immune function and the ability of the body to digest and use supplements and oils (see BODY pH ACID/ALKALINE BALANCE).

Immune Deficiency Syndrome

Single oils: Cistus

> **Blends:** Brain Power, Exodus, Valor, Thieves, and ImmuPower.
>
> Exodus II: 6-8 drops on spine alternating days with Raindrop Therapy.

Valor and Thieves: 4-6 drops on feet for 3 weeks.

ImmuPower: 6 drops daily in water and drink.

Rain Drop Therapy: 3 times weekly for virus.

Supplements: Cleansing Trio, JuvaTone, ImmuGel, Thyromin, ImmuneTune, VitaGreen, Sulfurzyme, Exodus, Super B, Ultra Young, Goji Berry Tea, and Vita Life Juice.

Cleansing Trio for 120 days with JuvaTone.

ImmuGel: 1/2 tsp. 3 times daily. Hold in mouth for better absorption.

Thyromin: Start by taking 2 at night and 1 in morning.

ImmuneTune: 6-8 capsules daily.

VitaGreen: 6-10 capsules daily.

Sulfurzyme: 1 tablespoon.

Exodus: Up to 18 capsules daily.

Super B: 1.

Ultra Young: 3 squirts on each inside of each cheek, 4-5 times daily.

Eat 5-6 mini-meals per day, primarily Power Meal (3 times daily) and fish for protein. Do not eat chicken for first 3-6 weeks to allow more energy for immune building.

Impotence

Single oils: Ylang ylang, clary sage, sandalwood, clove, ginger, nutmeg, rose, and pepper.

Nutmeg supports the nervous system to overcome impotence.

Supplements: EssPro 7 and ProGen.

Infection, Bacterial, Viral, Staph, Strep

Single oils:

- Cypress with rosemary, rose, lavender, lemongrass, basil, thyme, oregano, nutmeg, rosewood, mountain savory, frankincense, myrrh, cistus, or marjoram.

- Melaleuca or sage or rosemary with lemongrass, lemon, Idaho tansy, German chamomile, thyme, basil, lavender, clary sage, eucalyptus (globulus and radiata), geranium, bergamot, pine, spruce, or tarragon. Thyme with ravensara, melissa, petitgrain, oregano, frankincense, clove, cinnamon, or lavender.

Blends:

- Cypress with Purification, Melrose, or R.C.
- Melaleuca or rosemary with Thieves, Melrose, Purification, ImmuPower, R.C., or Di-Tone.
- Thyme or sage with Melrose, Purification, Exodus, Raven, Thieves, or 3 Wise Men.

Use: Add 1-3 drops of each single oil to the corresponding blends above (according to your sensitivity).

Supplements: Radex, Super C, Exodus, Immu-Gel, Royal Essence, VitaGreen, ImmuneTune, Rehemogen, and Colloidal Essence

Mountain savory, ravensara, and thyme applied by Raindrop Therapy on the spine is beneficial for any and all infections, particularly chest-related infections.

Thieves or Exodus II applied to bottom of feet, with ImmuPower on the throat and chest, helps the immune system. Also, 1 or 2 drops of Thieves in V-6 Mixing Oil or Massage Oil Base massaged on the thymus stimulates the immune system.

For prevention of and protection from airborne viruses, periodically alternate diffusing Immu-Power and Thieves.

Mix 1 drop melaleuca and 1 drop rosemary for antiseptic and healing benefits for infectious cuts, wounds, rashes, cleansing, and purifying.

Clean, healthy, and detoxified blood helps to overcome any disease. Rehemogen cleans and purifies blood so that nutrients and oxygen may be delivered to the cells.

Viral Infection in the Spine (see SPINE).

Viral Strep

Single oils:

- Melaleuca with cinnamon, clove, thyme, oregano, ravensara, or frankincense.

Use: Add 1-3 drops to the corresponding single oils above (according to your sensitivity).

Blends:

- Melaleuca with Thieves.

Use: Add 1-3 drops of each single oil to the corresponding blends above (according to your sensitivity).

Strep Throat

Single oils:

- Cinnamon with lavender, chamomile, hyssop, myrrh, myrtle, or nutmeg.

Use: Add 1-3 drops to the corresponding single oils above (according to your sensitivity).

Application:

Mix in order:
- 1 drop cinnamon
- 6 drops lavender or chamomile
- 2 drops hyssop

Use up to 3 drops neat on the Vita Flex points of the feet.

Mix into 1/2 oz. V-6 Mixing Oil or Massage Oil Base and apply topically on throat.

Blends:

- Cypress with Purification, Melrose, or R.C.
- Melaleuca or rosemary with Thieves, Melrose, Purification, ImmuPower, R.C., or Di-Tone.
- Thyme or sage with Melrose, Purification, Exodus, Raven, Thieves, or 3 Wise Men.

Use: Add 1-3 drops of each single oil to the corresponding blends above (according to your sensitivity).

Supplements: Radex, Super C, Exodus, Immu-Gel, Royal Essence, VitaGreen, ImmuneTune, Rehemogen, and Colloidal Essence

Mountain savory, ravensara, and thyme applied by Raindrop Therapy on the spine is beneficial for any and all infections, particularly chest-related infections.

Thieves applied to bottom of feet, with ImmuPower on the throat and chest, helps the immune system. Also, 1 or 2 drops of Thieves in V-6 Mixing Oil or Massage Oil Base massaged on the thymus stimulates the immune system.

For prevention of and protection from airborne viruses, periodically alternate diffusing Immu-Power and Thieves.

Mix 1 drop melaleuca and 1 drop rosemary for antiseptic and healing benefits for infectious cuts, wounds, rashes, cleansing, and purifying.

Clean, healthy, and detoxified blood helps to overcome any disease. Rehemogen cleans and purifies blood so that nutrients and oxygen may be delivered to the cells.

For prevention of and protection from airborne viruses, periodically alternate diffusing Immu-Power and Thieves.

Mix 1 drop melaleuca and 1 drop rosemary for antiseptic and healing benefits for infectious cuts, wounds, rashes, cleansing, and purifying.

Whooping Cough

A contagious disease affecting the respiratory system mainly in children. Lungs are infected, and air passages are clogged with thick mucus. It starts like a cold, does not improve within a few days, and gets worse with coughing bouts of up to 1 minute in length. Breathing is difficult during the coughing bout, and the face turns red or even blue from lack of oxygen. A wheezing noise is made when trying to catch his/her breath.

Single oils:

- Cypress with rosemary, rose, lavender, lemongrass, basil, thyme, oregano, myrtle, or nutmeg.

- Melaleuca or sage or rosemary with lemongrass, lemon, Idaho tansy, Roman chamomile, thyme, basil, lavender, eucalyptus, geranium, or bergamot.

- Thyme with ravensara, melissa, petitgrain, oregano, frankincense, clove, cinnamon, lavender, myrrh, or ginger.

Use: Add 1-3 drops to the corresponding single oils above (according to your sensitivity).

Blends:

- Cypress with R.C.

- Eucalyptus ericifolia or rosemary with Thieves, Melrose, Purification, ImmuPower, R.C., or Di-Tone.

- Thyme or sage with Melrose, Purification, Thieves, or 3 Wise Men.

Use: Add 1-3 drops of each single oil to the corresponding blends above (according to your sensitivity).

Supplements: Radex, Super C, ImmuGel, Royal Essence, VitaGreen, ImmuneTune, Rehemogen, and Colloidal Essence

CAUTION: Whooping cough usually affects children. Always dilute in massage oil or V-6 Mixing Oil or Massage Oil Base when applying essential oils. Start with low concentrations until response is observed. Diffuse intermittently in bedroom. Again observe reaction. Do not overdo.

Infertility

Supplements: EssPro 7, VitaGreen, Ultra Young, and Thyromin.

Inflammation

Single oils:

- Birch with helichrysum, frankincense, hyssop, myrrh, marjoram, ravensara, lavender, oregano, Roman chamomile, cypress, peppermint, spearmint, or spruce.

- Mountain savory, clary sage, lemongrass, sandalwood, rose, spikenard, or fir.

- Melaleuca with German chamomile, tangerine, thyme, hyssop, eucalyptus radiata, jasmine, pepper, petitgrain, Idaho tansy, tarragon, yarrow, citronella, or coriander.

Use: Add 1-3 drops to the corresponding single oils above (according to your sensitivity).

Blends:

- Birch with Purification, PanAway, Aroma Siez, Exodus II, Melrose, Abundance, Relieve It, or ImmuPower.

Use: Add 1-3 drops of each single oil to the corresponding blends above (according to your sensitivity).

Supplements: EssPro 7, Ortho Ease, Relaxation, and Ortho Sport Massage Oils.

Any time there is tissue damage, there is always inflammation. There are many oils that have anti-inflammatory properties: Helichrysum, spruce, birch, vetiver, hyssop, and valerian

There are different types of inflammation for which one oil might be better than another.

Myrrh: Tissue and capillary damage, bruising or loss of oxygen.

Roman chamomile and lavender: Inflammation due to infection.

Ravensara, hyssop, or oregano: Viral.

Peppermint: Reduce fever.

For inflammation:
- 10 drops fir
- 6 drops melaleuca
- 4 drops German chamomile
- 2 drops peppermint
- 2 drops lemongrass

Mix in 2 oz. massage oil or V-6 Mixing Oil or Massage Oil Base.

Supplements: EssPro 7, Ortho Ease, Relaxation, and Ortho Sport.

Any time there is tissue damage, there is always inflammation. There are many oils that have anti-inflammatory properties: Helichrysum, spruce, birch, vetiver, hyssop, and valerian

There are different types of inflammation for which one oil might be better than another:

Myrrh: Tissue and capillary damage, bruising or loss of oxygen.

Roman chamomile and lavender: Inflammation due to infection.

Ravensara, hyssop, or oregano: Viral.

Peppermint: Reduce fever.

For inflammation:
- 10 drops fir
- 6 drops melaleuca
- 4 drops German chamomile
- 2 drops peppermint
- 2 drops lemongrass

Mix in 2 oz. massage oil or V-6 Mixing Oil or Massage Oil Base.

Mix:
- 6 drops frankincense
- 6 drops fir
- 6 drops eucalyptus citriodora
- 4 drops ravensara
- 3 drops birch
- 1 drop peppermint

Mix in 1/2 to 1 oz. massage oil or V-6 Mixing Oil or Massage Oil Base.

Injury

Bone: Birch, spruce, fir, PanAway, Relieve It on location, multiple times daily.

Muscle: Basil, marjoram, lavender, Relieve It, PanAway.

Ligament: Lemongrass, lavender (equal parts), PanAway, Relieve It, elemi, Idaho tansy.

Spasms: Aroma Siez with Ortho Ease or Ortho Sport Massage Oils.

Insect Bites, Bee and Wasp Stings

Single oils:

- Lavender with melaleuca, rosemary, Idaho tansy, clary sage, Roman chamomile, German chamomile, basil, patchouly, or bergamot.

Use: Add 1-3 drops to the corresponding single oils above (according to your sensitivity).

Blends:

- Lavender with Purification, R.C., PanAway, or Melrose.

Use: Add 1-3 drops of each single oil to the corresponding blends above (according to your sensitivity).

Application: Remove stinger with tweezers or scrape out with a knife so as to not squeeze the venom sack. Immediately apply Purification and Melrose with 1-2 drops lavender or Idaho tansy, neat, on site. Repeat until the venom spread has stopped. Then apply lavender with or without one or more of the single oils above, 2 - 3 times daily until redness abates. PanAway may be substituted for Purification.

Stings:
- 2 drops lavender
- 1 drop helichrysum
- 1 drop chamomile
- 1 drop birch

Stings and bites:
- 1 drop thyme
- 10 drops lavender
- 4 drops eucalyptus
- 3 drops chamomile

Mix in 1 Tbsp. massage oil or V-6 Mixing Oil or Massage Oil Base.

Black Widow Spider Bite

Rub 1 drop lavender every 2 to 3 minutes over the bite until you reach the hospital.

Brown Recluse Spider Bite

Purification neutralizes the venom of this spider's bite.

- 1 drop lavender
- 1 drop helichrysum
- 1 drop Melrose
- Cover with oatmeal poultice.

After poultice is removed, apply Purification.

Chigger Bites

Rub lavender or R.C. neat on site.

Ticks

Rub thyme on the tick and it will release its bite. Then apply Purification neat on site to detoxify the wound. Or rub 1 drop lavender every 5 minutes for a total of 10 drops to avoid pain and infection (see LYME DISEASE).

Insect Repellent

Single oils: Peppermint, eucalyptus, lemon, lime, lavender, melaleuca, cedarwood, geranium, bergamot, Idaho tansy, rosemary, patchouly, citronella, lemongrass, and thyme.

Blends: Purification, Thieves, Melrose

Skin Care: Sunsation Suntan Oil.

Diffuse oils in a room to keep insects out. Put on cotton balls or cedar chips in closets or drawers, etc.

Mix:
- 6 drops peppermint
- 6 drops melaleuca
- 9 drops eucalyptus

Mix in 2 oz. of sweet almond oil with the oil from 1 capsule of Vitamin E (to keep blend fresh). Shake well. Rub on exposed skin.

Lemon and peppermint repel mosquitoes.

Put lemon and peppermint in water in a spray bottle and mist over exposed skin.

Patchouly is used in Asia as a moth repellent.

Lemongrass with citronella makes an insect repellent.

Idaho tansy floral water is used as a mosquito repellent and to repel horse flies.

House and greenhouse plants:

Mix:
- 2 drops spearmint
- 3 drops orange

Mix in 2 quarts water, shake well, and spray on plants to keep bugs and aphids away. Diffuse in greenhouse.

Cockroaches:

Mix:
- 10 drops peppermint
- 5 drops cypress

Mix in 1/2 cup water. Shake well. Spray where roaches run and live.

Insomnia

Single oils:

- Lavender with Roman chamomile, marjoram, myrtle, German chamomile, ravensara, basil, ylang ylang, tangerine, bergamot, mandarin, orange, or valerian.

- Cypress with marjoram, lavender, basil, geranium, rosemary, clary sage, German chamomile, rosewood, or angelica.

Use: Add 1-3 drops to the corresponding single oils above (according to your sensitivity).

Blends:

- Lavender with Peace & Calming, Valor, Aroma Siez, Present Time, Motivation, Harmony, Surrender, or White Angelica.

- Cypress with Peace & Calming, Valor, 3 Wise Men, Gentle Baby, or Citrus Fresh.

Use: Add 1-3 drops of each single oil to the corresponding blends above (according to your sensitivity).

Lavender with Roman chamomile is excellent for insomnia.

Lavender with marjoram and Peace & Calming diffused in the bedroom aids in reducing restlessness and insomnia.

Rub Peace & Calming or Dream Catcher across the shoulders along with a little lavender or Roman chamomile if desired.

Rub on the bottom of the feet, on stomach, and around the navel.

Diffuse in the bedroom.

Place a drop of Dream Catcher on your pillow and a few drops around hotel or motel room.

Insomnia:
- 12 drops orange
- 8 drops lavender
- 4 drops bergamot
- 3 drops geranium
- 2 drops Roman chamomile

Mix in 1/2 to 1 oz. massage oil or V-6 Mixing Oil or Massage Oil Base.

Insomnia:
- 9 drops lavender
- 3 drops tansy
- 3 drops marjoram

Mix in 1/2 to 1 oz. V-6 Mixing Oil or Massage Oil Base.

Calming:
- 15 drops lavender
- 15 drops Peace & Calming

Mix in 1/2 oz. V-6 Mixing Oil or Massage Oil Base.

If a person is sleeping too much, possibly from not being able to release negative memories, diffuse Motivation, Aroma Life, or Clarity or your favorite blend in the bedroom. Six to eight hours of sound sleep is normal for a healthy person. Bowel toxicity may also be a factor in insomnia. A colon and liver cleanse may be required.

HRT or CardiaCare may be needed to support heart function. (see HEART).

Put 1 drop of Harmony on energy meridians to help balance the energy flow in the body. (1 drop on stomach, navel, thymus, throat, forehead, crown of head).

Other Products: AuraLight, Evening Peace Bath and Shower Gel, Relaxation Massage Oil, Super Cal, Thyromin, and EssPro 7.

Evening Peace makes a relaxing bubble bath. Add 10 drops of lavender or geranium in 1/2 cup bath or Epsom salts. Run bath water through the salts and soak.

Indigestion causes gas, and toxins in the intestines and the liver will produce insomnia, frequent recurring migraine headaches, skin eruptions, discoloration, change in pigmentation, acne, and bumpy skin (like turkey skin).

Influenza

(See COLDS.)

Irritable Bowel Syndrome

(See COLON.)

Single oils: Peppermint

Blends: Di-Tone

Supplements: Royaldophilus, I.C.P., and ComforTone.

Use yogurt, kefir, Royaldophilus, I.C.P., and ComforTone.

Use Di-Tone (2-3 drops in distilled water) and peppermint.

Itching

Single oils: Lavender, valerian, and patchouly.

Blends: Aroma Siez

Supplements: Super B, JuvaTone, and ComforTone.

Jaundice

Single oils: Carrot seed, Roman chamomile, German chamomile, and geranium.

Blends: JuvaFlex and Release.

Supplements: Cleansing Trio, Juva Tone, and Rehemogen.

Joints

Single oils: Spruce, elemi, Idaho tansy, basil, rosemary, oregano, fir, and birch.

- Black pepper with rosemary, marjoram, lavender, nutmeg, or vetiver.
- Spruce with sandalwood, fir, hyssop, lemongrass, birch, helichrysum, German chamomile, Idaho tansy, or vetiver.

Use: Add 1-3 drops to the corresponding single oils above (according to your sensitivity).

Supplements and Skin Care: Power Meal, Ultra Young, PanAway, Aroma Siez, Relieve It, Ortho Sport and Ortho Ease Massage Oils.

Stiffness

Sulfurzyme:1-2 Tbsp. 2-3 times daily, Power Meal, Ultra Young.

Topically: PanAway, Aroma Siez, spruce, elemi, tansy, basil, rosemary, oregano, fir, birch, vetiver, Relieve It, Ortho Sport and Ortho Ease Massage Oils.

Stiff Joints:
- 10 drops black pepper
- 2 drops rosemary
- 5 drops marjoram
- 5 drops lavender

Mix in 1/2 oz. V-6 Mixing Oil or Massage Oil Base.

Pain Relief:
- 8 drops spruce
- 8 drops sandalwood
- 7 drops fir
- 5 drops hyssop
- 4 drops lemongrass
- 5 drops helichrysum
- 4 drops birch
- 2 drops blue chamomile
- 3 drops vetiver
- 1 drop tansy

Mix in 1/2 to 1 oz. V-6 Mixing Oil or Massage Oil Base.

Ortho Ease and Ortho Sport Massage Oils are very soothing to ligament/cartilage damage (see ARTHRITIS and CONNECTIVE TISSUE).

Juvenile Dwarfism

Blends:

Brain Power stimulates the limbic system.

Use Power Meal and 3 squirts of Ultra Young 3 times a day.

Kidneys

Stones

Damage to the glomeruli (tiny filtering units in the bladder and the kidneys, caused by bacteria infections of the urine or kidneys, is called pyelonephritis. The source of the bacteria can be from other parts of the body through the blood stream, or most often from poor hygiene in the area of the urethral opening.

Abnormal proteins trapped in the glomeruli cause inflammation and damage to these tiny filtering units. This is called glomerulonephritis. This diseases may be mild or severe, acute (flaring up in a few days), or chronic (taking months or years to develop). The mildest forms may not show any symptoms except through a urine test. At more advanced stages, small amounts of blood appear in the urine (smoky looking). In severe cases of glomerulonephritis, the urine appears bright red as large amounts of blood are passed.

In severe cases a person may feel generally unwell, drowsy, nauseous, and may also vomit. These are symptoms of impending kidney failure.

High blood pressure can be a cause and a result of chronic kidney failure, since kidneys are central to blood regulation (see BLOOD PRESSURE).

With poor kidney function, smaller amounts of urine are produced, and fluids tend to accumulate in the tissues. Edema (swelling) under the skin is noticeable, mostly around the ankles.

Fluid may also accumulate in the chest, making breathing difficult.

Capillaries Being Attacked in the Kidneys

Blends:

- Aroma Life with JuvaFlex, cypress, or juniper.

Use: Add 1-3 drops of each single oil to the corresponding blends above (according to your sensitivity).

Supplements: K & B Tincture, Master HIS/HERS and CHILDREN'S Multiple Vitamin, VitaGreen, ImmuneTune, Radex, Super C, K & B Tincture, and Rehemogen.

Support the body with VitaGreen and Power Meal.

Cleanse the body with colon and liver cleanse.

Rehemogen: 3 droppers (75 drops) 3 times daily.

Drink 1/2 gallon Goji Berry (wolfberry) Tea daily.

Apply Aroma Life and JuvaFlex over the kidneys, on kidney Vita Flex points of the feet, and around the navel.

After 10 days add ImmuneTune, Radex and Super C.

Diuretic, Increase Urine Flow

Single oils:

- Birch with rosemary, juniper, fennel, eucalyptus radiata, grapefruit, geranium, or sage.

- Lemongrass with juniper, fennel, rosemary, geranium, or marjoram.

Use: Add 1-3 drops to the corresponding single oils above (according to your sensitivity).

Blends:

- Birch with EndoFlex, Di-Tone or Acceptance.

- Lemongrass with EndoFlex.

Use: Add 1-3 drops of each single oil to the corresponding blends above (according to your sensitivity).

Application: Massage over the kidney area or apply a compress. (see MASSAGE AND COMPRESSES).

Juniper leaf oil is toxic to the kidneys; juniper berry oil is not. The highest quality juniper oil is derived from juniper berries, plus some branches. This combination has shown no toxicity and is more effective than straight juniper berry oil.

Cleanse colon and liver with Cleansing Trio, JuvaTone, and JuvaFlex.

Supplements: K & B Tincture, Cel-Lite Magic Massage Oil, and JuvaTone

CAUTION: Do not use fennel longer than 10 days at a time, since it excessively increases flow through the urinary tract.

Edema

This condition appears when fluids accumulate in the tissue, making a noticeable puffiness under the skin. It is more predominate around the ankles and perhaps the knees at the end of the day when fluids settle to the lowest part of the body.

Single oils:

- Tangerine with cypress or orange.

- Cypress with tangerine, juniper, orange, lemon, fennel, geranium, or cedarwood.

Use: Add 1-3 drops to the corresponding single oils above (according to your sensitivity).

Blends: Aroma Life

Supplements: Cel-Lite Magic Massage Oil, Essential Manna, and Super Cal

Potassium deficiency can cause edema. Increase potassium intake by taking Super Cal.

Rub 2-3 drops of Aroma Life on heart Vita Flex point on left foot and over the heart to balance heart.

Recipe 1:
- 6 drops tangerine or orange
- 2 drops cypress

Mix in V-6 Mixing Oil or Massage Oil Base and massage into affected area.

Recipe 2:
- 10 drops tangerine
- 5 drops cypress
- 10 drops lemon

Mix V-6 Mixing Oil or Massage Oil Base and massage into affected area.

Recipe 3:
- 10 drops tangerine
- 5 drops cypress
- 3 drops juniper

Rub on bladder Vita Flex area, which is outside and inside of the feet and ankle bone and up the achilles tendon. Results should be noticed in 2 to 3 minutes. Inhale the same oil mix blend at the same time for more positive results.

Recipe 4 – To tighten skin and move water:
- 10 drops tangerine
- 10 drops cypress

Mix in 1/2 oz. V-6 Mixing Oil or Massage Oil Base. Rub on legs from the feet up the legs in the morning.

At night do the same using:
- 8 drops geranium
- 5 drops cypress
- 5 drops helichrysum

Seal with Cel-Lite Magic Massage Oil.

Thyroid and liver functions are factors for causing edema (see THYROID and LIVER AILMENTS).

It was reported that a man who had a heart bypass used a vein removed from his leg. The leg swelled up from fluid retention and could be moved around like jelly. The leg was massaged with 4 drops cypress mixed into Cel-Lite Magic Massage Oil. Then the leg was massaged with 4 drops fennel and 4 drops geranium mixed into the same massage oil. Both applications were massaged from the foot up. The leg was massaged for 15 to 20 minutes, and in 30 minutes the fluid was gone.

Single oils:

- Tangerine or lavender with orange, grapefruit, lemon, along with cypress, juniper, basil, fennel, or marjoram.

- Cypress with fennel, juniper, helichrysum, or lemongrass.

- Birch with rosemary, juniper, eucalyptus radiata, fennel, or geranium.

- Sage with cypress, tangerine, lemongrass, fennel, or orange.

Use: Add 1-3 drops to the corresponding single oils above (according to your sensitivity).

Blends:

- Lavender with Citrus Fresh, Aroma Life, or EndoFlex.

- Cypress with EndoFlex or Di-Tone.

- Birch with EndoFlex.

- Sage with Citrus Fresh or Cel-Lite Magic Massage Oil.

Use: Add 1-3 drops of each single oil to the corresponding blends above (according to your sensitivity).

Supplements: Cel-Lite Magic Massage Oil, Super C, K & B Tincture, Master HIS/HERS, and Master CHILDREN'S.

Application: Massage or apply a compress over the kidneys and rub on Vita Flex points on feet.

Recipe 1 – Kidney Compress:
- 5 drops juniper
- 5 drops tangerine
- 3 drops geranium
- 1 drop helichrysum

Place compress over kidney area for 1 night.

The next night make a compress with Immu-Power and place over kidneys. At the same time rub on the kidney vita flex points on the feet.

Recipe 2:
- 10 drops birch
- 6 drops fennel
- 2 drops tansy
- 3 drops patchouly
- 10 drops tangerine

Mix in 1/2 to 1 oz. massage oil or V-6 Mixing Oil or Massage Oil Base. Supports liver, kidneys, and decreases water retention.

Recipe 3: alleviate fluid retention.
- 1 drop lemon
- 1 drop tangerine

K & B Tincture: 3 droppers in 4 oz. distilled water, 3 times daily as required. Strengthen weak bladder, kidneys, and urinary tract. Drink plenty of liquids, preferably distilled water.

Drink 8 oz. water with about 10% cranberry juice and the juice of 1/2 lemon to help cleanse and strengthen.

Cleanse with colon and liver with Cleansing Trio to help balance body fluids.

Kidney Detoxification

Single oils:

Helichrysum with juniper or fennel.

Use: Add 1-3 drops to the corresponding single oils above (according to your sensitivity).

Blends:

- Helichrysum with Di-Tone, JuvaFlex or EndoFlex.

Use: Add 1-3 drops of each single oil to the corresponding blends above (according to your sensitivity).

Supplements: K & B Tincture, JuvaTone, Vita-Green, Wolfberry Power Bar, Goji Berry Tea, and Sulfurzyme.

Colon and liver cleanse: Cleansing Trio.

Add Sulfurzyme to further stimulate liver cleanse.

Wolfberry is used in China as a kidney tonic and detoxifier.

Kidney Infection

Single oils: Myrrh, cypress.

Blends:

- Cypress or marjoram with Thieves, JuvaFlex, or Inspiration.
- Juniper with EndoFlex.

Use: Add 1-3 drops of each single oil to the corresponding blends above (according to your sensitivity).

Inspiration helps overcome kidney infections. Apply as a compress over kidneys and also on kidney Vita Flex points on the feet.

Supplements:

K & B Tincture: 3 droppers 3 times daily.

Make a hot compress of juniper with EndoFlex over the kidneys and bladder.

Make a hot compress of cypress, marjoram and Thieves or JuvaFlex over kidneys and bladder.

Drink a gallon of water mixed with cranberry juice per day.

Kidney Stones

Single oils:

- Geranium with juniper and eucalyptus.
- Helichrysum with fennel.
- Rosemary with juniper, geranium, or lemongrass.

Use: Add 1-3 drops to the corresponding single oils above (according to your sensitivity).

Mix:
- 10 drops rosemary
- 10 drops geranium
- 10 drops juniper
- 1 Tbsp. honey
- 1/2 lemon
- 8 oz. distilled water

Mix and drink three glasses per day until the kidney stones pass.

For kidney blockage due to kidney stones, cleanse colon and liver with Cleansing Trio and JuvaTone.

JuvaTone: Start with a small amount, 1 tablet 3 times daily for the first week. Increase 2-3 tablets 3 times daily during the second week.

Increase 3-6 tablets 3 times daily and maintain for 90 days.

During this cleansing period one should also do the following:

- K & B Tincture: 1 dropper in water every 2 hours
- Drink 1/2 gallon of Gogi Berry Tea made with water every 2 hours.

Apply a hot compress:
- 10 drops juniper
- 10 drops geranium
- 10 drops lemongrass

Apply over kidneys once a day.

- Massage juniper and geranium on bottom of the feet twice a day.

Additional Application:
- 10 drops geranium
- 10 drops juniper
- 10 drops eucalyptus.

Apply as hot compress over kidneys and rub on kidney Vita Flex points on the feet.

Mix and Drink:
- 10 drops rosemary
- 10 drops juniper
- 10 drops geranium
- 1 tsp. honey
- Juice of 1 whole lemon
- 8 oz. distilled water

K & B Tincture helps strengthen weak bladder, kidneys, and urinary tract.

Juniper with lemongrass strengthens and tones the connective tissue in kidneys.

Carrot seed oil helps expel kidney stones.

Drink a lot of water when passing a kidney stone.

To help dissolve or partially dissolve stone so that it will pass, take 2 Tbsp. olive oil in 8 oz. apple juice, 2 to 3 times daily until the stone passes.

Supplement: K & B Tincture.

Ureter Infections

The ureter is the duct from the kidney to the bladder.

Single oils: Lemon and myrtle.

Knee Cartilage Injury

Single oils:

- Lavender with lemongrass, marjoram, or ginger.

Use: Add 1-3 drops to the corresponding single oils above (according to your sensitivity).

Blends:

Mix:
- 9 drops lemongrass
- 10 drops marjoram
- 12 drops ginger

In 2 oz. massage oil or V-6 Mixing Oil or Massage Oil Base. Massage 3 times daily.

For swelling, elevate and apply ice packs.

For inflammation, alternate with hot packs and ice packs.

Leukemia

(See CANCER.)

Leg Ulcers

(See SKIN CARE.)

Liver

Brown spots on the skin (back of hands arms, etc.), cracking around fingernails and rough, dry skin indicate liver toxicity and liver problems. (See SKIN CARE.)

The liver plays a major role in helping the body detoxify. The final products of digestion are transported through the portal vein from the colon to the liver to be cleansed.

Cleanse with Cleansing Trio.

Single oils:

- Rosemary with ravensara, geranium, German chamomile, Roman chamomile, frankincense, Idaho tansy, thyme, dill, helichrysum, or mandarin.

- Sage with geranium, German chamomile, Roman chamomile, frankincense, or thyme.

Use: Add 1-3 drops to the corresponding single oils above (according to your sensitivity).

Blends:

- Rosemary or sage with JuvaFlex or Di-Tone.

Use: Add 1-3 drops of each single oil to the corresponding blends above (according to your sensitivity).

Idaho tansy has been reported to help fade liver spots.

Helichrysum is very cleansing to the liver and gall bladder.

Mandarin affects hepatic duct function (bile duct leaving the liver).

JuvaFlex dilates biliary (bile) ducts.

Liver, kidney, and water retention:
- 10 drops birch
- 6 drops fennel
- 2 drops tansy
- 3 drops patchouly
- 10 drops tangerine

Mix in 1/2 to 1 oz. massage oil or V-6 Mixing Oil or Massage Oil Base and Massage over legs, ankles, and specific areas.

Supplements: JuvaTone, Rehemogen, Power Meal, and Sulfurzyme.

Wolfberry is used in China as a liver tonic and detoxifier. Rehemogen and JuvaTone together have been reported to regenerate liver function and have even altered the need for a liver transplant.

Babies with Poor Liver Function

Continuous crying may indicate poor liver function.

Blends: JuvaFlex

A baby that quits crying when JuvaFlex is massaged on the liver Vita Flex points on the feet may indicate a deficient liver. JuvaFlex applied to that area once or twice a day may bring relief.

Detoxification (Liver) - Jaundice

Single oils:

- Helichrysum with German chamomile, Roman chamomile, sage, geranium, Idaho tansy, blue tansy, or patchouly.

- German chamomile with cedarwood, orange, rosemary, or Roman chamomile.

Use: Add 1-3 drops to the corresponding single oils above (according to your sensitivity).

Blends:

- Helichrysum with Di-Tone, JuvaFlex, EndoFlex, or Acceptance.

Use: Add 1-3 drops of each single oil to the corresponding blends above (according to your sensitivity).

Supplements: JuvaTone, Rehemogen, Chelex, and Sulfurzyme Capsules.

French research has shown that helichrysum dilates the liver ducts, releases toxins and poisons, and helps expel them from the system, thereby stimulating greater healing. Carrot seed oil and geranium help liver detoxification.

Patchouly digests toxic wastes.

Liver detoxification:
- 2 drops German chamomile
- 3 drops helichrysum
- 10 drops orange
- 5 drops rosemary

Mix in 1 oz. massage oil or V-6 Mixing Oil or Massage Oil Base. Apply over liver.

Mix:
- 2 drops Roman chamomile
- 2 drops German chamomile

Massage over Vita Flex points on bottom of feet.

Rehemogen helps make or balance platelet production, more red blood cells, and enhances the blood.

JuvaTone, taken at the same time enhances the action of the tincture. This combination may help with liver regeneration.

Chelex draws heavy metals out of the blood.

Cardamom assists in drawing out heavy metals. and may be used when taking JuvaTone to assist in cleansing the liver.

Viral Hepatitis

Hepatitis A, B, and C are highly infectious infections of the liver. The virus is spread by contaminated food and water, and also through contact with blood or stools from an infected person. It may spread for 2 to 6 weeks before symptoms appear and for some time afterward. Symptoms may include jaundice, weakness, loss of appetite, nausea, brownish or tea colored urine, abdominal discomfort, fever and whitish bowel movements.

Begin colon and liver cleanse with Cleaning Trio. After 3 days add JuvaTone.

Single oils:

- Rosemary with ravensara, geranium, German chamomile, Roman chamomile, frankincense, Idaho tansy, or thyme.
- Sage with geranium, German chamomile, Roman chamomile, frankincense, thyme, clove, or myrrh.

Use: Add 1-3 drops to the corresponding single oils above (according to your sensitivity).

Blends:

- Rosemary verbenon or sage with JuvaFlex, Di-Tone, Release, ImmuPower, or Thieves.

Use: Add 1-3 drops of each single oil to the corresponding blends above (according to your sensitivity.

Supplements: Royaldophilus, Master HIS/HERS or CHILDREN'S, VitaGreen, JuvaTone, Exodus II, ImmuneTune, Super C, Radex, ImmuGel, Wolfberry Power Bar, Rehemogen, or Colloidal Essence.

Use 4-oz. of VitaLife Juice 4 times daily.

Daily Program:
- Super C: 6 tablets, 3 times daily.
- Radex: 3 tablets, 3 times daily.
- ImmuGel:1/2 tsp., 2 to 3 times daily.
- VitaGreen: 2 to 6 capsules, 3 times daily, according to blood type.
- Royaldophilus: 1 to 2 capsules at breakfast and bedtime.
- Master HIS/HERS: 2 to 6 tablets, 3 times daily, according to blood type.
- Exodus: 4 tablets, 4 times daily.

Apply a hot compress of JuvaFlex over the liver.

Rub 3-4 drops of Release on the bottom of the feet.

Alternate once a day with Release and JuvaFlex.

Rub ImmuPower, Exodux II, or Thieves up the spine or use Raindrop application method twice daily.

Rub Thieves on the feet, dilute in V-6 Mixing Oil or Massage Oil Base and rub on carotid arteries in the neck and behind the ears (carotid arteries are an excellent place to apply oils for fast absorption).

Ravensara is quite specific for hepatitis.

ImmuGel fights against infection. Do not mix with citrus juices.

Royaldophilus is good for viral conditions.

Rehemogen cleans and fortifies the blood.

317

Colloidal Essence is a powerful fighter of bacteria, fungus, and viruses and may be taken internally or applied externally as required.

Vomiting Bile

Blends: JuvaFlex: rub around navel.

Supplements: JuvaTone and Megazyme.

Liver Cancer

(See CANCER.)

Lou Gehrig's Disease

(See NEUROLOGICAL DISEASES.)

Supplements: JuvaTone, Chelex, Power Meal, Ultra Young, and water create a better firing of the synapse.

Lumbago - Backache in Small of Back

(See SPINE.)

Lupus

There are 3 kinds of lupus.

Lupus vulgaris is tuberculosis of the skin. Brownish lesions may form on the face and become ulcerous and form scars. This is possibly caused by tuberculosis elsewhere in the body (see TUBERCULOSIS).

Lupus erythematosus often has scaly red patches on the skin and has two forms; the discoid (mild) type shows round or butterfly-shaped lesions on the face. It is best to stay out of the sun or at least use a good sunscreen (see SUNBURN under SKIN CARE).

The systemic (more serious) type inflames the connective tissue in any part of the body. Most commonly the inflammation occurs in the joints, muscles, skin, blood vessels, the membranes surrounding the lungs and heart, and sometimes the kidneys and brain.

Single oils: Cypress and lemongrass.

Blends: ImmuPower, Valor, EndoFlex, Joy, Acceptance, and Present Time.

EndoFlex, and nutmeg support adrenal glands so they can produce hormones, cortisone, ephedrine, adrenaline, etc.

ImmuPower applied on liver Vita Flex areas on feet and over the liver, 3 times daily may give relief.

Put 30 drops of Endo lex in a Bath Gel Base and soak in a bath for 30 minutes every day.

Massage EndoFlex on bottom of the feet. Two hours later rub on Thieves.

ImmuPower:10-15 drops over the liver and on bottom of the feet 2-3 times daily.

Recipe:
- 30 drops cypress
- 30 drops lemongrass
- 30 drops EndoFlex

Mix in 4 oz. massage oil or V-6 Mixing Oil or Massage Oil Base.

Massage entire body with mixture every day.

Rub Valor on bottom of the feet.

Adrenal Glands:
- 3 drops clove
- 3 drops nutmeg
- 7 drops rosemary

Mix in 20 drops massage oil or V-6 Mixing Oil or Massage Oil Base.

Use a hot compress on adrenal glands, which are on top of the kidneys on your back,

2 inches above a line through the elbows.

Supplements:

Therapeutic program for first 90 days.

Support program for following 30 days.

Maintenance program after 120 days.

Colon and liver cleanse with Cleansing Trio. (See COLON.)

ImmuGel: 1/2 tsp. 2-3 times daily. Supports immune function.

Super Cal: 2-3 capsules 2-3 times daily.

Super C: 2-4 tablets 2-3 times daily

ImmuneTune: 2-4 capsules 2-3 times daily.

Megazyme: 2-6 tablets 2-3 times daily.

Sulfurzyme: 1-2 Tbsp. in water 1-2 times daily. (For arthritic symptoms)

AlkaLime: 1 Tbsp. in water 1-2 times daily.

VitaGreen: 2-4 capsules 2-3 timesdaily,

Ultra Young: 3 squirts in mouth 2-3 times daily.

Thyromin: 1 capsule morning, noon, and bedtime. If the temperature drops, delete the supplement at lunch or morning (see THYROID) Monitor basal temperature. If it does not rise in 3 days, increase the amount of Thyromin or Ultra Young. The endocrine system, particularly the pituitary, may need boosting.

Lyme Disease - Rocky Mountain Spotted Fever

Caused by the bite of an infected tick.

Blends: PanAway, Melrose, Thieves, Exodus II, and Immupower.

Supplements: Body Balance, Power Meal, ImmuneTune, Radex, and Exodus II, Thyromin.

Colon and liver cleanse: Cleansing Trio.

Body Balance provides the minerals and enzymes necessary to fight the disease.

(See TICK BITES under INSECT BITES.)

Lymphatic System

Single oils:

- Sandalwood with helichrysum, myrtle, lemon, grapefruit, lemongrass, rosemary, lavender, or rose.
- Cypress with helichrysum, bergamot, grapefruit, lemon, orange, tangerine, rosemary, thyme, or lavender.
- Lemongrass or sage with helichrysum, lemon, grapefruit, basil, cypress, rosemary, spruce, lavender, or tangerine.

Use: Add 1-3 drops to the corresponding single oils above (according to your sensitivity).

Blends:

- Helichrysum with Di-Tone, JuvaFlex, EndoFlex, Thieves, Acceptance, or Raven.
- Cypress with Citrus Fresh or Aroma Life.
- Lemongrass or sage with Citrus Fresh or En-R-Gee.

Use: Add 1-3 drops of each single oil to the corresponding blends above (according to your sensitivity.

Massage oils on sore spots.

Then apply Cel-Lite Magic and essential oils, such as grapefruit and cypress. Grapefruit and cypress help to digest chemicals stored in body fat. This encourages the body to discharge chemicals and stimulate the lymphatic system.

Helichrysum is a powerful lymphatic decongestant. Others are grapefruit, myrtle, orange, tangerine, lemon, cypress, and lemongrass. Experiment by massaging other oils in the manner stated above, to find which gives the best relief. Mix 1 or 2 drops of the oil or oil blend that works best in V-6 Mixing Oil or Massage Oil Base and massage in the armpits to stimulate lymphatics. Thieves is good for this purpose but should always be diluted.

Lymphatic Cleanse:
- 3 drops cypress
- 1 drop orange
- 2 drops grapefruit

Mix in 1/2 gallon distilled water. Grade C maple syrup may be added. Drink daily.

Supplements and Skin Care: Cel-Lite Magic Massage Oil, Morning Start Bath Gel, Super C, Radex, ImmuGel, Royal Essence, VitaGreen, and Goji Berry Tea.

Colon and liver cleanse: Cleansing Trio.

Goji Berry Tea helps cleanse the lymphatic system.

Lymphatic Pump Therapy

This will assist in clearing a sluggish lymphatic system. The lymphatic system pump is performed as follows:

- Have the person lie on his/her back or sit in a comfortable chair.

- With one hand support one foot by lifting just above the heel.

- Grasp the toes of that foot by clamping your other hand over them (cover both sides of the toes).

- Bend the toes up as far as is comfortable and hold the toes in that position; pull the foot down as far as is comfortable.

- Then bend the toes down as far as is comfortable. Holding the toes like this, push the foot up as far as is comfortable.

- Bend the toes up as far as is comfortable and repeat.

Pump like this 2 to 6 times. Less for the first time and more as the lymph system clears. Repeat on the other foot.

Lymphoma

(See CANCER.)

M.C.T. (Mixed Connective Tissue Disease)

M.C.T. acts much like lupus in that the connective tissue in the body becomes inflamed and achy. The problem is poor assimilation of protein. Smoking also blocks protein assimilation.

Researchers have linked most degenerative diseases to lack of nutrients in the body. Insufficient minerals and trace minerals account for most of the nutritional deficiencies.

Single oils:

- Rosemary with nutmeg and clove.

- Lemongrass with marjoram or peppermint.

- Basil with birch, cypress, or peppermint.

Use: Add 1-3 drops to the corresponding single oils above (according to your sensitivity).

Blends:

ImmuPower, Valor, Present Time, Joy, and Acceptance.

For aches and discomfort:
- 10 drops basil
- 8 drops birch
- 6 drops cypress
- 3 drops peppermint

Apply neat on location, massage larger areas mixed with V-6 Mixing Oil or Massage Oil Base. For general aching, do Raindrop Therapy.

Rub ImmuPower over the liver and on liver Vita Flex Points on the bottom of the right foot. This has been reported to help lupus, which is similar to M.C.T. (see LUPUS).

Valor helps the other oils work better. Rub on the bottom of the feet.

Present Time gives emotional strength.

Joy and Acceptance help overcome impressions of low self-worth, low self-esteem, and self-distrust that come with disease.

Adrenal support:
- 3 drops clove
- 3 drops nutmeg
- 7 drops rosemary
- 20 drops Massage Oil or V-6 Mixing Oil.

Use as a hot compress over the adrenal glands

Supplements: ImmuGel, Master HIS/HERS, Super C, Super B, VitaGreen, ImmuneTune, ArthroTune, Super Cal, Thyromin, Rehemogen, and EssPro 7.

Stay away from acid foods. Eat alkaline foods, such as barley or wheat sprouts.

VitaGreen: 2 to 6 capsules 3 times daily for alkaline balancing.

Use Cleansing Trio to expel toxins. It is important to quit smoking and keep away from contaminants, such as chemical industries, auto garages, paint shops, cleaning products, etc.

Amino acids are generally lacking in people with connective tissue problems. ImmuGel is a powerful source of amino acids. (See BODY pH, ACID/ALKALINE BALANCE.)

Rehemogen purifies and fortifies the blood.

- Super C: 1-3 tablets 2-3 times daily.
- Super Cal: 2-4 capsules 1-2 times daily.
- ImmuneTune: 2-4 capsules 2-3 times daily.
- Super B: 1 tablet 3-4 times weekly.
- Master HIS/HERS: 3-6 tablets 2-3 times daily.
- ArthroTune: 2-3 capsules 2-3 times daily.

Malaria

Single oils: Lemon and ylang ylang

Lemon oil in water with honey, sip when feeling an attack coming.

Also see INSECT REPELLENT and INSECT BITES.

Measles

Single oils:

- Lavender with Roman chamomile, melaleuca, or German chamomile.

Use: Add 1-3 drops to the corresponding single oils above (according to your sensitivity).

Recipe #1:
- 15 drops lavender
- 15 drops Roman chamomile
- 5 drops melaleuca

Mix 4 drops into 1 pint of water, shake well, and sponge child down once a day.

Recipe #2:
- 5 drops lavender
- 5 drops German chamomile

Add to 4 oz. of body lotion, shake well, and dab on spots.

Recipe #3:
- 2 drops lavender
- 1 drop Roman chamomile

Added to 1 cup Epsom salts in a bath twice a day.

Memory

(See MEMORY under BRAIN FUNCTION.)

Menopause - Hormone Imbalance, Hot Flashes, Night Sweats, PMS (Premenstrual Syndrome)

(See Chapter on Hormones.)

PMS is one of the most common hormone-related conditions in otherwise healthy women. Women can experience a wide range of symptoms for 10 to 14 days before menstruation, and even 2 to 3 days into menstruation. These symptoms include mood swings, fatigue, headaches, breast tenderness, abdominal bloating, anxiety, depression, confusion, memory loss, sugar cravings, cramps, low back pain, irritability, weight gain, acne, pimples, and oily skin and hair. Causes include hormonal, nutritional, psychological, and stress of the western culture.

Ultra Young and Thyromin (start with 2 capsules before bedtime). Add ImmuneTune.

Single oils:

- Basil with clary sage, sage, fennel, bergamot, rosemary, rose, neroli, jasmine, ylang ylang, peppermint, tarragon, spikenard, vitex, marjoram, or hyssop.

- Sage with clary sage, fennel, basil, bergamot, yarrow, German chamomile, Roman chamomile, pine, anise, or orange. Lavender and geranium are secondary.

Use: Add 1-3 drops to the corresponding single oils above (according to your sensitivity).

Blends:

- Basil or Aroma Siez with Dragon Time, Mister, EndoFlex, Acceptance, or Exodus II.

- Sage or EndoFlex with Mister.

Use: Add 1-3 drops of each single oil to the corresponding blends above (according to your sensitivity.

Supplements and Skin Care: Dragon Time Bath and Shower Gel, Master HERS, FemiGen, Thyromin, VitaGreen, Estro, Femalin, Royal Essence, Super B, Body Balance, ArthroTune, EssPro 7, Super Cal, Mineral Essence, A. D. & E. Liquid, and Exodus.

Essential oils help in balancing hormones and emotions. For this, diffusing is most efficient.

Rub 2 to 6 drops of Dragon Time, Mister (sometimes works better in winter time) or EndoFlex on reproductive Vita Flex areas on hands and feet. Some people have had results applying to the crown of head and forehead. Also apply on the groin and across the lower back. Hot compresses can be added if desired.

Put 1 drop of EndoFlex on the tongue and roof of the mouth or apply as above. For hot flashes, apply oils on feet, solar plexus, tongue, and crown of head.

Fennel contains sclareol, which is an estrogen-like property that helps balance hormones.

Sage and clary sage are estrogen-like and help improve estrogen, progesterone, and testosterone balance.

1 drop bergamot and 1 drop geranium may help hormone balance.

Hormone Balance:
• 10 drops basil
• 10 drops marjoram
• 8 drops hyssop
• 4 drops helichrysum
• 6 drops ylang ylang

Mix in 1 oz. V-6 Mixing Oil or Massage Oil Base.

EssPro 7 is an excellent source of natural progesterone and may help balance hormone levels. Excellent results have been reported with younger women in reducing PMS and even to re-start monthly periods in cases in which they have been devoid for some time. The cream is used by menopausal women as a hormone support. Each person must determine by experimentation the amount required for her own body. Some will need 1 application per day. Others need 2 or 3 applications per day. Apply to soft tissue areas, such as inside thighs, upper arms, breast, lower abdomen, and buttocks. Rub until the skin completely absorbs the creams (no slippery feeling).

Femalin is designed to harmonize female hormone levels. This tincture is the perfect companion to EssPro 7.

The synergistic supplement is FemiGen. You may use up to 6 times a day, particularly during menstrual periods. Vitamins B6 and B12 are important for hormonal balance, so adequate B vitamins are required. Super B is a good source of all B vitamins.

Royal Essence helps hormonal balance and increases energy. Take 1 dropper in distilled water or directly under the tongue for the fastest results.

For PMS and cramping before and during the cycle, make a blend of 10 drops Dragon Time and 4 drops basil. Rub around your ankles, lower back and stomach. A week after cycle ends, take Master HERS along with VitaGreen.

The pollutants to which we are exposed are carried to the fatty tissue, such as the breasts, thyroid, ovaries, uterus, etc. Many chemicals mimic or imitate our natural hormones and can fit the hormone receptors, thus tricking or over-stimulating these organs. This may become a major source of cancers of the breast, uterus, etc. The soy in Body Balance helps protect the hormone (estrogen) receptors and therefore assists hormone regulation. Take Body Balance at least once a day.

Endometriosis

This is when the lining of the uterus develops in other places; for example, on the muscular wall of the uterus, ovaries, fallopian tubes, vagina, intestines, or scars in the abdominal wall. These fragments bleed like the lining of the uterus. Because the blood cannot escape, a fibrous cyst forms around the misplaced uterine tissue. Generally no corresponding symptoms appear, but symptoms can include abdominal or back pain during your period, a pain that often increases after the period is over. Other symptoms may include heavy periods and pain during intercourse.

Single oils: Eucalyptus

Blends: Melrose and Thieves.

Supplements: EssPro 7, ImmuGel, Super C, Femalin, and ProTec.

Douche with Femalin or Protec.

Protec implant may be very helpful.

Colon and liver cleanse: Cleansing Trio.

Hot compress of Melrose on the stomach.

Apply Thieves to bottom of the feet.

Menstrual Cramps - Irregular Periods

Single oils:

- Rosemary with basil, clary sage, sage, marjoram, lavender, Roman chamomile, cypress, tarragon, vitex, or Idaho tansy.

Use: Add 1-3 drops to the corresponding single oils above (according to your sensitivity).

Blends: Dragon Time and EndoFlex.

Supplements: FemiGen, EssPro 7, and Estro.

Apply oils to the reproductive Vita Flex points on the hands and feet. (See Vita Flex chart). Hot compresses may be used if desired.

Sage assists and promotes menstrual discharges.

Apply clary sage around ankles for cramps and PMS.

Jasmine helps menstrual problems.

Excessive hemorrhaging:
- 10 drops helichrysum

Mix in 1 tsp. V-6 Mixing Oil or Massage Oil Base; rub around ankles, lower back, and stomach.

For cramp relief:
- 10 drops chamomile
- 10 drops fennel

Mix in 1 oz. V-6 Mixing Oil or Massage Oil Base.

Mix:
- 3 drops helichrysum
- 1/2 tsp. cayenne
- 6-oz. water

Mix well, and drink all at once.

Period regulator:
- 5 drops peppermint
- 9 drops *Conyza canadensis*
- 16 drops clary sage
- 11 drops sage
- 5 drops jasmine

Mix in 1/2 to 1 oz. massage oil or V-6 Mixing Oil or Massage Oil Base.

When migraine headaches accompany monthly periods, a colon and liver cleanse may help by purging the body.

Hysterectomy

Supplements: FemiGen and EssPro 7.

Mold

Single oils: Cedarwood

Blends: Purification

Mono-Nucleosis (Mono)

Single oils:

- Ravensara with hyssop and frankincense.

Use: Add 1-3 drops to the corresponding single oils above (according to your sensitivity).

Blends:

- Thyme or ravensara and mountain savory with Thieves or R.C.

Use: Add 1-3 drops of each single oil to the corresponding blends above (according to your sensitivity.

Supplements: ImmuGel and Super C.

Colon and liver cleanse: Cleansing Trio.

Add ImmuGel and Super C to build the immune system.

Mix:
- 3 drops Thieves
- 3 drops thyme
- 3 drops mountain savory
- 2 drops ravensara

Rub over bottom of feet.

Morning Sickness - Nausea

(See PREGNANCY, BABIES AND CHILDREN.)

Massage 1 drop of Di-Tone on outer ear.

Motion Sickness

Single oils:

• Lavender with peppermint, ginger, juniper, rosemary, tarragon, or spearmint.

Use: Add 1-3 drops to the corresponding single oils above (according to your sensitivity).

Blends:

• Lavender with Di-Tone, Harmony, or JuvaFlex.

Use: Add 1-3 drops of each single oil to the corresponding blends above (according to your sensitivity.

Supplements: Mint Condition and Megazyme.

Place 1 drop on the end of the tongue or around the navel and on the thymus or rub behind the ears (on the mastoid). Diffuse or mix in water and sip slowly.

Mouth Wash

(See HALITOSIS.)

Single oils:

• Peppermint or spearmint with lemon, mandarin, or cinnamon.

Use: Add 1-3 drops to the corresponding single oils above (according to your sensitivity).

Supplements:

If one has persistent bad breath or gum disease, it may be a sign of poor digestion or other health problems. One should consult a physician (see DIGESTION PROBLEMS and GUMS).

A refreshing and disinfectant mouthwash or gargle that is effective against oral infections and gums:

Mix:
• 3 drops peppermint
• 2 drops lemon
• 1 drop mandarin

Mix in 2 Tbsp. honey and dilute in 16 oz. of hot water. For fresh breath, gargle or rinse mouth in the morning or after eating food such as garlic, onions, etc. This is meant as a mouthwash or gargle and could be swallowed.

Mucus

Most oils help tissues expel mucus. Using the oils both topically and by diffusing will get them into the tissues to help rid the body of excess mucus. If congestion occurs while inhaling a diffused oil, this is the oil to help your body release and discharge mucus. An expectorant discharges mucus, soft and hard plaque, and toxins out of the body.

Single oils: Frankincense, lavender, hyssop, helichrysum, fennel, eucalyptus, cypress, German chamomile, marjoram, mugwort, myrtle, pepper, patchouly, ravensara, rosemary, and sage.

Blends: Di-Tone, 3 Wise Men, Raven, R.C., and Purification.

Milk and milk products produce mucus. The pineols in lavender and chamomile help to reduce the over-production of mucus. Apply on the thoracic vertebrae, T4 and T5 (at the neck-to-shoulder intersection). Also apply on bottom of the feet to slow down the parasympathetic system and thus reduce the over-production of mucus.

Multiple Sclerosis (MS)

(See NEUROLOGICAL DISEASES.)

Mumps

Single oils: Oregano, thyme, mountain savory, myrrh, and cypress.

Blends: R.C., Raven, Thieves, and Exodus II.

Supplements: ImmuGel, Dentarome Plus, Fresh Essence, Super C, and Exodus.

Muscles - Sore, Spasmed, or Pulled

Single oils:

• Basil with marjoram, cypress, ginger, peppermint, spruce, vetiver, lavender or lemongrass.

• Rosemary with basil, marjoram, cypress, lemon, clary sage, lavender, German chamomile, Roman chamomile, ginger, vetiver, or elemi.

- Birch with basil or marjoram.

Use: Add 1-3 drops to the corresponding single oils above (according to your sensitivity).

Blends:

- Basil with Aroma Siez, PanAway, R.C., Relieve It, or M-Grain.

- Rosemary with Aroma Siez or Clarity.

Use: Add 1-3 drops of each single oil to the corresponding blends above (according to your sensitivity).

Supplements and Skin Care: Arthro Plus, Super Cal, ArthroTune, Royal Essence, Mineral Essence, Sulfurzyme, Relaxation, Ortho Ease and Ortho Sport Massage Oils.

Royal Essence is good for any muscular problems. Apply Ortho Ease Massage Oil to areas where muscles are over-exercised. This boosts oxygen and prevents tearing or other damages.

Make Ortho Ease a little stronger by adding to 4 oz bottle:

Recipe #1:
- 10 drops birch
- 10 drops peppermint
- 10 drops marjoram
- 8 drops elemi
- 8 drops vetiver
- 5 drops helichrysum
- 5 drops cypress

Recipe #2:
- 20 drops birch
- 15 drops marjoram
- 10 drops juniper
- 10 drops cypress
- 6 drops spruce

Mix in 4 oz. V-6 Mixing Oil or Massage Oil Base.

Lavender with Roman chamomile or birch with marjoram are excellent for tired muscles.

Elemi is for toning muscles.

Marjoram with lemongrass makes a great combination for torn ligaments/tendons or muscles.

Ortho Sport Massage Oil soothes ligament/tendon damage.

Aroma Siez has been very effective for sore, tired, spastic or tight muscles. Massage into affected muscle areas.

Relief for sore aching muscles due to over exertion or straining:

Recipe #3:
- 9 drops cypress
- 8 drops rosemary
- 8 drops lavender
- 2 drops elemi
- 2 drops valerian

Mix in 2 oz. V-6 Mixing Oil or Massage Oil Base. Massage into the affected area and then apply a hot pack to speed the results.

Cypress increases circulation, which is important for damaged tissue.

Circulation and Pain:
- 5 drops basil
- 8 drops marjoram
- 10 drops cypress
- 3 drops peppermint

Mix in palm of left hand. Mix clockwise with fingers of right hand, then massage on location. You can then further massage with Ortho Ease. It is best to mix with V-6 Mixing Oil or Massage Oil Base, since more than 3 drops of basil neat on the skin will sting due to the methyl chavicol content.

Circulation:
- 2 or 3 drops of basil
- 1 or 2 drops of marjoram
- 1 drop of peppermint

Mix in left hand and apply neat on location. Then massage with Ortho Ease over the general area.

Increase circulation:
- 3 drops basil
- 2 drops peppermint
- 4 drops cypress
- 8 drops marjoram
- 10 drops birch

Mix in 1 oz. V-6 Mixing Oil or Massage Oil Base.

Muscle and tissue regeneration:
- 8 drops spruce
- 8 drops sandalwood
- 7 drops fir
- 5 drops hyssop
- 4 drops lemongrass
- 5 drops helichrysum
- 4 drops birch
- 2 drops vetiver
- 1 drop Idaho tansy

Mix in 1/2 to 1 oz. V-6 Mixing Oil or Massage Oil Base.

Muscle tightness:
- 6 drops marjoram
- 4 drops cypress
- 4 drops birch
- 3 drops valerian
- 1 drop helichrysum

Mix in 1 oz. V-6 Mixing Oil or Massage Oil Base. Apply on location, then massage with Ortho Ease.

Sore muscle:
- 5 drops rosemary
- 10 drops juniper
- 10 drops lavender
- 10 drops marjoram
- 5 drops vetiver

Mix in 2 oz. V-6 Mixing Oil or Massage Oil Base.

Aching legs:
- 5 drops clary sage
- 5 drops lavender
- 5 drops chamomile
- 3 drops rosemary cineol

Mix in 1 oz. V-6 Mixing Oil or Massage Oil Base. In cold weather, add ginger and rub on knees.

For sports injury:
- 3 drops basil
- 5 drops Aroma Siez

Mix in 1 oz. V-6 Mixing Oil or Massage Oil Base and apply.

Muscle cold:
- 1 to 2 drops ravensara
- 4 to 5 drops Aroma Siez
- 1 drop black pepper

Mix in 1 oz. V-6 Mixing Oil or Massage Oil Base and apply.

When selecting oils, particularly for injuries, think through the cause and type of injury and select oils for each segment. For instance, whiplash could encompass muscle damage, nerve damage, ligament strain or tear, inflammation, bone injury, fever on location, and possibly an emotion. Select oils for each perceived problem and apply.

Any time there is tissue damage, there is always inflammation. Apply anti-inflammatory oils first in order of activity: hyssop, myrrh, birch, marjoram, ravensara, lavender, and Roman chamomile.

Myrrh, Roman chamomile, and lavender: Contusion to the tissue, such as damaged capillaries, bruising, or loss of oxygen.

Ravensara, hyssop, or oregano: Inflammation due to infection or virus.

Peppermint: Reduce fever.

Muscle inflammation and pain relief:
- 12 drops fir
- 10 drops melaleuca
- 8 drops lavender
- 6 drops marjoram
- 3 drops yarrow
- 3 drops spearmint
- 2 drops peppermint

Mix in 1 oz. V-6 Mixing Oil or Massage Oil Base.

Sore, tired muscles may be lacking in trace minerals. Royal Essence or Mineral Essence are excellent sources of trace minerals and good for all muscle conditions.

Bruised Muscles (see BRUISING).

Single oils:

- Birch with marjoram, basil, cypress, rosemary, vetiver, peppermint, spruce, fir, and oregano.

Use: Add 1-3 drops to the corresponding single oils above (according to your sensitivity).

Blends:

- Birch with Aroma Siez, PanAway, and Peace & Calming.

Use: Add 1-3 drops of each single oil to the corresponding blends above (according to your sensitivity).

When a bruise has a lot of black and blue discoloration and pain, you might start with helichrysum, birch, and oregano. Once the pain and inflammation starts to reduce, use cypress, then basil with Aroma Siez to further enhance the muscle relaxation. Follow with peppermint to stimulate the nerves and reduce fever in the tissue. Follow with cold packs to enhance oil absorption, to cool fever, and to continue healing (see COLD PACKS).

Cypress increases circulation. Apply on location.

Supplements and Skin Care: ArthroTune, Super Cal, Mineral Essence, and Ortho Sport, Relaxation, and Ortho Ease Massage Oils.

Cramps and Charley Horses - Night Leg Cramps

Some causes of cramps and charley horses are magnesium deficiency and fatigue.

Single oils:

- Rosemary with basil, clary sage, vetiver, cypress, marjoram, lavender, elemi or German chamomile.

Use: Add 1-3 drops to the corresponding single oils above (according to your sensitivity).

Blends:

- Rosemary with Aroma Siez or Relieve It.

Use: Add 1-3 drops of each single oil to the corresponding blends above (according to your sensitivity).

Supplements and Skin Care: Super Cal, ArthroTune, Mineral Essence, Relaxation, Ortho Ease, and Ortho Sport Massage Oils.

Super Cal: Provides magnesium and calcium.

ArthroTune: Helps reduce stiffness from sitting for long periods.

Mineral Essence: Makes up mineral deficiencies.

Relaxation and Ortho Sport Massage Oils: Help reduce tightness and cramping.

ArthroTune: 2-3 capsules morning and night help reduces night leg cramp.

Weakness - Fatigue

Single oils:

- Ravensara with lemongrass, juniper, and nutmeg.

Use: Add 1-3 drops of each single oil to the corresponding blends above (according to your sensitivity).

Blends: En-R-Gee

Supplements: VitaGreen, Royal Essence, and Seagal Power Meal.

Muscular Dystrophy

Single oils: Marjoram and lemongrass (equal parts of each), pine, and lavender.

Blends: Aroma Siez and Relieve It.

Supplements: Megazyme, Seagal Power Meal, Sulfurzyme, VitaGreen, Mineral Essence, Thyromin, Ultra Young, and Ortho Ease, and Ortho Sport Massage Oils.

Nails

Single oils: Frankincense, myrrh, and lemon.

Blends: Citrus Fresh

Supplements: Sulfurzyme: 2 Tbsp. in water 2 times daily, Super Cal, and Mineral Essence.

Poor or weak nails, often containing ridges, indicate a sulfur deficiency.

To strengthen nails:
- 2 drops Wheat Germ Oil
- 2 drops frankincense
- 2 drops myrrh
- 2 drops lemon

Rub on nails twice per week.

Nausea

(See MOTION SICKNESS, PREGNANCY.)

Nerve Itching

An itch for no obvious reason is possibly inflammation from chemicals.

Single oils: Melaleuca with Lavender (equal parts)**Blends:** Peace & Calming

Supplements: Super B, Super Cal, and Sulfurzyme.

Nerve Tissue

Single oils: Peppermint, geranium, juniper, helichrysum, and lavender.

Blends: Peace & Calming

Supplements: Super B, Super Cal, and Sulfurzyme.

Application: Raindrop Therapy.

Nerve-Ending Problems Caused by Metallic Shock

(See VASCULAR CLEANSING - CHELATING METALLICS.)

Single oils: Helichrysum, peppermint, juniper, geranium.

Helichrysum is a powerful chelator.

Blends: JuvaFlex

Supplements: Chelex, Radex, and JuvaTone.

Nerve Equilibrium

Single oils: Petitgrain and lavender.

Petitgrain helps re-establish equilibrium.

Supplements: Sulfurzyme and Mineral Essence

Nervous Fatigue

Can cause motor skill problems.

Single oils: Juniper, geranium, and helichrysum.

- Oregano with thyme, nutmeg, jasmine, and peppermint.

Use: Add 1-3 drops to the corresponding single oils above (according to your sensitivity).

Blends: Brain Power and Clarity.

Neuralgia

Pain from a damaged nerve; can be in the face or sciatica, or similar nerve damage.

Single oils: Marjoram, peppermint, and spearmint.

Blends: PanAway, Relieve It

Supplements: Ultra Young, EssPro 7, Sulfurzyme, Super B, and Ortho Ease and Ortho Sport Massage Oils.

Nutmeg supports the nervous system to overcome neuralgia.

Sulfurzyme and Super B work well together to repair nerve damage.

Neuritis, Nerve Inflammation from Virus, Neuropathy

Single oils:

- Lavender with juniper, oregano, thyme, geranium, peppermint, or clove.

Use: Add 1-3 drops to the corresponding single oils above (according to your sensitivity).

Blends:

- Lavender with Valor, Aroma Siez, or Peace & Calming.

Use: Add 1-3 drops of each single oil to the corresponding blends above (according to your sensitivity).

Diffuse Peace & Calming for any nervous problem or condition. This blend helps to sedate a hyper-intensive (over-active) nervous system. Valor supports the nervous system.

Supplements: Super Cal, VitaGreen, Sulfurzyme, and Ultra Young.

VitaGreen is very important for neurological problems.

Progesterone builds, repairs, and regenerates the myelin sheath around nerves. EssPro 7 is a good source of progesterone.

Super Cal provides calcium necessary to carry the electrical nerve signals along neurological pathways.

Nervous System Disorders

Single oils:

• Peppermint with lavender, cedarwood, basil, clary sage, sage, rosemary, spruce, tangerine, sandalwood, melaleuca, ravensara, marjoram, palmarosa, thyme, lemongrass, birch, cypress, and helichrysum.

Use: Add 1-3 drops to the corresponding single oils above (according to your sensitivity).

Blends:

• Lavender with Valor, Peace & Calming, or Citrus Fresh.

Use: Add 1-3 drops of each single oil to the corresponding blends above (according to your sensitivity).

Lavender, myrrh, Roman chamomile, marjoram, German chamomile, and tangerine all have a sedative effect on the nervous system.

Basil is a nerve stimulant, and a stimulator of the adrenal cortex.

Diffuse Peace & Calming for any nervous condition. It helps to sedate a hyper-intensive (over-active) nervous system.

Valor supports the nervous system.

For nerve problems:
• 2 drops peppermint
• 10 drops juniper
• 1 drop geranium
• 8 drops marjoram
• 4 drops helichrysum

Mix neat or in 1 oz. V-6 Mixing Oil or Massage Oil Base and apply.

Supplements: Super Cal, VitaGreen, Sulfurzyme, Seagal Power Meal, Super C, and Super B.

VitaGreen is very important for neurological problems.

Progesterone is very necessary in the building, repair and rejuvenation of the myelin sheath around nerves.

EssPro 7 is a good source of progesterone.

Super Cal offers the calcium necessary to carry the electrical nerve signals along neurological pathways.

Sulfur deficiency is very prevalent in nerve problems. Sulfur requires calcium and vitamin C for the body to metabolize. Super B and Sulfurzyme work well together to help repair nerve damage and the myelin sheath.

Bells Palsy or Facial Palsy

A type of neuritis, marked by paralysis on one side of the face and inability to open or close the eyelid.

Single oils:

• Peppermint with helichrysum and juniper.

Use: Add 1-3 drops to the corresponding single oils above (according to your sensitivity)

Blends: Aroma Siez and Relieve It.

Supplements: EssPro 7 and Ultra Young.

Rub Peppermint with helichrysum on the facial nerve, which is in front and behind the ear and on areas of pain.

Carpel Tunnel Syndrome

Nerves pass through a tunnel formed by wrist bones (known as carpals) and a tough membrane on the under-side of the wrist that binds the bones together. The tunnel is rigid, so if the tissues within it swell for some reason, they press and pinch the nerves creating a painful condition known as carpal tunnel syndrome. This condition is fairly common in pregnant and menopausal women, possibly due to hormone imbalance. It can also be sports-related or due to activities that involve strenuous or repeated use of wrists. A similar condition can occur in the ankle (tarsal tunnel syndrome), or even the elbow. These two are less common.

Single oils:

• Birch with cypress, peppermint, marjoram, or basil.

• Helichrysum with birch, lemongrass, cypress, or peppermint.

Use: Add 1-3 drops to the corresponding single oils above (according to your sensitivity).

Blends: PanAway and Relieve It.

One layered application of PanAway and Relieve It has been reported to relieve carpal tunnel syndrome.

Recipe:
- 5 drops birch
- 3 drops cypress
- 1 drop peppermint
- 2 drops marjoram
- 3 drops lemongrass

Mix neat or double quantities in 1 oz. V-6 Mixing Oil or Massage Oil Base. Also use ice pack.

Supplements and Skin Care: EssPro 7, Super C, Super Cal, Mineral Essence, and Ortho Sport Massage Oil.

Progesterone is very necessary in building, repairing, and regenerating the myelin sheath around nerves. EssPro 7 is a good source of natural progesterone.

Nervous System - Parasympathetic/Sympathetic

This is part of the autonomic nervous system. The nerves originate in the brain and sacral region of the spinal cord. It controls and regulates constriction of eye pupils, heartbeat, breathing, digestion, rate of glandular activity, contraction and dilation of blood vessels.

The other part of the autonomic nervous system is the sympathetic nervous system which reacts to aggression in an emergency, preparing the body to defend itself by fight or flight. The two systems check and balance each other.

Single oils: Lavender and marjoram.

Lavender helps regulate the parasympathetic nervous system.

Blends: Valor and Peace & Calming.

Supplements: Seagal Power Meal, Super Cal, Sulfurzyme, and Mineral Essence.

Neuropathy - Peripheral

Damage to peripheral nerves (other than spinal or those in the brain), generally starts as tingling in hands and feet and slowly spreads along limbs to the trunk.

Numbness, sensitive skin, neuralgic pain, weakening of muscle power can all develop in varying degrees. Most common causes include complications from diabetes (diabetic neuropathy), alcoholism, vitamin B12 deficiency, tumors, too many pain killers, exposure and absorption of chemicals, metallics, pesticides and many other causes.

Single oils:
- Juniper with geranium, helichrysum, peppermint, cypress, or lemongrass.

Use: Add 1-3 drops to the corresponding single oils above (according to your sensitivity).

Blends: JuvaFlex and Brain Power.

Supplements: Super B, Royal Essence, Mineral Essence, Super C, VitaGreen, Body Balance, Master HERS, and Master HIS.

Trace minerals need to be replaced. The body must be supported with sufficient supplements if there is a nutritional deficiency. In particular, the first 5 supplements listed above are extremely beneficial.

Recipe:
- 10 drops juniper
- 10 drops geranium
- 10 drops helichrysum

Mix in 1/2 oz. V-6 Mixing Oil or Massage Oil Base. Massage on location of tingling or numbness. Also massage cypress with peppermint or lemongrass mixed with body lotion.

Recipe:
- 15 drops geranium
- 10 drops helichrysum
- 6 drops cypress
- 10 drops juniper
- 5 drops peppermint

Mix in 2 Tbsp. V-6 Mixing Oil or Massage Oil Base. Apply oils on location and on the feet.

If paralysis is the problem, a regeneration of up to 60% may be possible. If, however, the nerve damage is too severe, treatment may not help. When the damage starts to reverse, there will be pain. Apply PanAway on location and on the feet.

If the person does not have diabetes, then toxic overload may be indicated. Cleanse colon and liver with Cleansing Trio.

Neurological Diseases

These diseases are mainly caused by metallics in the brain, causing misfiring of neurons (see BRAIN FUNCTION).

Single oils: Frankincense, helichrysum, oregano, sage, juniper, rosemary, clove, cardamom, and vitex.

Blends: Acceptance, Joy, Gathering, Brain Power, Clarity, and Forgiveness.

Cleanse colon and liver with Cleansing Trio.

Put the oils on directly as is practical. It is most important to apply on the brain on reflex points on the head, forehead, temples and mastoids (the bone just behind the ear). Use direct pressure application to the brain stem along the center of the backbone on the neck at the skull and down the spine. Put the oils on a loofah brush and rub along the spine as vigorously as desired.

CAUTION: Use a natural bristle brush, since the oils dissolve some plastics.

Apply oils through Raindrop Therapy application on the spine.

CAUTION: Never use hot packs on neurological problems. Always use cold packs to increase penetration of oils. In other words, reduce temperature of the damaged site.

Juniper promotes nerve function.

Frankincense may help clear the emotions of fear and anger, which is common with people who have these neurological diseases. When these diseases are contracted, people often become suicidal.

Hope, Joy, Gathering, and Forgiveness will help work through the psychological and emotional aspects of the disease.

Vitex has been shown to reduce the symptoms of Parkinson's disease by 89% in animal studies.

Recipe:
• 1 drop rosemary
• 1 drop helichrysum
• 1 drop ylang ylang
• 1 drop clove.

Supplements: JuvaTone, Ultra Young, Vita-Green, Seagal Power Meal, Rehemogen, EssPro 7, Chelex, Super Cal, Super C, and Super B.

Progesterone is very necessary in the building, repair and rejuvenation of the myelin sheath around nerves. EssPro 7 is a good source of progesterone.

Sulfur deficiency is very prevalent in these neurological diseases. Sulfur requires calcium and Vitamin C for the body to metabolize. Super B and Sulfurzyme work well together to help repair nerve damage and the myelin sheath.

Huntington's Chorea (Saint Vitus Dance)

A rare degenerative nerve disease that generally starts in middle age, often after child birth. Uncontrollable body movements gradually develop, followed by mental deterioration. Sometimes the mental deterioration occurs first.

Single oils:

• Peppermint with juniper or basil.

Use: Add 1-3 drops to the corresponding single oils above (according to your sensitivity).

Blends: Aroma Siez

Recipe:
• 5 drops peppermint
• 10 drops juniper
• 3 drops basil
• 5 drops Aroma Siez

Mix and apply in Raindrop Therapy application.

Multiple Sclerosis (MS)

This disease is a break-down the myelin sheath, caused from a neuralgia injury.

Single oils: Juniper, helichrysum, geranium, peppermint, thyme, oregano, birch, cypress, basil, marjoram, and rosemary.

Blends: Valor, Aroma Siez, Acceptance, and Awaken.

Apply oils by layering. Lightly massage oils in the direction of MS paralysis. For example: If it is lower down the spine, massage down, followed by cold packs. Apply also by Raindrop Therapy application.

Applying heat is the worst thing to do for MS. Drop body temperature 3° F by having the person lie on a table, cover them with a sheet, then cover them with ice, shower curtain and blankets. Work the feet with oils and watch for benefits. There have been individuals who within a few days have been able to get out of a wheel chair.

Layer helichrysum, juniper, geranium, and peppermint and apply cold packs for 30 minutes, then repeat cold packs.

Apply Valor on spine. If the MS is affecting the leg, rub down the spine moving the energy in the direction of the flow of the nerve signals; if it is affecting the neck, then rub up the spine.

Juniper promotes nerve function. Apply cypress and juniper as a base layer on back of the neck, then add Aroma Siez.

Recipe:
• 10 drops helichrysum
• 10 drops peppermint
• 10 drops rosemary

Mix and apply neat.

Supplements: Super Cal, Super B, Super C, VitaGreen, Master HERS, Master HIS, ImmuneTune, EssPro 7, Rehemogen, Chelex, ArthroTune, and Sulfurzyme.

Supplements are very important in working with MS. The following supplements should be divided between your daily meals: Super C, Super Cal, Super B, VitaGreen, ImmuneTune, Master HERS/HIS, Sulfurzyme.

Cleanse colon and liver with Cleansing Trio and JuvaTone.

Rehemogen helps clean the blood for better nutrient delivery.

Degenerative diseases, such as MS, respond well to hormone replacement therapy. EssPro 7 is a good source of progesterone. Progesterone is also necessary for building, repairing and restoring the myelin sheath around nerves.

To help the person emotionally with the MS symptoms, use Acceptance and Awaken. Be patient. Overcoming MS is a long-term endeavor.

Parkinson's Disease

Parkinson's disease involves the deterioration of specific nerve centers in the brain and affects more men than women by a ratio of 3:2. The main symptom is tremors, an involuntary shaking of hands, head, or both. Other symptoms include rigidity, slowed movement, gait disorder, and loss of balance. In many cases these are accompanied by a continuous rubbing together of thumb and forefinger, stooped posture, mask-like face, trouble in swallowing, depression, and difficulty performing simple tasks. These symptoms may all be seen at different stages of the disease. The tremors are most severe when the affected part of the body is not in use. There is no pain or other sensation, other than a decreased ability to move. Symptoms appear slowly, in no particular order and may elapse before they interfere with normal activities.

Single oils: Juniper, Peppermint, and Vitex.

Blends: Peace & Calming and Valor.

Supplements: Sulfurzyme and Super B.

Juniper promotes nerve function.

Vitex has been shown to reduce Parkinson's symptoms by 89% in animal studies. The sulfur found in the Sulfurzyme is necessary to rebuild the myelin sheath.

Night Sweats

(See MENOPAUSE, NIGHT SWEATS.)

Single oils: Sage, clary sage, and yarrow.

Blends: Mister and EndoFlex.

Supplements: EssPro 7, Estro, Femigen, Ultra Young, and Thyromin.

Nose

Bleeding

Nosebleeds are normally not serious. However, if bleeding does not stop in a short time or is excessive or frequent, consult your doctor.

Single oils: Helichrysum and lavender.

• Lemon with cypress.

Use: Add 1-3 drops to the corresponding single oils above (according to your sensitivity).

Mix:
• 2 drops helichrysum or lavender
• 2 drops cypress

Apply to the nose and back of neck. Repeat as needed.

Put 1 drop helichrysum, lavender, or cypress on a tissue paper and wrap the paper around a chip of ice about the size of a thumb nail, push it up under the top lip in the center to the base of the nose. Hold from the outside with lip pressure. This helps to stop bleeding in a very short time.

Dry

Single oils:

• Lavender with lemon or peppermint.

Use: Add 1-3 drops to the corresponding single oils above (according to your sensitivity).

Mixing:
• 2 drops lavender
• 1 drop myrrh
In 1 tsp. cold pressed olive oil.

Rub inside the nose when needed. It works well for a dry nose.

Supplements: A. D. & E. and EssPro 7.

Loss of Smell (Due to Chronic Nasal Catarrh)

Single oils: Basil and frankincense.

Supplements: ImmuneTune, Exodus, and Seagal Power Meal.

Nasal wash with Epsom salts.

Polyps In The Nose

Single oils: Citronella

Blends: Purification: apply neat with a cotton-tip swab.

Nursing

(See chapter on PREGNANCY.)

Single oils: Fennel and nutmeg.

Blends: Di-Tone

Supplements: VitaGreen and Seagal Power Meal.

Osteoporosis - Wasting or Deterioration of Bones

Researchers have linked most degenerative diseases to lack of nutrients in the body. Insufficient minerals and trace minerals account for most of the nutritional deficiencies.

Single oils:

• Birch with spruce, fir, pine, cypress, peppermint, marjoram, rosemary, vetiver, or basil.

• Elemi with birch, cypress, peppermint, rosemary, marjoram, or basil.

Use: Add 1-3 drops to the corresponding single oils above (according to your sensitivity).

Blends:

• Birch with Aroma Siez, Purification, Melrose, Sacred Mountain, Relieve It, or PanAway.

• Birch with PanAway or Aroma Siez.

Use: Add 1-3 drops of each single oil to the corresponding blends above (according to your sensitivity).

Supplements and Skin Care: Ortho Ease, Ortho Sport, and Relaxation Massage Oils, Super Cal, ArthroTune, Arthro Plus, Mineral Essence, EssPro 7, Seagal Power Meal, Sulfurzyme, Thyromin, and Ultra Young.

Massage oils on location.

Cypress increases circulation.

ArthroTune and Super Cal both help to maintain bone composition.

Mineral Essence is a good source of all trace minerals.

Carbonated drinks leach calcium out of the body.

Dr. John Lee, M.D., has found that EssPro 7 applied to the skin will prevent bone loss, even without additional estrogen. EssPro 7 is a good source of natural progesterone. Rub on soft tissue of the body, such as chest, breast, upper arms, inner thighs, and abdomen until absorbed.

Thyromin, EssPro 7, and Ultra Young help bring hormones into balance.

Super Cal, Seagal Power Meal, Sulfurzyme (minimum of 4 Tbsp. per day).

AlkaLime: 1 Tbsp. daily or as needed. Check pH levels.

Ovarian and Uterine Cysts

(See CANCER.)

Single oils:

- Frankincense with geranium, melaleuca, oregano, or cypress.

Use: Add 1-3 drops to the corresponding single oils above (according to your sensitivity).

Blends: Melrose, Dragon Time, and Mister.

Supplements: Master HERS, FemiGen, Femalin, and Protec.

Douche:
- 7 drops Purification
- 2 drops frankincense

Mix with 1 tsp. V-6 Mixing Oil

May be added to Protec for extra strength as a douche.

Protec may be use as a douche. It is already diluted.

If irritation occurs, discontinue use for 3 days before restarting.

Protec may also be used in a vaginal retention implant when mixed into 1 Tbsp. V-6 Mixing Oil or Massage Oil Base. Insert and retain overnight.

Vaginal Retention Implant:
- 5-10 drops frankincense
- 5 drops basil in a vaginal retention implant with 1 Tbsp. V-6 Mixing Oil or Massage Oil.

Implant:
- 5-10 drops frankincense
- 5-10 drops geranium
- 5-10 drops cypress
- 1 Tbsp. V-6 Mixing Oil

Apply as compresses on location and over the lower back in conjunction with Vita Flex application or alone.

They may also be applied on the Vita Flex points for the groin. These points are around and on the anklebone, inside and outside of the foot, and working down to the arch of the foot.

Pain

Chronic

Single oils: Helichrysum, spruce, birch, clove, elemi, rosemary cineol, and valerian.

Blends: Relieve It and PanAway.

Muscle (Analgesic Oils)

Single oils:

- Birch, basil, rosemary, eucalyptus, peppermint, marjoram, cypress, ginger, melaleuca, melissa, lemongrass, or Roman chamomile.
- Birch with clove, helichrysum, peppermint, or marjoram.
- Helichrysum with birch, clove, or peppermint.
- Spruce with helichrysum or pepper oil.
- Helichrysum with basil, cedarwood, geranium, Idaho tansy, fir, juniper, marjoram, or cypress.

Use: Add 1-3 drops to the corresponding single oils above (according to your sensitivity).

Blends:

- Lavender, birch, or helichrysum with Sacred Mountain, Relieve It, Release, PanAway, or Aroma Siez.

Use: Add 1-3 drops of each single oil to the corresponding blends above (according to your sensitivity).

Supplements and Skin Care: ArthroTune, Super Cal, Sulfurzyme, Ortho Ease and Ortho Sport Massage Oils.

The MSM found in Sulfurzyme equalizes fluid pressure inside cells by affecting the protein envelope of the cell so that water transfers freely in and out. When fluid pressure inside cells is higher than outside, it creates pain.

Find the best oil by the following method:

Bone-Related (hips, shoulder, etc): Use birch, cypress, pine, and helichrysum on Vita Flex points on bottom of feet; should work in approximately 2 minutes.

For direct application: birch, fir, spruce, cypress, and peppermint. If this does not work, the pain may be muscle related, the after-effects of an old injure or tissue-inflammation.

Muscle Related: Basil, rosemary verbenon, or marjoram.

Old Injury Related (probably nerves): Peppermint, lavender, nutmeg, and black pepper.

Inflammation: Helichrysum, melissa, vetiver, patchouly, spruce, and geranium.

Massage the oil found by this process on location of the problem and on Vita Flex points on feet. Repeat as pain returns, which may be in 2 hours or as much as 6 months.

PanAway is also powerful for pain reduction. When applied to Vita Flex points on the feet, it can act as fast as within 3 seconds. Alternate with Relieve It. These 2 blends are a powerful combination for deep tissue pain that is not bone-related.

Any oil found by the above selection process may be added to a blend, such as PanAway, to increase the effect.

Hot packs drive the oils faster and deeper when applied on location (see COMPRESS).

Sandalwood and geranium rubbed around hairline of the head and tips of the toes may help pain related to accidents, traumas, etc.

Pain relief:
- 12 drops fir
- 10 drops melaleuca
- 8 drops lavender
- 6 drops marjoram
- 3 drops spearmint
- 2 drops peppermint

Mix in 1 ounce V-6 Mixing Oil or Massage Oil.

Ortho Ease and Ortho Sport Massage Oils help relieve arthritic and rheumatic pain. ArthroTune helps to alleviate rheumatism and rheumatic conditions.

Pancreas

(see DIABETES MELLITUS.)

Pancreatitis

Single oils: Vetiver, peppermint, mountain savory, and oregano.

Blends: Exodus II, ImmuPower, and Thieves.

Supplements: Exodus, ImmuGel, VitaGreen, Super B, Megazyme, and Seagal Power Meal.

Parasites, Intestinal

Parasites can cause diarrhea, gas, bloating, cramping, and nausea, and in severe cases can even delay or stop bowel movements. Parasites can also give off toxins while using up needed nutrients, leaving the body nutritionally deficient. Parasites can lie dormant in the body and then be awakened by something one drinks or eats, giving the impression that the food is the problem. This can make it difficult to determine the cause of an upset stomach.

Parasite elimination and control, while very important, is not a total solution by itself. Always consider a balanced approach in applying health product solutions. Overall health improvement of the body should be addressed.

Single oils:
- Basil with tarragon, peppermint, ginger, spearmint, hyssop, fennel, or Roman chamomile.
- Cypress with tarragon, ginger, rosemary, anise, clove, lemongrass, nutmeg, caraway seed, fennel, lemon, juniper, rosewood, or mountain savory.

- Thyme with melaleuca, oregano, tarragon, peppermint, myrrh, mugwort, or helichrysum.

Use: Add 1-3 drops to the corresponding single oils above (according to your sensitivity).

Blends:

- Basil with Di-Tone.

- Cypress with Di-Tone or JuvaFlex.

- Thyme with Di-Tone or JuvaFlex.

Use: Add 1-3 drops of each single oil to the corresponding blends above (according to your sensitivity).

Supplements: Colloidal Essence, Megazyme, ComforTone, I.C.P., and ParaFree.

Di-Tone is excellent for parasite removal. Apply up to 6 drops to instep area on both feet (small intestine and colon Vita Flex points). This has helped in the passing of parasites within 6 to12 hours after application.

Alternate application: Place 10-15 drops of chosen oils in 100° F water. Lay cloth on water, then place cloth on stomach. Cover with plastic wrap, then with a heavy towel to keep in the heat.

Direct application: Place up to 15 drops in palm; rub over stomach and navel. Apply a hot compress over same area.

The most effective method is a combination of navel and foot applications.

Ginger is also a very specific and powerful anti-parasitic. Ginger with Di-Tone in a retention enema can be effective in 1 to 2 minutes. Use each night for 7 nights. Take 7 days off. Repeat this cycle 3 times to eliminate all stages of parasite development.

A colon parasite, *Cryptosporidium parrum*, that is spread by drinking water, is becoming more widespread, since current city water systems cannot filter it out. It takes either distillation or a 3 micron filter to filter it out. Colloidal silver, found in Colloidal Essence, poisons and inactivates the enzyme respiratory system of *Cryptosporidium parrum*. This may work as fast as within 3 minutes. A colon cleanse will then flush the organisms out of the colon. Do this at least 3 times for this organism after the cleanse (from the research of Terry Friedmann, M.D.).

Supplements to rid body of parasites:

- Colloidal Essence destroys parasites

- ComforTone dislodges plaque and debris from intestinal wall

- I.C.P. Fiber Cleanse scraps intestinal wall

- ParaFree Gel Caps aid in the elimination of parasites.

Perspiration Regulation

Single oils:

- Sage with nutmeg, rosemary, or basil.

Use: Add 1-3 drops to the corresponding single oils above (according to your sensitivity).

Blends:

- Sage with EndoFlex or En-R-Gee.

Use: Add 1-3 drops of each single oil to the corresponding blends above (according to your sensitivity).

Supplements: EssPro 7

Sage helps regulate sweating. Excessive perspiration may indicate adrenal, diabetes, or thyroid problems.

Pets - Dogs, Cats, etc.

(See VETERINARIAN MEDICINE.)

Fleas and Other Parasites

(See PARASITES.)

Single oils: Lemongrass, citronella, and peppermint.

Blends: Di-Tone Add 1 or 2 drops of lemongrass to pet shampoo. Oils repel fleas and other external parasites. Wash blankets with oils added to the wash water. Place 1-2 drops of lemongrass on collar to eliminate fleas.

For internal parasites, rub Di-Tone on the pads (bottom) of the feet. Many people have reported that they have seen the parasites eliminated from the animal.

Coughs, Colds, Flu, etc. (see COLDS)

Cuts, Scrapes, Wounds (see WOUNDS and BURNS)

CAUTION: When putting oils in pet ears, be careful to not drop onto the eardrum. Use a cotton swab.

Horses (To Calm)

Single oils: Add chamomile to feed.

Repel Flies from Horses and Other Animals

Single oils: Spray Idaho tansy floral water or Idaho tansy in water on animals to repel flies.

Skin Cancer (see CANCER)

Single oils: Frankincense, lavender, clove, and inula: Apply neat.

pH Balance

(See BODY pH ACID/ALKALINE BALANCE.)

Phlebitis - Thrombosis

(See CARDIOVASCULAR SYSTEM.)

Single oils: Idaho tansy followed with lavender: 5-10 drops each, layered 3 times directly towards the heart.

Supplements: Megazyme, Super Cal, and Seagal Power Meal.

Rehemogen: 3 droppers in water 3 times daily.

Pink Eye

(See EYES, CONJUNCTIVITIS.)

Diffuse: Purification, 3 Wise Men, or Immu-Power while sleeping.

Plaque

(See CARDIOVASCULAR SYSTEM.)

Pleurisy

Single oils: Ravensara, mountain savory, and thyme.

Blends: Raven, R.C., ImmuneTune, and Exodus II.

Supplements: Exodus, ImmuGel, Super C, Ultra Young, Mineral Essence, and Sulfurzyme.

Pneumonia - Emphysema - Pleurisy

Single oils:

- Frankincense with cypress, ravensara, sandalwood, eucalyptus (globulus and radiata), mountain savory, thyme, birch, or hyssop.

- Lavender with lemon, lemongrass, ginger, tarragon, peppermint, oregano, frankincense, thyme, clove, fennel, or spearmint.

- Melaleuca with fir, spruce, Idaho tansy, oregano, helichrysum, thyme, cinnamon, or cedarwood.

Use: Add 1-3 drops to the corresponding single oils above (according to your sensitivity).

Blends:

- R.C., Raven, Sacred Mountain, Inspiration, or Exodus II.

- Lavender with Melrose, ImmuPower, Di-Tone, or Thieves.

- Melaleuca with Melrose, Aroma Siez, Purification, R.C., Di-Tone, or Christmas Spirit.

Use: Add 1-3 drops of each single oil to the corresponding blends above (according to your sensitivity).

Application of oils:

- Massage on the Vita Flex points on the feet and hands.

- Apply 4 drops oregano and 4 drops thyme to Raindrop Therapy.

- Other oils and blends may be substituted for oregano and thyme (see RAINDROP THERAPY).

Diffuse Purification, ImmuPower, Melrose, R.C., or your other favorite blend to kill airborne germs and bacteria. Both Sacred Mountain and Inspiration are powerful antiseptics for the respiratory tract.

Mix R.C., frankincense, and lemon for congestion.

Peppermint removes mucous and reduces fever and throat infection.

Myrrh is very effective on throat troubles and phlegm.

Jasmine helps coughs, hoarseness, and laryngitis.

Myrtle is good for chronic coughs.

Hyssop for colds

Cedarwood for congestion and coughs.

For lung congestion:
- 2 drops sage
- 4 drops myrrh
- 5 drops clove
- 6 drops ravensara
- 15 drops frankincense

Mix in 1/2 oz. V-6 Mixing Oil or Massage Oil Base. Use in a rectal implant, hold as long as possible, and retain throughout the night.

For general relief of pneumonia, emphysema and pleurisy symptoms:
- 10 drops rosemary
- 8 drops ravensara
- 8 drops frankincense
- 2 drops oregano
- 2 drops peppermint

Mix oils and gargle 4 times daily.

Mix:
- 2 drops ravensara
- 1 drop thyme
- 3 drops frankincense
- 3 drops lemon
- 3 drops rosemary

Mix in 1/2 teaspoon honey. First week gargle 4 times daily, 2nd week 2 times daily, 3rd week 3 times daily, and 4th week 1 time daily. Stop for 1 month and repeat if necessary.

ImmuGel helps strengthen resistance to infection (do not mix with citrus juices). Royaldophilus is good for any viral condition and should be taken up to 4 times a day.

Exodus is proving to be a powerful body defense and immune builder that speeds the body's healing process. Exodus II is the companion product to Exodus.

Rosemary is good for colds, flu, and pneumonia. Anise and clove aid in strengthening the respiratory system. Clary sage relieves respiratory complaints. Fennel stimulates the respiratory system. Peppermint stimulates respiratory system, helps remove mucous, and reduces fever. Marjoram is calming to the respiratory system.

Chest Congestion:
- Ravensara
- Eucalyptus
- Frankincense
- Lemon

Congestion:
- ImmuPower
- Aroma Siez
- Exodus II

Apply on throat and chest to help release mucous.

Compress:
- Aroma Siez
- Birch
- Spruce

For long term chest congestion from welding, smoking, etc., use R.C. and myrtle in hot packs or compresses on chest and back and intense inhalation.

The antibacterial and antiviral oils, which are very powerful prophylactic agents for protection against colds, flu, etc., are basil, lavender, hyssop, frankincense, rosemary, bergamot, eucalyptus, melaleuca, clove, oregano, cistus, thyme, and mountain savory.

Bath for flu and colds:
- 2 oz. Evening Peace Bath Gel
- 2 drops eucalyptus
- 6 drops frankincense
- 3 drops helichrysum
- 6 drops spruce
- 15 drops ravensara
- 1 drop birch

Mix in bath and soak until cool.

Cough

Mix:
- 2 drops cypress
- 1 drop eucalyptus

Mix in 6 ounces of water, shake well and sip. Keep covered and shake before use.

Mix:
- 2 drops eucalyptus
- 2 drops lemon
- 2 Tbsp. honey.

Put 1 tsp. in glass of warm water and sip slowly.

Heavy, deep cough:
- 3 drops frankincense (known to alleviate coughs)
- 3 drops lemon
- 2 drops ravensara
- 1 drop thyme

Mix in 1/2 teaspoon honey and sip slowly.

Congestion and Coughing

- Raven or R.C. with 2 drops eucalyptus.

- Massage or apply hot compress over chest and back.

- Hold saturated wash cloth or towel over nose, on throat and neck glands.

- Diffuse.

- Mix in water and gargle.

Dry Cough

- 2 drops lemon
- 3 drops eucalyptus

Mix in 2 Tbsp. honey and dissolve 1 tsp. in 4 oz. of warm distilled water and sip slowly.

Sore Throat

Mix:
- 2 drops thyme
- 2 drops cypress
- 1 drop eucalyptus
- 1 drop peppermint
- 1 drop myrrh

Put in glass of water, mix well, and gargle as desired.

Mix:
- 2 drops eucalyptus
- 5 drops lemon
- 2 drops birch

Mix in 2 Tbsp. honey, dissolve in warm water, shake well, and gargle

Rub sage or Purification on throat area.

Strep Throat

Single oils: Oregano, thyme, frankincense, myrrh, and mountain savory.

Apply 1 to 2 drops on tongue.

Blends: Thieves, Exodus II.

Put 1 to 2 drops on tongue.

Supplements: ImmuneTune, Super C, Immu-Gel, and Royal Essence, Radex, Super C, Royal Essence, VitaGreen, Royaldophilus, Rehemogen, Colloidal Essence, Exodus, and Cleansing Trio.

- ImmuneTune: 2 to 4 capsules 3 times daily.

- Super C: 2 to 3 tablets 3 times daily.

- Radex: 2 to 4 tablets 3 times daily.

- Use Raindrop Therapy with ImmuPower and/or Exodus II on spine and back.

- Gargle every hour with Royal Essence.

Poisoning

(See CHEMICAL SENSITIVITY.)

Carbon Monoxide (Co) Poisoning

(See CHEMICAL SENSITIVITY.)

Blends:

- Myrtle with R.C., Inspiration, Sacred Mountain, Purification, Valor, or Harmony.

Use: Add 1-3 drops of each single oil to the corresponding blends above (according to your sensitivity).

Supplements: Master Formula HERS/HIS/CHILDREN'S, Royal Essence, VitaGreen, Super B, Super C, and Radex

Cleanse colon and liver with Cleansing Trio and JuvaTone.

Take a full compliment of vitamins and minerals daily as listed under supplements above.

Massage Valor on the bottom of feet.

Apply Purification through Raindrop Therapy on the spine and back.

Diffuse Purification, rub on the feet.

In an actual case of CO poisoning, one or more of the above was done every 3-4 hours.

After carbon monoxide poisoning, the electrical frequency tends to vary and go out of balance. Harmony may be used to bring the body back into balance. After a couple of days, one should start to feel better. If bronchial tubes become sensitive, alternate diffusing R.C. and Purification.

Inhaling R.C., Purification, Inspiration, and Sacred Mountain, and rubbing on the lung Vita Flex areas on bottom of the feet and on top of the feet at the base of the toes, helps the lungs open up and transfer more oxygen.

Polio – Effects on Tendons, Motor Nerves

Single oils:

- Lemon with ylang ylang, frankincense, birch, myrtle, cypress, myrrh, tarragon, or sage.

Use: Add 1-3 drops to the corresponding single oils above (according to your sensitivity).

Recipe:
- 2 drops lemon
- 10 drops ylang ylang
- 7 drops frankincense
- 10 drops birch
- 7 drops myrtle
- 8 drops cypress
- 15 drops myrrh
- 10 drops tarragon
- 6 drops sage

Mix in 1 ounce V-6 Mixing Oil or Massage Oil.

Pregnancy

(See chapter on PREGNANCY, BABIES, AND CHILDREN.)

Single oils:

- Jasmine with lavender, myrrh, or geranium.
- Helichrysum with fennel, peppermint, ylang ylang, or clary sage.

Use: Add 1-3 drops to the corresponding single oils above (according to your sensitivity).

Blends: Gentle Baby, Joy, Magnify Your Purpose, Envision, and Valor.

Rub Gentle Baby on lower stomach and lower back to help reduce cramping and discomfort and to improve elasticity of the skin reducing stretch marks. Lavender or myrrh will also help reduce stretch marks.

Use jasmine during childbirth for labor pains. Also rub Gentle Baby on perineum (tissue between vagina and rectum) to make it more elastic, preventing tearing or the need for an episiotomy (cutting the perineum) to allow enlargement of the vagina during birth. Geranium can also be used for this purpose.

To Use During Labor:
- 4 drops helichrysum
- 4 drops fennel
- 2 drops peppermint
- 5 drops ylang ylang
- 3 drops clary sage

Mix in 1 ounce of V-6 Mixing Oil or Massage Oil Base. Apply only after labor starts. Massage on reproductive Vita Flex areas on the ankles, which are the front of the ankle in line with the ankle bone and inside and outside of the foot just above the ankle bone and up along the achilles tendon and inside the little toes. Also rub on lower tummy and lower back.

Expectant fathers may also wear Gentle Baby to reduce anxiety while waiting for delivery.

After birth, diffuse Gentle Baby in home and nursery to soothe, relax, and comfort.

Constipation

This is a major problem for some women during pregnancy and a major cause of hemorrhoids and varicose veins. Cleanse colon and liver with Cleansing Trio. It might also be helpful to take ComforTone for maintenance of the colon and liver during pregnancy (see HEMORRHOIDS, VARICOSE VEINS).

Many babies are born with weak immune function. This comes in part from mothers having constipation and a toxic system that naturally backs up into the baby. A clean colon and liver will help alleviate this.

Lactation

Single oils: Fennel, geranium, lemongrass, and sage. Massage into breast.

Supplements: EssPro 7, VitaGreen, Seagal Power Meal, and Essential Manna.

Mix 20 drops fennel in 1 oz. V-6 Mixing Oil or Massage Oil Base and massage over breast and on Vita flex points of the feet. Geranium helps restore and increase milk.

CAUTION: Do not use fennel longer than 10 days at a time, as it will excessively increase flow through the urinary tract.

Mastitis (Caked Breast)

Single oils: Tangerine with lavender.

Blends: Citrus Fresh with lavender and Exodus II.

Supplements: ImmuGel and Exodus.

Mix:
- 10 drops tangerine
- 10 drops lavender

Mix in 1 ounce of V-6 Mixing Oil or Massage Oil. Rub on the breasts and under armpits twice per day.

Morning Sickness - Nausea

Single oils: Spearmint and peppermint.

Blends: Di-Tone

Supplements: Mint Condition and Megazyme.

Apply 1 drop of Di-Tone on the mastoid bone under and behind each ear and a couple of drops around the navel. Mint Condition has been helpful.

Psoriasis

(See SKIN CARE.)

Single oils: Roman chamomile, melaleuca, and patchouly.

Blends: Melrose

Supplements: Cleansing Trio, JuvaTone, Sulfur-zyme, and Rehemogen.

To sooth cracking skin, cover with Rose Ointment to keep soft.

Prostate, Enlargement, Decongestant

(See CANCER.)

Due to the research conducted by Jerilynn Prior, M.D., an endocrinologist at the university of British Columbia, it was discovered that ovarian, prostate, or reproductive cancer is directly related to petrochemicals ingested and stored in the reproductive organs. These petro-chemicals interfere with the follicle of the hormone, rendering them unable to function properly. This causes inflammation in the endocrine gland that leads to cancer.

Single oils: Cypress with helichrysum, frankincense, myrtle, peppermint, myrrh, sage, juniper, yarrow, or spruce.

Use: Add 1-3 drops to the corresponding single oils above (according to your sensitivity).

Blends:

- Cypress with Mister, Dragon Time, or EndoFlex.

Use: Add 1-3 drops of each single oil to the corresponding blends above (according to your sensitivity).

Supplements: ProGen, Master HIS, Royal Essence, EssPro 7, Protec, Dragon Time Bath and Shower Gel.

Mix 3 to 5 drops of oil in 1 tsp. V-6 Mixing Oil or Massage Oil Base. Apply as a rectal implant at bed time and retain all night.

Protec may be used as a rectal implant. Start with 2 Tbsp. for 7 consecutive days and 7 consecutive nights. Rest for 3 nights and then repeat until you have used it for 21 nights. Then rest 4 days. If irritation occurs, discontinue use for 3 days, before restarting.

Oils may be applied topically in the region between the rectum and the scrotum. Mister works well here.

You can also rub oils on reproductive Vita Flex areas.

Recipe:
- 10 drops frankincense
- 5 drops myrrh
- 3 drops sage

Mix in 1 Tbsp. V-6 Mixing Oil or Massage Oil Base.

Zinc helps reduce prostrate swelling. Royal Essence and Master HIS are good sources of zinc (and all minerals).

Adding natural progesterone to the body helps normalize levels of zinc, copper, and hormones, which in turn helps prostate problems. EssPro 7 is a good source of natural progesterone.

Peppermint acts as an anti-inflammatory to the prostate.

Prostate Cancer

(See CANCER, PROSTATE.)

Prostatitis, Inflammation of Prostate

Single oils:

- Rosemary with myrtle, clary sage, sage, mountain savory, fennel, bergamot, sandalwood, ylang ylang, geranium, yarrow, or peppermint.
- Thyme with rosemary, tarragon, lavender, eucalyptus, spruce, clove, or cinnamon.

Use: Add 1-3 drops to the corresponding single oils above (according to your sensitivity).

Blends:

- Aroma Siez with Mister or Dragon Time.
- Thyme with Melrose, Purification, R.C., or Di-Tone.

Use: Add 1-3 drops of each single oil to the corresponding blends above (according to your sensitivity).

Supplements: Colloidal Essence

Mix 3 or 5 drops of oil in 1 tsp. V-6 Mixing Oil in a rectal implant at bed time.

Oils may also be applied topically in the region between the rectum and the scrotum. Mister works well here.

You can also rub oils on reproductive Vita Flex areas on the feet.

Colloidal Essence has powerful antibacterial, antifungal, and antiviral properties. It may be taken internally or applied externally as required. Peppermint is anti-inflammatory to the prostate.

Psoriasis

(See SKIN CARE.)

Radiation Damage
(From cancer treatments, etc.)

Single oils: Melaleuca

Blends: Melrose

- Melaleuca or neroli with Melrose.

Use: Add 1-3 drops of each single oil to the corresponding blends above (according to your sensitivity).

Supplements: Radex, Super C, Seagal Power Meal, and Essential Manna.

For external damage mix Melrose with melaleuca. Apply neat or mix equal part with V-6 Mixing Oil and massage directly. Mix in 1 oz. V-6 Mixing Oil or Massage Oil Base; spread on location.

For colon or bowel damage take Radex daily.

Raynaud's Disease

Single oils: Helichrysum and cypress.

Blends: PanAway

Supplements: JuvaTone, ComforTone, Ultra Young, Brain Power, and PanAway.

Full body massage with helichrysum, cypress, or PanAway diluted with V-6 Mixing Oil or Massage Oil Base.

Restlessness
Restless Leg Syndrome

Single oils: Oregano, basil, marjoram, lavender, cypress, Roman chamomile, and peppermint.

Blends: Peace & Calming and Aroma Siez

Supplements: Mineral Essence, Thyromin, and VitaGreen.

Do Raindrop Therapy using the essential oils of oregano, basil, marjoram, lavender, cypress, and peppermint.

Rheumatic Fever

Single oils: Mountain savory, peppermint, thyme, and oregano in Raindrop Therapy application.

Blends: Thieves, Exodus II, and ImmuPower.

Supplements: Exodus, ImmuneTune, Super C, and Goji Berry Tea.

Rheumatism

Inflammation of joints may develop because of microbes and toxins, which react within the joint. Researchers have linked most degenerative diseases to lack of nutrients in the body. Minerals and trace minerals account for most of the nutritional deficiencies.

Single oils:

- Birch with spruce, fir, pine, cypress, peppermint, vetiver, mountain savory, marjoram, rosemary, basil, oregano, or vitex.

- Lavender with birch, cypress, peppermint, rosemary, marjoram, basil, ginger, pepper, or tarragon.

- Cypress with spruce, fir, pine, cedarwood, juniper, rosemary, peppermint, helichrysum, birch, basil, lemon, Idaho tansy, or nutmeg.

- Thyme with birch, basil, rosemary, cypress, melaleuca, spruce, peppermint, or oregano.

Use: Add 1-3 drops to the corresponding single oils above (according to your sensitivity).

Blends:

- Birch with Aroma Siez, PanAway, Relieve It, or Peace & Calming.

- Lavender or thyme with PanAway or Aroma Siez.

- Cypress with Aroma Life, PanAway, Purification, Melrose, Aroma Siez, or Sacred Mountain.

Use: Add 1-3 drops of each single oil to the corresponding blends above (according to your sensitivity).

Supplements and Skin Care: Ortho Ease, Relaxation, and Ortho Sport Massage oils, Super Cal, ArthroTune, Royal Essence, Mineral Essence EssPro 7, Rehemogen, Colloidal Essence, Goji Berry Tea, Exodus, and Sulfurzyme.

Detoxification of the body and particularly the joints is important, as is eradication of all of the infection.

Massage oils on location.

Cypress increases circulation.

Birch and Oregano work well together to reduce rheumatoid pain. For sharp rheumatic pain, use lavender with marjoram.

Vetiver is rubefacient (induces local warming).

PanAway and Relieve It, which relieve rheumatoid pain, have cortisone-like action without the cortisone side effects.

ArthroTune: take up to 3 times daily (Terry Friedmann, M.D.). This supplement increases circulation, helps alleviate arthritis, rheumatic conditions, and damage from old injuries, and reduces stiffness from sitting long periods, such as driving, sitting in front of computers, etc. Exodus provides the pantothenic acid complex needed by those who suffer from rheumatism.

Rehemogen cleans and fortifies the blood.

Rhinopharyngitis

Single oils: Eucalyptus radiata, thyme, and ravensara.

Blends: Raven, R.C., Thieves, and Exodus II.

Supplements: Exodus, ImmuGel, Dentarome, and Fresh Essence.

Ringworm

(See FUNGUS.)

Saint Vitus Dance (Chorea)

(See NEURITIS, SAINT VITUS DANCE.)

Scabies

Single oils: Citronella, lavandin, Roman chamomile, black pepper, and ginger.

Blends: Di-Tone, Purification, and Peace & Calming.

Supplements and Skin Care: ParaFree and Lavender Hair and Scalp Wash.

Scarring

Single oils: Helichrysum, lavender, frankincense, myrrh, and sandalwood.

Blends: 3 Wise Men and Inspiration.

Supplements: A. D. & E., Super C, Radex, Seagal Power Meal, and Essential Manna.

Sciatica

(See SPINE.)

Single oils: Pine and nutmeg.

Schizophrenia

Single oils: Cardamom, melissa, frankincense, rosemary, basil, and peppermint.

Blends: Brain Power, Clarity, and M-Grain.

Supplements: Mineral Essence and Ultra Young.

Sclera Derma

Single oils: Frankincense, Roman chamomile, lavender, patchouly, sandalwood, and myrrh

Blends: Melrose

Supplements: Cleansing Trio, JuvaTone, Thyromin, Mineral Essence, Seagal Power Meal, and Sulfurzyme.

For scar tissue in advanced stages: R.C. diffused and in a rectal implant with frankincense.

Topical application: Roman chamomile, lavender, and patchouly in equal portions over location with V-6 Mixing Oil to eliminate dryness. Alternate with equal portions of sandalwood and myrrh with V-6 Mixing Oil or Massage Oil Base.

Scoliosis

Single oils: Oregano, thyme, basil, birch, cypress, marjoram, and peppermint

Blends: Aroma Siez and PanAway.

Supplements: Mineral Essence, Super Cal, Essential Manna, Seagal Power Meal, Sulfurzyme, and Ortho Sport Massage Oil.

Scurvy

Single oils: Ginger, lemon, and orange.

Supplements: Super C and Power Meal.

Seizures

(See BRAIN FUNCTION.)

Single oils: Frankincense, sandalwood, melissa, and basil.

Blends: Valor, Aroma Siez, and Exodus II.

Supplements: Mineral Essence, A. D. & E., and Goji Berry Tea.

Remove all forms of sugar from diet.

Sexual Diseases

Genital Herpes

This is similar to cold sores and is caused by herpes simplex virus type 2, transmitted by sexual contact. Four to seven days after contact with an infected partner, tingling, burning, or persistent itching usually heralds an outbreak. One or two days later, small pimple-like bumps appear over reddened skin. The itching and tingling continue, and the pimples turn into painful blisters, which burst, bleeding with a yellowish pus. Five to seven days after the first tingling, scabs form, and healing begins.

Alternate Melrose, Hope, or Melissa (inject 10-15 drops with ear bulb syringe or saturated in a tampon). If burning sensation lasts longer than 3-5 minutes, dilute with V-6 Mixing Oil or Massage Oil Base.

Single oils:

- Lavender with peppermint, melaleuca, Idaho tansy, melissa, ravensara, bergamot, clary sage, or lemon.

Use: Add 1-3 drops to the corresponding single oils above (according to your sensitivity).

Blends:

- Lavender with Melrose, Thieves, Exodus II, ImmuPower, and Purification.

Use: Add 1-3 drops of each single oil to the corresponding blends above (according to your sensitivity).

As soon as a lesion is noticed or suspected, apply neat:
- 1 drop lavender
- 1 drop melaleuca or Melrose

CAUTION: Peppermint stings on an open sore, so wait until sore is closed, dilute in V-6 Mixing Oil, or mix 10-15 drops of lavender with 1 drop of peppermint.

Supplements: ImmuGel, Super C, Immune-Tune, Radex, Exodus, Royal Essence, VitaGreen, and ArthroTune.

If drying lesions cause discomfort, mix 10% of the essential oil in V-6 Mixing Oil or Massage Oil Base.

Recipe:
- 2 drops sage
- 2 drops neroli
- 4 drops ravensara
- 2 drops lavender

Mix in 1 oz. V-6 Mixing Oil or Massage Oil Base. Pat around outside of lesions. For body massage, use 10 drops frankincense in 1/2 oz. V-6 Mixing Oil or Massage Oil Base once a day.

Cleanse colon and liver with Cleansing Trio.

Single oils: Oregano, mountain savory, clove, and cinnamon. Black cumin seed oil has an 88% to 92% inhibitor effect against HIV (from the work of Dr. Farag of Cairo University, May 1994).

Blends: Thieves and Exodus II.

Supplements: Exodus, ImmuGel, Immune-Tune, ImmuPower, Sulfurzyme, Seagal Power Meal, Essential Manna, Super C, Super B, Vita-Green, Master Formula, and Mineral Essence.

Genital Warts

Single oils: Melissa, thyme, tansy, melaleuca, and lavender.

Blends: Melrose, Thieves, and ImmuneTune.

Supplements: A. D. & E., ImmuGel, Cleansing Trio, and JuvaTone.

Gonorrhea and Syphilis

Single oils: Oregano, melissa, thyme, mountain savory, and cinnamon.

Blends: Thieves and Exodus II.

Supplements: Exodus, ImmuGel, Mineral Essence, and Radex.

Sexual Frigidity

Single oils: Geranium, ylang ylang, jasmine, clary sage, nutmeg, and rose.

Blends: Joy, Passion, Sensation, Mister, and Dragon Time.

Supplements: Ultra Young, EssPro 7, Sensation Moisture Cream, VitaGreen, FemiGen, ProGen, and Sulfurzyme.

Ylang Ylang helps balance sexual emotion and sex drive problems. Its aromatic influence elevates sexual energy and enhances relationships.

Clary sage helps with frigidity, regulates and balances hormones.

Nutmeg supports the nervous system to overcome frigidity.

Sulfurzyme provides MSM (sulfur), which can help the libido.

Sexual Suppression

Marjoram reduces and suppresses sexual appetite.

Sexual Stimulation

Single oils: Cinnamon, myrrh, black pepper, pine, ylang ylang, ginger, nutmeg, and rose.

Blends: Sensation and Passion.

Supplements: FemiGen, ProGen, Ultra Young, and Sensation Massage Oil.

CAUTION: When diffusing cinnamon, be aware that it can irritate nasal passages. Always dilute cinnamon in V-6 Mixing Oil or Massage Oil Base or blend with 20 parts or more of lavender to 1 part cinnamon.

Shingles (Herpes Zoster)

An active (generally short-lived) viral infection of the central nervous system that affects certain areas of the skin. This usually starts with fatigue, fever, chills, and at times intestinal upset. On the third to fourth day, skin area becomes excessively sensitive. On the fourth or fifth day, small blisters, which crust over and are painful, erupt along the nerve pathway. Normally these heal in about 5 days without further problems. One attack usually gives immunity for life. However, with some, particularly the elderly, pain can persist for months, even years.

The virus that causes shingles is varicella zoster, which also causes chicken pox. A childhood bout with chicken pox leaves some viruses dormant in sensory (skin) nerves. If the immune system is compromised from things such as severe emotional stress, severe illness, or long term use of corticosteroids, the dormant viruses may start to infect the pathway of the skin nerves.

CAUTION: Occurrences of shingles around the eyes or on the forehead can cause blindness. Consult an ophthalmologist (eye doctor) immediately if such outbreaks occur.

Single oils: Elemi, tansy, clove, oregano, mountain savory, thyme juniper, geranium, and peppermint.

- Ravensara with *Calophyllum inophyllum* (an oil related to St. John's wort).

- Melaleuca with lemon, geranium, bergamot, eucalyptus, lavender, peppermint, or chamomile.

Use: Add 1-3 drops to the corresponding single oils above (according to your sensitivity).

Blends:

Supplements: ArthroTune, Super Cal, Colloidal Essence, and EssPro 7.

Equal amounts Ravensara and *Calophyllum inophyllum L.* applied to a shingles outbreak has produced dramatic improvement and complete remission within 7 days (from *Alternative Medicine, The Definitive Guide,* pages 56 and 971). Peppermint helps calm nerves.

Raindrop Therapy (layer in order): Oregano, mountain savory, and thyme (warm pack for 30 minutes between each oil application). Be sure to place a towel between the skin and hot pack. Continue with juniper, geranium, and peppermint with an ice pack for 30 minutes between each oil application.

On location:
- 5 drops elemi
- 5 drops tansy
- 2 drops clove

CAUTION: Peppermint stings on open sores or sensitive skin. Apply diluted with Lavender, V-6 Mixing Oil, or Massage Base Oil along the nerve pathway ahead of the lesion.

Recipe:
- 10 drops chamomile
- 5 drops lavender
- 4 drops bergamot
- 2 drops geranium

Mix in 1 oz. V-6 Mixing Oil or Massage Oil Base. Apply on location and also apply a cold or body temperature compress.

Colloidal Essence is powerful in fighting bacteria, fungus, and virus. It may be taken internally or applied externally as required.

Shock - Refresh & Revitalize

If a wound is large or if it occurs from an accident or traumatic event, the person may be in shock. Inhale oils to reduce shock.

Single oils:

- Melaleuca with frankincense, lavender, sandalwood, or rosemary.

- Helichrysum with basil or peppermint.

Use: Add 1-3 drops to the corresponding single oils above (according to your sensitivity).

Blends:

- Melaleuca with Trauma Life, Clarity, 3 Wise Men, Valor, Harmony, or Present Time.

- Helichrysum with Clarity.

Use: Add 1-3 drops of each single oil to the corresponding blends above (according to your sensitivity).

Helichrysum lessens the effects of shock.

If a person has passed out from shock due to an accident or traumatic event, such as emotional shock, Clarity and Valor will help return them to consciousness.

3 Wise Men is very good for emotional shock.

Sinusitis

Single oils:

- Melaleuca and helichrysum with ravensara, lemongrass, myrtle, spruce, frankincense, cedarwood, hyssop, or pine.

- Ravensara with eucalyptus (globulus or radiata), rosemary, peppermint, frankincense, lemon, clove, fir, birch, or cypress.

Use: Add 1-3 drops to the corresponding single oils above (according to your sensitivity).

Blends:

- Helichrysum with R.C., Raven, or Thieves, ImmuPower, and Purification.

Use: Add 1-3 drops of each single oil to the corresponding blends above (according to your sensitivity).

Mix:
- 3 drops melaleuca ericifolia
- 3 drops R.C.

Use cotton swab to apply and keep away from eye.

Mix:
- 10 drops peppermint
- 5 drops eucalyptus radiata
- 2-3 drops melaleuca

Put in a capsule and take internally.

Swab nasal cavity with Purification.

Ravensara with eucalyptus, frankincense, and lemon helps with congestion.

Ravensara strengthens the respiratory system, dilates and opens the pulmonary tract, and fights respiratory infection.

Inhaling spruce or peppermint helps open the sinuses.

Rub myrtle over the nose and sinus cavities and inhale.

Recipe:

- 1 drop lemon

- 2 drops eucalyptus

- 3 drops rosemary

- 2 drops peppermint

Mix in 1 tsp. V-6 Mixing Oil or Massage Oil Base. Massage on sinuses (forehead, nose, under cheekbones) and on chest and upper back.

Skin Disorders

Our skin is our armor and the largest absorbent organ of the body. Protecting its environment is most important. Many chemical molecules are too large to absorb and lay on the surface of the skin, causing irritation, resulting in rashes, itching, blemishes, flaky and dry skin, dandruff, and allergies. Essential oils are soluble with the lipids in the skin and are easily absorbed. They are absorbed into the blood stream and are able to carry nutrients and oxygen through the cell wall into the cell nucleus to feed the cells.

All skin conditions, such as blemishes, brown spots, eruptions, acne, pimples, pigmentation, moles, and warts, are related to the liver. One must therefore work at cleansing, stimulating, and conditioning the liver. Indigestion causes gas and toxins in the intestines and the liver. Gas and toxins in the liver produce insomnia, frequent recurring migraine headaches, skin eruptions, discoloration, change in pigmentation, acne, and bumpy skin (like turkey skin).

A colon and liver cleanse should be done for 30 to 90 days before the skin begins to improve.

Helichrysum improves skin conditions, such as chronic dermatitis, eczema, and psoriasis.

Jasmine has anti-inflammatory properties for skin conditions, such as dry, greasy, irritated, sensitive skin, and skin candida.

Therapeutic qualities of specific oils and oil blends:

- Lavender is very helpful on rashes, diaper rash, acne, psoriasis, and many other skin problems. Lavender, spikenard, and myrrh are excellent for chapped and cracked skin, wrinkles, and stretch marks.

- Myrrh soothes and helps with eczema, chapped and cracked skin, wrinkles, and stretch marks.

- Sage firms and helps skin conditions.

- Tarragon is cooling and soothing to skin.

- Roman chamomile is very mild and non-toxic. It is an excellent pain reliever and skin remedy for scratches, bruises, wounds, and chapped and dry skin.

- Spikenard is regenerating, balancing, and may soothe allergic reactions.

- Rosewood is soothing, healing, and rejuvenating to skin and restores skin elasticity

- Ylang ylang with lavender is excellent for the skin.

- Geranium is an excellent tissue regenerator and has been used for centuries for skin care.

- Helichrysum regenerates tissue.

- Jasmine, lavender, and mandarin help restore skin elasticity.

- Gentle Baby contains oils that regenerate skin and help prevent and retard wrinkles. It makes a wonderful aftershave, particularly for chapped or rough skin.

- Sensation leaves skin silky and youthful.

- Sensation Moisturizer and Lotion are very beneficial for skin problems.

- Colloidal Essence is a powerful bacterial, fungal, and viral fighter.

- Stevia extract heals blemishes of various types. Apply a couple of drops directly on the spot. For more serious cases, apply as a facial mask by spreading over the face, and let dry for 30 to 60 minutes. As it dries, the skin will feel tighter and tighter. Rinse off with water by patting skin with wet face cloth.

Acne

Blocked hair follicles allow bacteria to multiply, causing inflammation that may become puss-filled black heads. The blockage may be from over-production of sebum (an oily substance that lubricates the skin), from sebaceous glands in the hair follicles, or from excessive greasy makeup. This is more pronounced in adolescents because of the increase that stimulates the production of sebum in the sebaceous glands. According to research conducted by Dr. Asawa in Japan, acne and other skin problems are a direct result of the physical and spiritual body being out of balance.

Single oils: Blue tansy, Roman chamomile, geranium, rosewood, cedarwood, juniper, palmarosa, lemongrass, sage, clove, jasmine, eucalyptus radiata, patchouly, and vetiver.

- Frankincense with melaleuca.

- Melaleuca with lemon, lemongrass, thyme, basil, rosemary lavender, eucalyptus, geranium, neroli, and spikenard.

- Lavender with Roman chamomile (both extremely beneficial to skin), geranium, rosewood, cypress, palmarosa, myrrh, patchouly, melaleuca, mountain savory, rose, rosemary, sandalwood, cedarwood, sage, tarragon, or ylang ylang.

- Helichrysum or thyme with rosewood, patchouly, geranium, lavender, juniper, mountain savory, jasmine, carrot seed, myrrh, peppermint, Roman chamomile, and Blue tansy.

Use: Add 1-3 drops to the corresponding single oils above (according to your sensitivity).

Blends:

- Lavender with Purification, Sensation, Melrose, or Gentle Baby.
- Lemongrass with Purification, Melrose, or Gentle Baby.
- Helichrysum with Gentle Baby.
- Thyme with JuvaFlex, Gentle Baby, or Forgiveness.
- Frankincense with JuvaFlex or EndoFlex.

Use: Add 1-3 drops of each single oil to the corresponding blends above (according to your sensitivity).

Supplements: Master Formula HIS/HERS or CHILDREN'S, Seagal Power Meal, Mineral Essence, Exodus, Stevia, Rehemogen, Colloidal Essence, EssPro 7, and VitaGreen.

Skin care products: Rose Ointment, Mint Facial Scrub, Orange Blossom Facial Wash, Sandalwood or Sensation Moisturizing cream, Morning Start Bath and Shower Gel, Rawhide and Pharaoh Aftershaves, Dragon Time Bath and Shower Gel, Evening Peace Bath and Shower Gel, and Lavender hair and scalp wash.

Application:1 drop on location. Inhale on a daily basis to help balance the skin.

Cleansing the skin: Aroma Silk Sandalwood Toner, Purification, geranium, lemon, orange are excellent astringents.

Lemongrass reportedly clears acne and balances oily skin conditions. Lemongrass is the predominate ingredient in Morning Start Bath and Shower Gel, which can be used to balance the pH of the skin, decongest the lymphatics and stimulate circulation.

Dry skin: Chamomile, neroli, rose, palmarosa, sandalwood.

Oily skin: Cedarwood, cypress, geranium, lavender, lemon.

Puffy and greasy skin: lavender, lemon.

Sensitive skin: Chamomile, jasmine, neroli, rose.

Chapped or Cracked Hands

Single oils:

- Rosewood with patchouly, geranium, Roman chamomile, rose, sandalwood, or helichrysum.

Use: Add 1-3 drops to the corresponding single oils above (according to your sensitivity).

Skin Care Products: Sandalwood Moisterizer Cream, AromaSilk Satin Body Lotion, and Rose Ointment.

Body lotions with essential oils are very effective on chapped hands and aid in maintaining the natural pH balance of the skin. These lotions work to oxygenate, hydrate, and protect the skin.

Recipe:
- 1 drop rosewood
- 1 drop patchouly
- 1 drop geranium

Alternate oils of rose, chamomile, or sandalwood to body lotion.

Bath and shower gels, such as Dragon Time, Evening Peace, Morning Start, and Sensation, are formulated to help balance the acid mantel of the skin.

Orange Blossom Facial Wash:

Mint Scrub contains oat bran and corn flower, which are mild abrasives to help remove dirt, black heads, old pimple cores, and stimulate cell regeneration. If the texture is too abrasive, mix half and half with Orange Blossom Facial Wash. This is excellent for teenage skin, providing soothing relief to those with acne or just a little problem.

Spread over face and let dry for perhaps 5 minutes to draw out impurities, pulling and toning the skin at the same time. Put a hot towel over face for greater penetration. Wash off with warm water by gently patting skin with warm face cloth. If you do not have time to let mask dry, then just gently massage in a circular motion for 30 seconds.

Afterwards, apply Sandalwood Moisture Cream or AromaSilk Satin Body Lotion. This also works well underneath foundation makeup.

Men may apply Rawhide or Pharaoh Aftershaves.

Rawhide Aftershave may also remove cell melanoma.

To Tighten Skin and pull excess fluids out of tissue:

Single oils: Grapefruit, lavender, helichrysum, patchouly, and cypress.

Personal Care Products: Cel-Lite Magic and Massage Oil

Morning:
- 10 drops tangerine
- 10 drops cypress

Mix with 1/2 oz. V-6 Mixing Oil or Massage Oil Base and begin massaging feet and then legs.

Night:
- 8 drops geranium
- 5 drops cypress
- 5 drops helichrysum
- 1 drop peppermint

Mix with 1/2 oz. V-6 Mixing Oil or Massage Oil Base and massage beginning at the feet and legs. Seal with Cel-Lite Magic Massage Oil.

Freckles

Single oils: Idaho tansy: Apply 2-4 drops and spread over face. Mix with lotion if it is too drying or stings. Use 2-3 times a week.

Fungus

Single oils: Oregano: 1-2 drops 3-4 times daily.

Blends: Melrose: 1-2 drops 3-4 times daily.

Itching

This may be a result of a toxic or congested liver. It may be necessary to go into cleansing program for liver, blood, and bowels.

Single oils:

- 3 drops rosemary with 6 drops lavender

- 10 drops patchouly with 4 drops lavender, 2 drops blue chamomile, and 5 drops lemon, 2-4 drops each use.

- Melrose 2-4 drops with lotion

Mix with 1/2 to 1 ounce of V-6 Mixing Oil or Massage Oil Base.

Supplements: Sandalwood Moisturizer Cream and Rose Ointment.

Melanoma (see CANCER)

Frankincense neat, 1 to 2 drops on location, 2 or 3 times a day. To be sure to catch any impending melanoma, apply frankincense to any odd lumps, rough moles, or red rough lesions that develop on the skin. Idaho Tansy has been reported to help reduce odd lumps and growths on the skin and to help liver spots to fade.

Moles (Rough Scabby Kind)

Single oils: Frankincense, geranium, birch, lavender, and oregano.

Blends: Melrose

Skin care products: EssPro 7 and Rose Ointment.

Oregano has helped to heal and reduced pain and itching. Apply one or two drops neat (undiluted) directly on the mole, one or two times a day until it falls off.

EssPro 7, applied to moles and skin bumps, has been reported to help the process of ridding them from the body.

Poison Oak - Poison Ivy

Single oils:

- Frankincense, melaleuca with lemon, lemongrass, thyme, basil, rosemary, lavender, eucalyptus, geranium, and orange.

- Lavender with German chamomile, Roman chamomile (both are extremely beneficial to skin), geranium, Idaho tansy, fennel, rosewood, lemongrass, patchouly, rosewood and myrtle.

- Frankincense with melaleuca, lemongrass, or vetiver

Use: Add 1-3 drops to the corresponding single oils above (according to your sensitivity).

Blends:

- Melaleuca with Thieves.

- Lavender or lemongrass with Purification, Sensation, Melrose, Gentle Baby, or Raven.

- Frankincense with Release, JuvaFlex, Endo-Flex, or Purification.

Use: One drop, neat, on location.

Supplements: Master Formula HIS/HERS/CHILDREN'S and Stevia.

Skin Care Products: Rose Ointment, Stevia, AromaSilk Satin Body Lotion, Morning Start Bath and Shower Gel.

Lemongrass reportedly clears acne and balances oily skin and scalp condition, and is the predominate ingredient in the Morning Start Bath and Shower Gel. It balances the pH of the skin, decongests the lymphatics, and stimulates circulation. Some people use Morning Start as a shampoo because they have excessively oily hair.

Psoriasis

Psoriasis, eczema, dermatitis, dry skin, allergies, and similar problems indicate an excessive acid pH of the body. The more acid in the blood and skin, the less effect the oils will have. People who have a strong reaction to oils are usually highly acidic. We must maintain an alkaline balance in our blood and skin for the oils to work the best. AlkaLime and VitaGreen are both helpful for this balancing. (See pH OF BLOOD.)

Blends:

- 2 drops patchouly
- 2 drops Roman chamomile
- 2 drops lavender
- 2 drops Melrose

Add to Rose Ointment or body lotion and gently spread over affected area.

Skin Grafting

Single oils: Melaleuca, patchouly, lavender, helichrysum, frankincense.

Blends: Melrose and Rose Ointment.

Melrose and Rose Ointment regenerate tissue without scarring.

Cleanse wounds and maintain freshness.

Skin Care Products

- LavaDerm Cooling Mist, lavender with Sunsation Suntan Oil, or with AromaSilk Satin Body Lotion. Use Rose Ointment to keep tissue soft after it has scabbed over.

Application: Spray immediately with LavaDerm Cooling Mist and continue misting when necessary to cool the burn. Spray 4-5 times every hour. After misting apply 2-3 drops of lavender over burn area.

For third degree burn, spray every 10 minutes for the first 24 hours until the tissue appears to be well rehydrated. Apply a few drops of lavender oil after misting after the first 10 minutes. Spray with or without other oils, neat, by direct application 2 or more times per day for 3 or 4 days. To re-hydrate and heal the skin, apply extra lavender or apply by layering lavender first and then cover with Rose Ointment or body lotion.

Skin Tags

Single oils: Oregano

Blends: Thieves and Purification.

Apply oils neat on location, two or three times a day.

Stretch Marks

Single oils: Lavender, frankincense, spikenard, geranium, and myrrh.

Blends: Gentle Baby

Supplements: A. D. & E. and Sulfurzyme.

Sun Filter

Single oils:

- Helichrysum with lavender or peppermint.

Use: Add 1-3 drops to the corresponding single oils above (according to your sensitivity).

Supplements: A. D. & E.

- Helichrysum with Sunsation Suntan Oil.

Use: Add 1-3 drops of each single oil to the corresponding blends above (according to your sensitivity).

Helichrysum is a good sun filter and may be added to Sunsation Suntan Oil to increase the filtering protection. The ingredients in Sunsation Suntan Oil help filter out ultraviolet rays without blocking the absorption of Vitamin D, which is important in skin and bone development. The essential oils accelerate tanning, and lemongrass and citronella make a natural insect repellent.

CAUTION: Sunsation Suntan Oil will not prevent sunburn by itself. However, it works as a sun filter and promotes tanning: 15-20 minutes the first day, a little longer the next day, etc., with ample Sunsation Suntan Oil.

Sunburn

Single oils:

- Lavender, helichrysum, peppermint with LavaDerm Cooling Mist.

Use: Add 1-3 drops to the corresponding single oils above (according to your sensitivity).

Test 1 drop of peppermint oil mixed with AromaSilk Body Lotion, V-6 Mixing Oil, or Massage Oil Base. Peppermint is cooling and soothing to tissue and reduces inflammation (fever) in damaged tissue.

Blends:

- Lavender with Gentle Baby or Melrose.

Use: Add 1-3 drops of each single oil to the corresponding blends above (according to your sensitivity).

Ulcers, Skin

Single oils: Bergamot, clove, helichrysum, Roman chamomile, patchouly, myrrh, and lavender.

Blends: Melrose, Relieve It, 3 Wise Men, and Gentle Baby.

Supplements and Skin Care: Super C, Radex, Exodus, Cleansing Trio, AromaSilk Satin Body Lotion, and Boswellia Wrrinkle Cream.

Ulcers, Leg

Single oils: Lavender with both Roman and German chamomile, geranium, rosewood, or patchouly.

Use: Add 1-3 drops to the corresponding single oils above (according to your sensitivity).

Blends:

- Lavender with Purification, Sensation, Thieves, or Gentle Baby.

Use: Add 1-3 drops of each single oil to the corresponding blends above (according to your sensitivity).

Supplements and Skin Care: Super C, Radex, Exodus, Cleansing Trio, AromaSilk Satin Body Lotion, and Boswellia Wrrinkle Cream.

Wrinkles - Rough Skin -Aging

Single oils:

- Frankincense with helichrysum, cypress, rose, lavender, ylang ylang, patchouly, sage, geranium, lemon, lemongrass, clary sage, rosewood, sandalwood, jasmine, neroli, palmarosa, spikenard, and mandarin.

Use: Add 1-3 drops to the corresponding single oils above (according to your sensitivity).

Blends:

- Frankincense with Gentle Baby; or lavender with Sensation.

Use: Add 1-3 drops of each single oil to the corresponding blends above (according to your sensitivity).

Supplements: Ultra Young, Master HIS/HERS/ CHILDREN'S, Thyromin, Stevia, and Exodus.

Skin Care Products: EssPro 7, AromaSilk Satin Body Lotion, Rose Ointment, Pharaoh and Rawhide Aftershaves, Mint Scrub, and Sandalwood Moisture Cream.

AromaSilk Satin Body Lotion is very effective on chapped hands and rough skin. It softens and protects skin from harsh weather, work chemicals, household cleaners, etc.

For soft skin and to smooth out wrinkles:
- 5 drops sandalwood
- 5 drops helichrysum
- 5 drops geranium
- 5 drops lavender
- 5 drops frankincense

Mix with lotion and apply to skin.

Sandalwood or Sensation Moisturizer Cream is excellent for dry or prematurely aging skin. Rose Ointment was developed to feed and rehydrate the skin and to supply nutrients necessary to slow down the aging process. This lotion leaves the skin velvety smooth and feeling brand new, with no chemicals to cause irritation. EssPro 7 cream is great in reducing wrinkles and for hydrating the skin. Rub around eyes, on neck, and wherever needed.

To reduce wrinkles, add 10 drops of frankincense to the Pharaoh Aftershave and use on face. You can also use a topical application of frankincense with helichrysum, possibly in V-6 Mixing Oil or Massage Oil Base for premature aging of the skin and for the reduction of maturing lines. Patchouly helps reduce wrinkles, particularly around the eyes. It is best to mix with V-6 Mixing Oil or Massage Oil Base.

Recipe:
• 6 drops rosewood
• 4 drops geranium
• 3 drops lavender
• 2 drops frankincense

Mix in 1 oz. V-6 Mixing Oil or Massage Oil Base.

Thyromin capsules have been reported to help reduce wrinkles and alleviate dry skin. This supplement strengthens the thyroid, which is an important gland in so many body functions that affect the skin.

Sleep Disorders

Single oils: Lavender, valerian, marjoram, Roman chamomile, and orange.

Blends: Peace & Calming, Surrender, Inspiration, Hope, and Humility.

Supplements: AuraLight, Megazyme, and Mineral Essence.

Sores

Single oils: Roman chamomile, lavender, patchouly, and vetiver.

Blends: Melrose, Gentle Baby, Valor, and Harmony.

Supplements: Super C and Ultra Young.

Sore Throat

(See COLDS.)

Spina Bifida

Single oils: Mountain savory, helichrysum, thyme, and melaleuca.

Blends: Melrose, Thieves, and Exodus II.

Supplements: ImmuGel, Super C, and Radex.

Sprain

Single oils: Lemon, birch, basil, pine, spruce, cypress, and peppermint.

Blends: PanAway or Relieve It with lemongrass.

Supplements: Ortho Sport Massage Oil, Sulfurzyme, and Mineral Essence.

Stress

Single oils: Lavender, chamomile, Blue Tansy, marjoram, rose, sandalwood, frankincense, and cedarwood.

Blends: Humility, Harmony, Valor, and Joy .

Supplements: Super B, Ultra Young, Super C, Radex, VitaGreen, and Master Formula.

Smoking (Quitting)

Single oils: Cinnamon, clove, nutmeg.

Blends: Harmony, Peace & Calming, Thieves, Exodus II.

Supplements: Cleansing Trio, Rehemogen, JuvaTone, and Stevia.

Application of Harmony: Put 1 drop on each foot; have another person cross his/her arms and pull slightly on the heels for 2-3 minutes or until it "feels right". Anoint the crown of the head with 1 drop. Rub 1 drop over the heart. Rub 1 drop around the navel.

Alternate with Peace & Calming.

Cleanse colon and liver cleanse with Cleansing Trio and JuvaTone.

353

The liver cleanse detoxifies the liver and helps to remove the cravings for nicotine, caffeine, sugar, chocolate, etc. It may be necessary to take 3 tablets of JuvaTone up to 3 times daily.

Rehemogen cleans and detoxifies the blood and works synergistically with JuvaTone, rebuilding the liver and erasing the addiction blueprint in the liver (see ADDICTIONS).

Stevia has been reported to decrease cravings for tobacco and alcohol.

Snake Bikes

(See BITES.)

Sore Feet

Single oils: Peppermint, lavender, patchouly, myrrh, frankincense, sandalwood, and vetiver.

Blends: Melrose, PanAway, and Relieve It.

Supplements: A. D. & E., Essential Manna (potassium is extremely important), Super Cal, Master Formula, and Mineral Essence.

Mix peppermint in footbath; keep water agitated while soaking feet.

Spine (Straightening), Injuries, Problems

Single oils: Birch, spruce, peppermint, marjoram, and basil.

Blends: Valor, Aroma Siez, Thieves, Immu-Power, and PanAway.

Supplements: Super C, Mineral Essence, Royal Essence, and ArthroTune.

To effect a back (spinal) adjustment: Have the person lie flat on his/her back. Rub Valor (3 to 6 drops) on shoulders and on spinal Vita Flex points on feet. Some people have added Immu-Power, reporting good results. If available, have a second person hold his/her hands on the shoulders of the person being treated. Cross your hands and hold the patient's right foot with your right hand and the left foot with your left hand. Place hands so that palm covers as much of the bottom center and ball of the feet as possible. Hold and gently pull the feet, until the patient says that it "feels right". This may take 3-5 minutes or up to 10 minutes.

Sometimes you can even feel the movement, but this is not necessary for success. Always check the heels for alignment. To relax the spine and let it adjust itself, first use Valor on feet as noted above. Then apply birch, spruce, marjoram, or Aroma Siez and stimulate with a pointer as explained under Nerve Damage. After stimulating, spread Ortho Ease Massage Oil over the entire back. Follow with a warm towel being placed over the whole back and then covering with another dry towel to keep the heat in.

Chiropractors have found that by applying Valor on the bottom of the feet, spinal manipulations take 60% less time and work, and the results last 75% longer.

Aching Back

Single oils: Clary Sage with lavender and chamomile, basil, peppermint, geranium, or elemi.

Use: Add 1-3 drops of each single oils above (according to your sensitivity).

Blend:

- 5 drops clary sage
- 5 drops lavender
- 5 drops chamomile

Mix in 1 oz. V-6 Mixing Oil or Massage Oil Base (see MUSCLES, SORE, SPASMED, OR PULLED).

Calcification of Spine

Single oils: Geranium with rosemary, eucalyptus radiata, ravensara, oregano, vetiver, or elemi.

Use: Add 1-3 drops of R.C.

Use: Add 1-3 drops of each single oils above (according to your sensitivity).

Supplements: ArthroTune, Sulfurzyme, Super Cal, and Ortho Ease Massage Oil.

Apply oils directly on the spine and on the spinal Vita Flex areas on bottom of the feet by massage and Raindrop Therapy.

Chronic Lower Back Pain

This can be digestion related and the result of a congested colon or a damaged or pinched nerve (neuralgia).

Cleanse colon and liver.

Single oils: For neuralgia: Marjoram, nutmeg, basil, Roman chamomile, elemi, and peppermint.

Blends: For digestion: Di-Tone.

Rub Di-Tone on colon, stomach, and small intestine Vita Flex areas on the feet. Also apply around the navel. In severe cases use compresses or hot packs.

Herniated Disk and Deterioration

For this situation, it is best to consult a specialist. It is not likely that this situation may be helped with oils although with continued use, there would mostly likely be some relief.

For temporary relief until medical attention can be given:

Single oils: Helichrysum, pine, basil, thyme, melissa (Use with cold compress).

Blends: Relieve It, PanAway, Aroma Siez.

- Basil with Aroma Siez, or Spruce with Relieve It.

Use: Add 1-3 drops of each single oil to the corresponding blends above (according to your sensitivity).

Supplements: Sulfurzyme, ArthroTune, Super Cal, Ortho Sport and Ortho Ease Massage Oils.

Apply oils to back with Raindrop Therapy, then apply basil along the sides of the spine. Stimulate with the "pointer technique" as described under Nerve Damage. This has been very effective for disk problems.

Lumbago - Backache in Small of Back

Single oils:

- Lavender with spruce, fir, birch, helichrysum, basil, peppermint, cypress, or sandalwood.

Use: Add 1-3 drops to the corresponding single oils above (according to your sensitivity).

Blends:

- Lavender with Relieve It or PanAway.

Use: Add 1-3 drops of each single oil to the corresponding blends above (according to your sensitivity).

Supplements: ArthroTune, Sulfurzyme, Ortho Sport and Ortho Ease Massage Oils, Super C, and Super Cal.

Nerve Damage and Fever

If there is nerve damage and fever, apply about 6 drops of peppermint starting at the hips and finishing at the neck. Do Raindrop Therapy. Starting at the bottom of the spine, use a small-nosed pointer (about the size of a pencil but with a round end). Stimulate each vertebra between each rib on the vertebra knuckles all the way up on each side of the spine. Use medium pressure and a rocking motion for 1-10 seconds at each location. Then follow the same procedure once more up the center of the spine directly on each vertebra.

The above "pointer technique" may also be used on the Vita Flex points and areas on the feet.

Neck Pain and Stiffness

Single oils:

- Basil with marjoram and lavender or helichrysum with birch, nutmeg, pine, spruce, elemi, cypress, basil, or peppermint.

Use: Add 1-3 drops of each single oils above (according to your sensitivity).

Recipe 1:
- 5 drops basil
- 5 drops marjoram
- 3 drops lavender

Mix in 1/2 to 1 oz. V-6 Mixing Oil or Massage Oil Base.

Recipe 2:
- 2 drops helichrysum
- 10 drops birch
- 8 drops cypress
- 15 drops basil
- 4 drops peppermint

Mix in 1 oz. V-6 Mixing Oil or Massage Oil Base.

Sciatica

Characterized by pain in the buttocks and down the back of the thigh. The pain worsens when coughing and sneezing or bending the back. The pain is caused by pressure on the sciatic nerve as it leaves the spine in the lower pelvic region. This nerve is the largest in the body, with branches throughout the lower body and legs.

Single oils:

- Thyme with birch, basil, rosemary, cypress, spruce, peppermint, sandalwood, or oregano.

- Helichrysum with birch, clove, peppermint, or tarragon.

- Hyssop with birch, Roman chamomile, or Idaho tansy.

Use: Add 1-3 drops to the corresponding single oils above (according to your sensitivity).

Blends:

- Thyme with Aroma Siez or PanAway.

- Helichrysum with PanAway or Aroma Siez.

Use: Add 1-3 drops of each single oil to the corresponding blends above (according to your sensitivity).

Supplements: Ortho Ease or Ortho Sport Massage Oils, ArthroTune, Sulfurzyme, and Super B.

Hyssop with birch or Roman chamomile is very powerful.

Birch with oregano is very powerful for bruised and damaged sciatica.

Use 2 drops of oil in left palm; circulate clockwise with right hand thumb. Rub on low end of spine and on sciatica Vita Flex points on feet. Always do both feet.

Sulfurzyme and Super B work well together to help rebuild nerve damage and the myelin sheath.

Sports Aches & Pains

(See specific indication.)

Single oils: Rosemary, nutmeg, black pepper, basil, spruce, and fir.

Blends: Valor, Peace & Calming, En-R-Gee, Passion, and Clarity.

Supplements: Royal Essence, VitaGreen, Ultra Young, Be-Fit, and Seagal Power Meal.

Apply Valor on bottom of feet, Peace & Calming on back of neck, and Clarity on crown of head.

Single oils: Juniper, birch, lemon, rosemary, and lavender.

Recipe:
- 4 drops juniper
- 5 drops birch
- 4 drops lemon
- 2 drops rosemary
- 5 drops lavender

Mix in 1 oz. V-6 Mixing Oil or Massage Oil Base.

Sprains

(See CONNECTIVE TISSUE and MUSCLES.)

Stomach

(See DIGESTIVE DISORDERS.)

Stretch Marks

(See PREGNANCY.)

Stroke

(See BRAIN FUNCTION.)

Sunburn

(See SKIN CARE.)

Tachycardia

(See CARDIOVASCULAR SYSTEM.)

Tendonitis, Tenosynovitis

(See CONNECTIVE TISSUE.)

Testicular Regulation

Single oils:

- Rosemary with clary sage, sage, fennel, bergamot, sandalwood, ylang ylang, geranium, yarrow, or pine.

Use: Add 1-3 drops to the corresponding single oils above (according to your sensitivity).

Blends:

- Aroma Siez with Mister or Dragon Time.

Use: Add 1-3 drops of each single oil to the corresponding blends above (according to your sensitivity).

Supplements: EssPro 7

Teeth Grinding

Single oils: Lavender

Blends: Peace & Calming

Try diffusing Peace & Calming in the bedroom or rubbing lavender on the feet.

Thrush

(See FUNGUS.)

Thyroid

Hypothyroid

The vast majority of people suffer from hypothyroidism and do not realize it. People with low thyroid are often victims of hypoglycemia, candida, and fungal infections. The thyroid balances or controls digestion, circulation, immune functions, hormones (including sexual hormones), energy level, fatigue, body thermostat, and the emotions; so the thyroid is an important gland to take care of in order to have good health. People with type A blood have more of a tendency to have weak thyroid function.

The Barnes Basil Temperature Test is for checking thyroid function and is conducted as follows: Shake down a thermometer before going to bed at night and leave it on the bedside table. Immediately upon awakening in the morning, insert the thermometer snugly in the armpit and lie quietly for ten minutes. In normal thyroid function, the temperature range is 97.8 to 98.2° F, 36.5 to 36.7° C. A lower temperature indicates probable hypothyroidism. The test should be done on at least 2 consecutive days and repeated after a week. Women obtain the most accurate readings if not menstruating or on the second and third day of menstruation. The symptoms of hypothyroidism can mimic many of the physiological discomforts people experience. For example, people with recurring infections, which are chronically treated with antibiotics, frequently have hypothyroidism (see HYPOGLYCEMIA).

Chlorine inhibits thyroid function and therefore slows down metabolism, circulation and immune function.

Single oils:

- Lemongrass with myrtle, peppermint, spearmint, myrrh, or clove.

Use: Add 1-3 drops to the corresponding single oils above (according to your sensitivity).

Blends:

- Lemongrass with EndoFlex.

Use: Add 1-3 drops of each single oil to the corresponding blends above (according to your sensitivity).

For low or sluggish (hypo) thyroid, use lemongrass with Myrtle. Myrtle helps hypothyroid conditions (boosts the thyroid) or normalizes hormones.

For high or overactive (hyper) thyroid, use lemongrass with myrrh. Myrrh treats conditions of thyroidism (calms down thyroid).

EndoFlex possesses the correct frequency to stimulate the thyroid. Place 1 drop of EndoFlex on back (top) of large toes.

Thyromin is the best food to feed the thyroid gland and to help rebuild it. To receive the most benefit, take this supplement at bedtime. Start with 1 capsule before retiring. If the Basil Temperature indicates no improvement, add 1 capsule in the morning. If still no significant change, go to 2 capsules at night and 1 in the morning. Use this stepped approach until temperature is in correct range (see above). VitaGreen enhances the effect of the Thyromin and may be helpful to take along with it.

Supplements: Thyromin, VitaGreen, and EssPro 7.

CAUTION: Be sure to divide the total amount of the Thyromin taken between night and morning.

EssPro 7 helps improve thyroid hormone action and overall body hormone balance and also helps restore proper cell oxygen levels.

Since chlorine shuts down thyroid function by preventing absorption of iodine and the amino acid tyrosine, try to drink chlorine-free water. Distill drinking water or at least let stand unsealed and add a drop of lemon, peppermint, or spearmint to lower the chlorine levels. Chlorine-free water for showering and bathing is more difficult to achieve. Carbon filters remove chlorides from water (see WATER).

Hyperthyroid

Single oils: Myrrh, spruce, Blue Tansy

Blends: EndoFlex

Supplements: Thyromin: 1 only in the morning, VitaGreen, and Mineral Essence .

Myrrh normalizes hyperthyroid problems. For high or overactive (hyper) thyroid, use spruce with myrrh.

Toothache

(See GUMS.)

Single oils: Clove, birch, Blue Tansy melaleuca, and Idaho tansy.

Blends: Thieves and Exodus.

Supplements: Dentarome, Dentarome Plus, and Fresh Essence.

Application: Rub oil on gums at location of pain or dental infection. Dentists have used clove for many years. German chamomile can be used for teething pains.

CAUTION: For small children, dilute oils in V-6 Mixing Oil or Massage Oil Base.

Tonsillitis

Single oils: Clove, oregano, mountain savory, ravensara, and thyme.

Blends: Exodus II (massage outside of throat and put in water for a mouth wash) and Fresh Essence (gargle).

Supplements: ImmuGel and Super C.

Toxemia

Single oils: Fennel, tangerine, orange, and cypress.

Blends: Citrus Fresh, Inner Child, and Purification.

Supplements: I.C.P., ComforTone, Exodus, Super C, and Essential Manna (extremely important because of high potassium level).

Tuberculosis - Pulmonary Phthisis (of the lungs)

Single oils:

- Cypress with ravensara, rosemary, lemon, cinnamon, sandalwood, or eucalyptus (all varieties).
- Frankincense with ravensara, thyme, eucalyptus, cypress, rosemary, birch, rose, myrtle and Idaho tansy.
- Thyme with eucalyptus, ravensara, birch, chamomile, lemon, lemongrass, cinnamon, clove, oregano, peppermint, or spearmint.
- Sage with mountain savory or spruce.

Use: Add 1-3 drops to the corresponding single oils above (according to your sensitivity).

Blends:

- Cypress with Raven, R.C., or Sacred Mountain.

- Thyme with R.C., Raven, or Thieves.

- Frankincense with R.C., ImmuPower, Raven, or Inspiration.

Use: Add 1-3 drops of each single oil to the corresponding blends above (according to your sensitivity).

Supplements: ImmuGel, Radex, Super C, Royal Essence, VitaGreen, ImmuneTune, Rehemogen, and Colloidal Essence.

Application of oils: Diffused or massaged on the lung Vita Flex points on the feet and hands.

Raven and R.C. work very well when alternating in diffuser for any respiratory complaint.

Mix myrtle, mountain savory, eucalyptus and ravensara in 1 Tbsp. of V-6 Mixing Oil and apply as a rectal implant.

Raven: Put 20 drops in a capsule and swallow 3 times daily.

Diffuse Raven during the day.

Rectal implants of Raven at night.

Apply a hot compress of Exodus II on the spine and Raven on the back.

Rub Thieves on the bottom of the feet.

Exodus: 3-4 capsules 3 times daily for 21 days and rest for 7 days.

Mix in sequence:
- 2 drops sage
- 4 drops myrrh
- 5 drops clove
- 6 drops ravensara
- 15 drops frankincense

Mix in 1/2 oz. V-6 Mixing Oil or Massage Oil Base. Apply as rectal implant.

Rub ImmuPower up the spine daily and apply as a compress on back and chest twice a day and for Raindrop Therapy application.

Rose helps chronic tuberculosis.

Colloidal Essence is a powerful bacteria, fungus, and virus fighter. It can be taken internally or applied externally as required.

Cleanse colon and liver with Cleansing Trio and JuvaTone.

Rehemogen cleans and detoxifies blood.

Trauma

Blends: Trauma Life, Hope, Forgiveness, Release, Envision, and Valor.

Supplements: Super C and Mineral Essence.

Tumors

(See CANCER.)

Typhoid Fever

Single oils: Ravensara, cinnamon, peppermint, black pepper, and mountain savory.

Urinary Tract, Bladder Infection, Cystitis

Inflammation of the bladder, caused by bacteria that travel up the urethra. Symptoms include frequent urge to urinate with only a small amount of urine coming out. This urine may have a strong smell, may have blood in it, and may sting or burn as it passes. This disorder is more common in women than men because of the woman's shorter urethra.

Single oils:

- Sage with mountain savory, juniper, cedarwood, fennel, rosemary, melaleuca, lavender, sandalwood, hyssop, German chamomile, or lemongrass.

- Thyme with oregano, rosemary, tarragon, lavender, spruce, eucalyptus (all varieties), clove or cinnamon.

Use: Add 1-3 drops to the corresponding single oils above (according to your sensitivity).

Blends:

- Sage with Purification, Inspiration, or Melrose.

- Thyme with Melrose, Purification.

- Oregano with Thieves.

- R.C. or Di-Tone.

- Juniper with EndoFlex.

Use: Add 1-3 drops of each single oil to the corresponding blends above (according to your sensitivity).

Purification and Inspiration are very effective for bladder infections. Just rub over bladder.

Juniper with EndoFlex may be applied as a hot compress.

Colloidal Essence is a powerful bacteria, fungus, and virus fighter. It may be taken internally or applied externally as required.

K & B Tincture helps strengthen and tone week bladder, kidneys, and urinary tract (see KIDNEY DISORDERS).

Supplements: Colloidal Essence, K & B Tincture, and AlkaLime.

Vaginal Infection

Single oils: Myrrh, mountain savory, oregano, melaleuca, and thyme.

Blends: Melrose, 3 Wise Men, and Inspiration.

- Oregano and Thyme with Melrose.

Use: Add 1-3 drops of each single oil to the corresponding blends above (according to your sensitivity).

Do Raindrop Therapy with Thyme and Oregano. Douche with a mixture of 2 drops Oregano, 1 drop Thyme and 5 drops Melrose in 1 Tbsp. V-6 Mixing Oil or Massage Oil Base. Shake well and douche, or mix into 1 Tbsp. of V-6 Mixing Oil or Massage Oil Base and do a vaginal retention implant.

Vaginal Yeast Infection, Candida, Vaginitis

Candida is a fungus that is naturally occurring in the gut and is with us at all times. Our immune systems control candida and normally prevent its overgrowth. It grows from the fermentation of yeast and sugar (not the sugar or the yeast as individual agents). Symptoms can include indigestion, upper and lower gas, poor assimilation, poor electrolyte balance, allergic reaction to foods and other substances, along with emotional mood swings, fatigue, irritability, lack of motivation, discipline, and creativity.

Poor digestion is a major factor (see DIGESTION PROBLEMS). Work at getting digestion back on track by doing a colon and liver cleanse (see COLON).

Researchers have linked most degenerative diseases to lack of nutrients in the body. Insufficient minerals and trace minerals account for most of the nutritional deficiencies.

Hypoglycemia is a precursor and causes candida overgrowth. Candida is basically an exaggerated hypoglycemic condition. A person who is hypoglycemic is a candidate for candida. Once hypoglycemia is corrected, the candida becomes controlled (see HYPOGLYCEMIA).

One must also have good thyroid function because the thyroid secretes antibodies that regulate candida overgrowth (see THYROID). The endocrine system in general is also a factor in regulating candida (see ENDOCRINE SYSTEM). Stress should be controlled and reduced as much as possible.

Single oils:

- Lavender with melaleuca, frankincense, rosemary, Roman chamomile, thyme, geranium, bergamot, patchouly, ravensara, tarragon, hyssop, jasmine, rosewood, peppermint, spearmint, or laurus nobilis.

- Melaleuca with lemon, thyme, lemongrass, basil, rosemary, tarragon, lavender, spruce, eucalyptus (all varieties), geranium, bergamot, clove, or cinnamon.

- Thyme with rosemary, tarragon, lavender, spruce, cinnamon, eucalyptus (all), myrrh, or clove.

- Rosemary with clary sage, sage, mountain savory, fennel, bergamot, sandalwood, ylang ylang, geranium, or yarrow.

Use: Add 1-3 drops to the corresponding single oils above (according to your sensitivity).

Blends:

- Lavender with Melrose, Purification, Mister, Di-Tone, ImmuPower, Thieves (well diluted), or Exodus II.

- Melaleuca with Thieves (well diluted), Melrose, Purification, RC, or Di-Tone.

- Thyme with Melrose, Purification, R.C., or Di-Tone.

- Aroma Siez with Dragon Time, or Mister.

Use: Add 1-3 drops of each single oil to the corresponding blends above (according to your sensitivity).

Supplements: Femigen, Femalin, Estro, Thyromin, Royal Essence, Mineral Essence, Master Formula HERS/HIS, Royaldophilus, Megazyme, ImmuGel, ImmuneTune, VitaGreen, Super C, Radex, ArthroTune, Colloidal Essence, AlkaLime, and Exodus

Fungus grows in an acid environment. By balancing the body's pH and making it a more alkaline environment, the microbial overgrowths are controlled, and the production of disease-causing mycotoxins is choked off (see BODY pH, ACID/ALKALINE BALANCE).

VitaGreen is a food for alkaline balancing. AlkaLime is a precisely-balanced, acid-neutralizing mineral formula that can preserve the body's pH balance and thus combat yeast/fungus overgrowth.

Avoid yeast- and fungus- promoting (acidic) foods, such as meats, sugars, dairy products, mushrooms, and pickled and malted products. Garlic is excellent for controlling fungi and yeast. Other high-alkaline, fungus-inhibiting foods are green and yellow vegetables, beans, and whole, uncracked nuts.

The natural ratio in our diet should be 4 parts alkaline food to 1 part acid food. Dr. Morton Walker outlines some antifungal diets in his book, *Yeast Syndrome.*

Over-use of antibiotics increases the resistance of pathogenic microorganisms that kill the beneficial bacteria in our bodies and leaves the mycotoxin-generating yeast and fungi intact (see ANTIBIOTICS).

Candida infections can clear up and appear to be gone, only to erupt again in a few weeks. This is because the fungus (candida) may be lying dormant in the lymphatic system (not clearing well) or the spinal fluid. Sexual partners can also carry a candida infection and give it back. So both partners should try to rid their systems of the fungus at the same time.

Lymphatic pump therapy will assist in clearing a sluggish lymphatic system and thus help clear dormant funguses out. Keep working at cleansing the digestive system in order to clear these dormant fungi out of the body. (See Lymphatic System.)

Heartburn is a possible indication of candida. Fermentation of sugars is what feeds candida. A healthy, full-functioning digestive system will not allow this fermentation, and thus candida will not develop or progress. Royaldophilus will help provide the friendly intestinal flora to aid digestion. You should take 1 capsule of this supplement before each meal 3 times daily.

Candida will not grow in the presence of sufficient trace minerals (electrolytes) and enzymes. Royal Essence and Mineral Essence provide the necessary trace minerals. Megazyme, 3 times daily, is very important because it provides the required enzymes.

Excellent results have been reported with ImmuGel: teaspoon in water after each meal 3 times daily.

ArthroTune helps flush fungus out of the system. A one-day flush of 30 capsules of this supplement and 15 tablets of Megazyme, spread throughout the day, has produced very positive results.

ImmuneTune puts back the nutrients required to rebuild the immune system.

Thyromin helps the endocrine glands.

Super C provides bioflavonoids in addition to vitamin C.

Radex is necessary for antioxidant and free radical scavenging.

Colloidal Essence is a powerful fungus fighter.

Apply oils neat on location as well as to spinal Vita Flex points on feet and hands and around the heel, up to the anklebone. This is because fungus tends to reside long-term in the spinal fluid.

Thyme, Oregano, or Hyssop spread along the spine via Raindrop Therapy helps to drive the dormant fungus out of the spinal fluid.

Apply Thieves to the bottom of the feet.

ImmuPower on throat and chest, helps the immune system. Sip 3 drops in 2 oz. of water 3 times daily after meals.

Also, 1-2 drops of Thieves in V-6 Mixing Oil or Massage Oil Base massaged on thymus stimulates the immune system.

Alternate diffusing Thieves and ImmuPower for prevention of and protection from airborne viruses.

CAUTION: Do not diffuse Thieves for more than 15 minutes at a time as cinnamon may irritate the nasal passages.

Di-Tone enhances digestion. Rub 5-10 drops around navel and 3 drops on stomach Vita Flex areas on bottom of each foot.

Recipe 1:
- 1 drop bergamot
- 1 drop lavender
- 2 drops melaleuca

Mix in 1 Tbsp. olive oil. Use as a vaginal retention implant.

Recipe 2:
- 7 drops Purification
- 2 drops frankincense

Mix into 1 Tbsp. V-6 Mixing Oil or Massage Oil Base. Shake well and use as a douche, and vaginal retention implant.

Recipe 3:
- 2 drops juniper
- 2 drops lavender
- 2 drops melaleuca

Mix in 1 oz. V-6 Mixing Oil; apply as a vaginal retention implant.

Recipe 4:
- 12 drops melaleuca
- 12 drops Purification
- 12 drops juniper

Mix in 1-2 Tbsp. V-6 Mixing Oil or Massage Oil Base for a douche or as a vaginal retention implant every night.

For full body massage:
- 10 drops cinnamon
- 10 drops clove
- 10 drops melaleuca

Mix in 1 oz. (or more for delicate skin) V-6 Mixing Oil or Massage Oil Base. Massage and rub on bottom of feet once a day.

Royaldophilus provides friendly bacteria to help keep candida (fungus) in check. Good results have been reported from inserting a capsule of this supplement into the vagina after douching.

(See FUNGUS INFECTION.)

Uterine Cancer

(See CANCER, Uterine.)

Varicose Veins - Spider Veins - Strengthen Vascular Walls

The blue color of varicose veins is congealed blood in the surrounding tissue from hemorrhaging of capillaries around the veins. This blood has to be dissolved and re-absorbed.

Single oils:

- Basil with cypress, birch, helichrysum, peppermint, or Idaho tansy.

- Cypress with helichrysum, lemongrass, tangerine, lavender, bergamot, or lemon.

Use: Add 1-3 drops to the corresponding single oils above (according to your sensitivity).

Blends:

- Basil with Citrus Fresh, Aroma Life, or Aroma Siez.

- Cypress or lemongrass with Aroma Life.

Use: Add 1-3 drops of each single oil to the corresponding blends above (according to your sensitivity).

Supplements: Cel-Lite Magic, VitaGreen, Super B, and Royal Essence.

Since constipation is a major cause of varicose veins, do a colon and liver cleanse (see under COLON).

Helichrysum helps dissolve the coagulated blood in the surrounding tissue and makes it more easily dissolve into the tissue.

Cypress helps strengthen and regenerate capillary walls.

Idaho tansy helps weak veins.

Mix:
- 3-4 drops basil
- 1 drop birch
- 1 drop cypress
- 1 drop helichrysum

Apply neat on location. Rub very gently towards heart with smooth strokes along the vein, then up and over the vein until dry. Do this twice.

Follow with a soft massage of the whole leg using Citrus Fresh, Aroma Life, or Cel-Lite Magic Massage Oil. This activates the entire vascular and limbic systems. Wrap the leg to hold and support it. Elevate the leg to allow the vein and capillary walls time to regenerate. It is best to do this at night and to elevate the foot of the bed, an inch at a time, until it is 4 inches higher than the head. Wear support hose during daytime. Be patient. It may take up to a year to regenerate the cellular wall and prevent further hemorrhaging.

If at home, use 6 drops of tangerine with 6 drops of cypress over the area. Then do lymphatic pump (see under LYMPHATIC SYSTEM).

You may also use 2 drops helichrysum with 2 drops of cypress. Apply twice, followed by Cel-Lite Magic Massage Oil. Follow the directions above or apply by layering. For example, rub on 1-3 drops of helichrysum, then 1-3 drops of cypress, followed by Cel-Lite Magic. Follow directions above.

Recipe:
- 2 drops basil
- 2 drops Idaho tansy
- 8 drops sage
- 3 drops sandalwood

Mix in 1/2 oz. V-6 Mixing Oil or Massage Oil Base and apply as above.

If a clot develops in a vein, use cypress with helichrysum neat to dissolve it.

Vascular Cleansing - Chelating Metallics and Heavy Metals - Plaque Removal

Amalgam fillings in teeth contain mercury. People who are extremely sensitive to these metals may want to consider amalgam removal. However the process is expensive, and the replacement is not always without problems, since the compounds in the new fillings can still cause reactions.

We absorb heavy metals from air, water, food, skin care products, mercury fillings in teeth, etc. These chemicals lodge in the fatty tissues of the body, which in turn give off toxic gases that may cause allergic symptoms. Ridding our bodies of these heavy metals is extremely important in order to have healthy immune function, especially if we have amalgam fillings.

Single oils:

- Helichrysum with German chamomile, Roman chamomile, frankincense, cypress, lemongrass, geranium, or cardamom.

Use: Add 1-3 drops to the corresponding single oils above (according to your sensitivity).

Blends:

- Helichrysum with Aroma Life, Di-Tone, Thieves, JuvaFlex, EndoFlex, or Release.

Use: Add 1-3 drops of each single oil to the corresponding blends above (according to your sensitivity).

Supplements: JuvaTone, VitaGreen, Radex, Super C, ImmuneTune, ImmuGel, Royal Essence, Chelex, Kidney and Bladder Tincture (K & B), HRT, Rehemogen, Vitamin A., D. & E Liquid, Megazyme, and Cel-Lite Magic Massage Oil.

Aroma Life works very well for heart and vascular cleansing.

Helichrysum is a powerful chelator and anticoagulant.

Frankincense, cypress, helichrysum, and lemongrass strengthen the vascular walls.

There are 3 dietary supplements that are particularly useful in cleansing the vascular system and chelating heavy metals, metallics, and plaque out of the body. These supplements are JuvaTone, VitaGreen and Radex.

Clean, healthy and detoxified blood, helps fight disease.

Rehemogen cleans and fortifies the blood.

Intervenes chelation causes scar tissue on the vascular walls. The following supplements provide a natural method:

- A., D. & E. liquid vitamins
- Megazyme
- Rehemogen
- Cleansing Trio

This method takes longer, but there are no side effects.

Chelex, 1 dropper in 4 ounces of water 2 times daily, helps to remove metallics from the system. Cardamom and VitaGreen enhance the action. Massage the body with Aroma Life and 1-2 drops of helichrysum, followed by Cel-Lite Magic Massage oil. These oils are dilators and help with the chelation of metallics.

Recipe:
- 10 drops juniper
- 10 drops cypress
- 10 drops lemongrass

Mix in 1 oz. V-6 Mixing Oil or Massage Oil Base. Rub on arm pits, kidneys, and bottoms of feet.

To help pull mercury from the teeth out of the gum tissue, mix 3 drops helichrysum and 4 drops Thieves and put on a rolled gauze and place next to the gums. Only apply to one area at a time; for example, do the lower left one night, then upper left the next night and so on.

CAUTION: For very sensitive gums or on children, dilute with V-6 Mixing Oil or Massage Oil Base.

A reaction to metals, such as gold, composites, mercury in teeth, etc., indicates a body imbalance. A healthy body can handle metallic reactions. People who get an instant headache from diffusing Clarity have a blockage related to metallics or chemicals in the brain. The main oil in Clarity is cardamom, which contains high levels of trans-phenols. These are very high in oxygen molecules and will create almost instant headaches when there are chemical or metallic blockages in the brain (other oils can cause these headaches also). Such headaches indicate the need to chelate these blockages out of the tissues.

(See BLOOD CIRCULATION, CLEANSING, and DETOXIFICATION.)

Distilled water helps remove inorganic minerals and chemicals out of the body. Therefore, drink plenty of water when doing cleansing work. (See WATER.)

Vomiting - Flu

(See FLU.)

Warts

Warts are a form of skin candida fungus (see FUNGUS INFECTION).

Single oils: Oregano, thyme, melaleuca, frankincense, and hyssop

Blends: Thieves, and Melrose.

Supplements: A. D. & E Liquid Vitamin and Colloidal Essence.

Application of oils: 1 or 2 drops neat on site. Use Frankincense for stubborn warts.

Weight - Reduction/Gain

(See chapter on WEIGHT MANAGEMENT.)

Whooping Cough

(see COLDS, INFECTION.)

Wounds, Scrapes, Cuts

Single oils:

- Lavender with melaleuca, neroli (melaleuca), rosemary, Idaho tansy, eucalyptus (globulus and radiata), German chamomile, Roman chamomile, helichrysum, peppermint, clove, sandalwood, rose hip seed oil, ravensara, patchouly, geranium, rose, or palmarosa.

- Birch with melaleuca, neroli (melaleuca), lavender, lemon, frankincense, grapefruit, rosemary, thyme, or Roman chamomile.

- Thyme with melaleuca, rosemary, oregano, Roman chamomile, German chamomile, patchouly, lavandin, cedarwood, or lemon.

- Sage with hyssop, melaleuca, rosemary, Roman chamomile, German chamomile, mountain savory, myrrh, or patchouly.

- Lemongrass with peppermint, melaleuca, or bergamot.

Use: Add 1-3 drops to the corresponding single oils above (according to your sensitivity).

Blends:

- Lavender or birch with Purification, Raven, or Melrose.

- Thyme with Melrose, Purification, Thieves, or 3 Wise Men.

- (Any blend is beneficial and can be used in an emergency).

Use: Add 1-3 drops of each single oil to the corresponding blends above (according to your sensitivity).

Supplements, skin and hair care: Colloidal Essence, Rose Ointment, and Stevia.

Colloidal Essence is a very powerful bacteria, virus, and fungus killer. It can be applied externally or taken internally as required.

First Aid Spray

In a sterile spray bottle, mix 5 drops lavender, 3 drops melaleuca, and 2 drops cypress in 8 ounces of distilled water. Clean wound thoroughly. Shake well and spray the area. The area may then be covered with sterile gauze on which 1-3 drops of lavender have been placed. This should be repeated 2 times daily as necessary. After 3 days the cut or abrasion should be exposed to the air if possible. A drop of oil 1-2 times daily will promote healing until all of the skin is regenerated.

Bleeding from Open Wounds

Compress:
- 1 drop geranium
- 1 drop lemon
- 1 drop chamomile.

Alternate with hyssop, cypress, rose, and palmarosa.

Neat or direct application: 2 or more times daily for 3 or 4 days. Afterwards this can be reduced to 1-2 times daily until wound is healed.

A spray syringe works well on large wounds.

Lavender is very mild and may be used neat on children. It is a very good all-around disinfectant and healing promoter. It is an ideal first aid for wounds, scrapes, cuts, etc.

Roman chamomile is also very mild and non-toxic; it is an excellent pain reliever and skin remedy for scratches, wounds, chapped and dry skin. Add Roman chamomile to Rose Ointment for a wonderful first aid salve.

Bruises and wounds: (may be used on babies and small children):
- 3 drops helichrysum
- 3 drops lavender

Mix in 1/8 oz. V-6 Mixing Oil or Massage Oil Base.

Infected or fresh cuts:
- 7 drops lemongrass
- 5 drops peppermint
- 10 drops melaleuca
- 8 drops bergamot

Apply neat.

CAUTION: Peppermint stings when applied to a fresh open wound. Either wait a day or so or use 1 drop with 20 drops lavender or dilute in V-6 Mixing Oil or Massage Oil Base. After a couple of days, peppermint may be applied to the sealed-over wound. This will soothe, cool, and reduce inflammation in damaged tissue.

Benefits of various oils:

* Rose hip seed oil and rose prevent scarring and are anti-hemorrhaging and anti-infectious.

* Frankincense and hyssop also prevent scarring.

* Helichrysum stops bleeding quickly and reduces scarring and discoloration. It stings, however, and should be applied sparingly or diluted with lavender.

* Rose Ointment makes a wonderful synergistic ointment for all wounds.

* Stevia produces rapid healing without scaring. Apply a few drops of water-based Stevia extract directly on wound. This stings for a few seconds, followed by significant lowering of pain.

* Lemon stops bleeding.

* Patchouly stimulates cell rejuvenation as does lavender and helichrysum.

* Neroli is a strong tissue regenerator.

* Myrrh is a healer of all skin problems and scars.

* Sandalwood helps wounds heal faster and reduces or takes away lumps (proud flesh) from healing of wounds.

* Liquid lecithin and 1-2 drops each of lavender and helichrysum is very good on scar tissue.

* A blend of lavender, lemongrass, and geranium is also good for scar tissue.

* Oregano counteracts proud flesh; add lavender if used on open wounds, as oregano can sting.

* Thyme is a powerful disinfectant and germicide.

* Idaho tansy has been reported to disinfect and aid healing of abrasions.

* Hyssop is a very powerful antiviral disinfectant and is ideal for sterilizing instruments used for working on wounds or for vaginal and rectal implants, etc.

* Melaleuca is antimicrobial and antiseptic

* Thyme is antimicrobial, strengthens nervous system, helps overcome fatigue and exhaustion.

* German chamomile helps skin conditions and stress.

* Mountain savory is antimicrobial and a general tonic for the body

Scar tissue:
* 10 drops helichrysum
* 6 drops lavender
* 8 drops lemongrass
* 4 drops patchouly

Mix in 1/2 to 1 oz. V-6 Mixing Oil or Massage Base and apply.

During WW II melaleuca was found to have very strong antibacterial properties and worked well in preventing infection in open wounds. Melrose is a blend containing both types of melaleuca oil; it is a particularly good antiseptic and tissue regenerator. A very good combination is Melrose with Rose Ointment, which disinfects and promotes fast healing.

When selecting oils, particularly for injuries, think through the cause and type of injury and select oils for each aspect of the trauma. For instance, a wound could encompass muscle damage, nerve damage, ligament damage, inflammation, infection, bone injury, fever, and possibly an emotion. Therefore, select an oil or oils for each of the perceived problems.

Examples of oil application for wounds:

A person's finger was cut deeply and was bleeding badly, apparently needing stitches. 3 drops of helichrysum and 1 drop of clove were applied. This stopped the bleeding and pain. Next, 1 drop each of lavender, Melrose, and lemongrass were applied. The wound was covered with Rose Ointment and a band-aid. When changing it in the night and morning, myrrh and patchouly were added each time. The wound was healing well but then became infected.

Thieves was applied above the infected area. The redness started to reduce, and the infection was gone by night. In 2 weeks it was healed. 2 months later there was not even the slightest scar.

Surgical wound:
- 24 drops lavender
- 18 drops helichrysum
- 18 drops frankincense

Apply with 2 Tbsp. V-6 Mixing Oil or Massage Base.

Worms

(See PARASITES under CLEANSING.)

Wrinkles

(See SKIN CARE.)

Yeast Infection

(See HORMONES.)

References

Hirsch, Alan. A Scentsational Guide to Weight Loss. Rockport, MA: Element, 1997.

Young, Robert O. Sick and Tired. Alpine, UT, 1977.

Valnet, Jean. The Practice of Aromatherapy. Rochester, NY: Healing Arts Press, 1990

Privitera, James. Silent Clots. Covina, CA: 1996

Bernardis LL, et al. "The lateral hypothalamic area revisited: ingestive behavior." *Neurosci Biobehav Rev.* 20(2):189-287 (1996).

Pénoël, Daniel and P. Franchomme. L'aromatherapie exactment. France, 1990: Roger Jallois

Gattefossé, René-Maurice. Gattefossé's Aromatherapy. Saffon Waldon, UK: C.W. Daniels & Co., 1993.

Pénoël, Daniel. Natural Home Health Care Using Essential Oils. Salem, UT: Essential Science Publishing, 1998.

Compendium of Olfactory Research. Edited by Avery N. Gilbert. Dubuque, IA: Kendall Hunt Publishing, 1995.

Maury, Marguerite. The Secret and Life of Youth. Saffon Waldon, UK: C.W. Daniels & Co., 1995.

Hirsch, Alan. "Inhalation of 2 acetylpyridine for weight reduction." *Chemical Senses* 18:570 (1993).

Brodal A. Neurological Anatomy in Relation to Clinical Medicine. New York: Oxford University Press, 1981.

Fleming, T., Ed. PDR for Herbal Medicines, Medical Economics Company, Inc., Montvale, NJ (1998)

Murray, M. Encyclopedia of Nutritional Supplements, Prima Publishing, Rocklin, CA (1996)

Gumbel, D. Principles of Holistic Therapy with Herbal Essences, Haug International, Brussels, Belgium (1993)

Tisserand, R. and T. Balacs Essential Oil Safety, Churchill Livingstone, New York, NY (1996)

Pedersen, M. Nutritional Herbology, A Reference Guide to Herbs, Wendell W. Whitman Company, Warsaw, IN (1998)

Montagna, F. J. HDR Herbal Desk Reference Kendall/Hunt Publishing Company, Dubuque, IA (1979)

Tyler, V. E. Herbs of Choice Pharmaceutical Products Press, Binghamton, NY (1994)

McGuffin, M., et al. Botanical Safety Handbook, CRC Press, Boca Raton, FL (1997)

Tyler, V. E. The Honest Herbal, Lubrect & Cramer, Ltd., Port Jervis, NY (1995)

Appendix

AFNOR/ISO Standards for Therapeutic-Grade
Chamomaelum Nobilis

Gas Chromatograph profile 4.10

CONSTITUENTS	Min %	Max %
Isobutyl angelate + Isoamyl methacrylate	30	45
Isoamyl angelate	12	22
Methyl allyl angelate	6	10
2-methyl butyl angelate	3	7
Isoamyl isobutyrate	3	5
Trans-pino-carveol	2	5
Isobutyl n-butyrate	2	9
α-pinene	1.5	5
Pinocarvone	1.3	4
Isobutyl methacrylate	1	3
2-methyl butyl methacrylate	.5	1.5

AFNOR/ISO Standards for Therapeutic-Grade
Lavendula Angustifolia

Gas Chromatograph profile 4.10

CONSTITUENTS	Min %	Max %
Linalol	25	38
Linalyl acetate	25	45
cis-β-ocimene	4	10
trans-β-ocimene	1.5	6
terpinen-4-ol	2	6
Lavendulyl acetate	2	—
Lavendulol	.3	—
β-phellandrene	traces	.5
α-terpineol	—	1
Octanone-3	traces	2
Camphor	traces	.5
Limonene	—	.5
1,8 cineole	—	1

AFNOR/ISO European and World Standards
for Therapeutic-Grade
Eucalyptus globulus

Gas Chromatograph profile 4.11

CONSTITUENTS	Pure Essential Oil		Rectified Essential Oil	
	crushed raw	traditional	70%-75%	80%-85%
1,8 cineol min %	48	58	70	80
α-Pinene min %	10	20	Traces	Traces
max %	20	22	20	12
Aromadendrene min %	6	1	—	—
max %	10	5	traces	traces
Limonene min %	2	1	2	2
max %	4	8	15	15
p-cymene min %	1	1	1	1
max %	3	5	6	10
trans-pinocarveol min %	1	1	traces	traces
max %	4	5	10	6
Globulol min %	.5	.5	—	—
max %	2.5	1.5	traces	traces

AFNOR/ISO European and World Standards for
Therapeutic-Grade
Salvia sclarea
Gas Chromatograph profile 4.10

CONSTITUENTS	Traditional	Crushed Green
Linalyl acetate		
min %	62	56
max %	78	70.5
Linalol		
min %	6.5	13
max %	13.5	24
Sclareol		
min %	.4	.4
max %	2.6	2.6
d-germacrene		
min %	1.5	1.2
max %	12	7.5
α-terpineol		
min %	traces	1
max %	1.2	5

AFNOR/ISO Standards for Therapeutic-Grade
Cupressus Sempervirens
Gas Chromatograph profile 4.11

CONSTITUENTS	Min %	Max %
α-pinene	40	65
δ-3-carene	12	25
limonene	1.8	5
α-Terpenyl acetate	1	4
Myrcene	1	3.5
Cedrol	.8	7
β-pinene	.5	3
D-germacrene	.5	3
Terpinen-4-ol	.2	2

AFNOR/ISO Standards for Therapeutic-Grade
Basilicum Ocimum
Gas Chromatograph profile 4.8

CONSTITUENTS	Min %	Max %
Methyl chavicol	75	85
1,8 cineol	1	3.5
Trans-beta ocimene	.9	2.8
Linalol	.50	.30
Methyl eugenol	.3	2.5
Terpinen-4-ol	.20	.60
Camphor	.15	.50

AFNOR/ISO Standards for Therapeutic-Grade
Syzygium Aromaticum
Gas Chromatograph profile 4.8

CONSTITUENTS	Min %	Max %
Eugenol	80	92
B-caryophyllene	4	17
Eugenyl acetate	.2	4

Index